Many Voices

Interpretive Studies in Healthcare and the Human Sciences

VOLUME 3

Many Voices

Toward Caring Culture in Healthcare and Healing

Edited by

Kathryn Hopkins Kavanagh

and

Virginia Knowlden

THE UNIVERSITY OF WISCONSIN PRESS

The University of Wisconsin Press
1930 Monroe Street
Madison, Wisconsin 53711

www.wisc.edu/wisconsinpress/

3 Henrietta Street
London WC2E 8LU, England

5   4   3   2   1

Printed in the United States of America

Library of Congress Cataloging-in-Publication Data

Many voices : toward caring culture in healthcare and healing / edited
by Kathryn Hopkins Kavanagh and Virginia Knowlden.
p. ;   cm. — (Interpretive studies in healthcare and the human sciences ; v. 3)
Includes bibliographical references and index.
ISBN 0-299-19760-3 (cloth : alk. paper) — ISBN 0-299-19764-6 (pbk : alk. paper)
1. Nursing—Psychological aspects. 2. Caring. 3. Nurse and patient. 4. Transcultural nursing.
[DNLM: 1. Nursing Care—psychology. 2. Empathy. 3. Nurse-Patient Relations.
4. Transcultural Nursing—methods. WY 87 M295 2004] I. Kavanagh, Kathryn Hopkins.
II. Knowlden, Virginia. III. Series.
RT86.M367 2004
610.73'06'99—dc22
2003022355

To Nancy L. Diekelmann,
whose boundless caring and ceaseless efforts
keep open possibilities otherwise unimagined
as she wonders with us

like the question no one
poses, as to what we're,
any of us, doing
here: what is this
elbowed, unsheltering,
obtrusively
concatenated fiefdom
we poor, cliff-dwelling
pseudo-pioneers
have somehow
blundered into?

Amy Clampitt, "Progress at Building Site with (Fewer) Pigeons"

Contents

Foreword   ix
    Nancy L. Diekelmann and Pamela M. Ironside
Acknowledgments   xv
    Kathryn Hopkins Kavanagh and Virginia Knowlden

An Introduction: Caring and Culture in Interpretation
and Practice   3
    Virginia Knowlden and Kathryn Hopkins Kavanagh

1. Difference, Dialogue, Dialectics: A Study of Caring
    and Self-Harm   21
    Andrew Estefan, Margaret McAllister, and Jennifer Rowe
2. "These Are the Children We Hold Dear"   62
    Jacqui Kess-Gardner (with introduction and conclusion
    by Kathryn H. Kavanagh)
3. Personal Dialogue on Connecting Caring: A Journey   105
    Joanna Basuray
4. Prejudice, Paradox, and Possibility: The Experience
    of Nursing People from Cultures Other Than
    One's Own   140
    Deb Spence
5. Cultivating Stories of Care   181
    Billie M. Severtsen

6. Preceptors as the Champions of the New Nurse:
The Context in Which Student Nurses Learn the
Culture of Caring   218
   Louise G. Rummel

Contributors   263
Index   267

Foreword

Nancy L. Diekelmann and Pamela M. Ironside

Many Voices lays bare a neoteric path to thinking and understanding caring and culture. Standard approaches to caring and culture are familiar as core concepts to practitioners in the health and human sciences, and it is rare to have another view of caring and culture proffered, one that is multiperspectival and reflective. The volume editors, Kathryn Kavanagh and Virginia Knowlden, have brought together studies in which originary approaches to understanding caring and culture in interpretation and practice are explicated. Perhaps humans do not have a culture but rather are cultures in which caring as concern is constitutive of being human. Understood in this way, caring is not a positive human attribute or characteristic but a kind of culturally embedded concern that can be lived out in either empowering or oppressive ways.

It seems imperative with a rapidly evolving healthcare system and community-based care that caring and culture are *enjoined into converging conversations*. That is exactly what these volume editors have created with the selection and juxtaposition of interpretive studies in caring and culture. Perhaps for too long, healthcare professionals have viewed these two areas as separate and discrete, two phenomena of interest and concern. Yet, as lived, they are experienced inseparably. Humans are always their cultures, and caring as concern is constitutive of being—one is only understood in light of the other.

This volume challenges healthcare professionals to explore the commonly taken neutral stance of "protecting patients from *other* professionals who are insensitive and uncaring." The possibility that one could *personally* be uncaring or culturally insensitive (albeit unintentionally) is rarely explored. What are brought to bear in this book are studies that make explicit how *intentions*, though they matter, are not the sole arbiters of how caring and culture are experienced. Rather it is reflecting and learning how to interpret situations from a variety of perspectives and always holding understandings open and problematic that give caring and culture meaning and significance. This is the first step toward a new caring culture in healthcare wherein all actions or interventions themselves are open, problematic, and always evolving.

The common stance of "*I intend* to be culturally sensitive and caring, therefore *I am*" is challenged by these studies. In this volume, narrative interpretations that extend current epistemological and ontological understandings as the "invisible obvious" are explored and explicated. Some of the insights explored in these studies are familiar and at-hand. They stand in front of healthcare professionals, so familiar (the nearness of the near) that they are invisible. Yet this book goes beyond critique of these oversights to explore ways in which the caring comportment both shapes and is shaped by culture. These studies reveal new possibilities for professionals providing culturally sensitive healthcare that is reflective of an ethic of caring culture.

The interdisciplinary and global perspectives the authors bring to this volume reflect how cultural differences, even when seen, are often ignored in the global community of healthcare professionals. And the silence of care and caring is broken in this book by sharing difficult stories—stories that healthcare professionals often do not want to hear. Kavanagh and Knowlden explicate in their introduction how the call to understanding care and culture is an interpretive practice. Through this new lens, this collection of interpretive studies explores the meaning and significances of caring cultural practices in the lives of patients and their families. As we listen to the voices that break our silence, new ways to keep open a future of possibilities to care for patients and their families show up.

This book, which is much more than an indictment of contemporary healthcare, makes a positive contribution to the literature in the health and human sciences. It points to a new future for healthcare professionals by illuminating how caring practices and culturally sensitive care can be learned through dwelling in thoughtful and thought-provoking narrative exegeses. Narrative research makes us *mindful*, enhancing our understanding of how uncaring and culturally insensitive care comes to be and is experienced by people in our contemporary society. It creates a research-based literature for future students in the healthcare professions that is rich with food for thought. These studies also show how providing culturally sensitive care is often learned "with a high price." That is, healthcare professionals often make costly mistakes before learning to provide care that is culturally sensitive. As students study the experiences of caring culture laid bare in these chapters, new ways of being-in-the-world open up for them as future practitioners.

Reflecting is a central practice advocated for healthcare practitioners. This vanguard book elucidates how reflecting, rethinking, and reinterpreting the nature or the intersections and co-occurrences of caring and culture provide new approaches for teaching, practice, and research. Issues of culture, like language, are *always* interpretive and the contexts in which humans read situations. Concern is how the world shows up with some issues of more interest than others. Caring as concern is thus always situated, temporal, and historical. In this approach to research, contexts are explicated that are familiar and at hand as well as evocative and thought provoking. The studies in this volume make us mindful while they show and safeguard practices and approaches that often are nuanced yet hold within them revolutionary ways of attending to care and culture in the contexts of contemporary healthcare. Both practical and theoretical insights into caring are afforded in particular cultural contexts. Each study provides readers with both theoretical and practical examples of how theoretical positions can be worked out in practice and educational settings.

Health professions courses in research, multiculturalism, and professional issues are enriched by this book, which provides rigorous interpretive studies, reflecting a plurality of approaches from hermeneutics to post-structuralism and autoethnography. Although these studies examine familiar constructs (caring and culture), the methodological pluralism embraced by the authors adds richness and complexity to contemporary understanding of the nexus of caring and culture in the human sciences. For instance, Estefan, McAllister, and Rowe explicate how the language of healthcare and the predominant biomedical approach to mental illness covers over possibilities for caring. What is most striking about this study is the paradox of how current approaches to caring for self-harmers emphasize behavioral and control issues overlooking the mental and psychological. The authors show how ineffective such an exclusionary approach is as lived. This study also challenges and extends extant research. For example, current approaches to the development of expertise in which guided intuition develops in practitioners of care over time are challenged by narratives revealing the intuition that novices bring to the clinical situation. Furthermore, in the context of a post-structural analysis of caring for persons who self-harm, the authors delineate educational implications for teaching students to resist assimilation within the dominant (oppressive) biomedical practices.

A mother's personal struggle with caring for a child with severe disabilities reveals the cultural issues of difference, tolerance, and "nonengagement." In this study by Kess-Gardner and Kavanagh, a mother's voice shapes our understanding of an unexpected, tragic, and culturally "forbidden" view of a less than perfect child and reveals how she and her family keep open a future of new possibilities for all. Basuray uses autoethnography to illuminate the multileveled experiences and responses, examples and discourses, that reveal constructions of culture and how they influenced her experiences. Her analyses have significant implications for teaching students, particularly, how constructions of culture and caring are never simple and straightforward, nor are their influences always clear.

In the Spence hermeneutic study the nursing of people from cultures other than one's own is explicated—in this instance, caring that attempts to "reconcile interpersonal aspects of nursing within a highly political, sociocultural context and illuminate some of the prejudices influencing nursing practice." In this study new possibilities lie in examining the ways in which healthcare providers' understanding of those to whom they provide care shapes, disrupts, and facilitates effective practice.

The possibilities in using narratives to teach caring, culture, and healing is explicated in the Severtsen study. Learning and practicing interpretive skills assists students in developing their healing practices while being mindful of how caring and culture co-occur. Rummel uses interpretive phenomenology and Heideggerian hermeneutics to describe and open up for critical review how nurse preceptors transmit and co-create the nursing culture with students. The common practice of instructing students in the health professions is made transparent, and thought-provoking pedagogical commentary is proffered.

Volume editors Kathryn Kavanagh and Virginia Knowlden are to be commended for the extraordinary converging conversations of caring and culture this book creates. The insights provided elicit healthcare providers to persistently question how caring and culture shape and are shaped by their day-to-day practice and interactions with patients. True to its interpretive title, the *many voices* speaking reveal the nexus of caring and culture toward creating a caring culture in healthcare and healing.

Acknowledgments

Kathryn Hopkins Kavanagh and Virginia Knowlden

A community of scholars gathers annually at the University of Wisconsin–Madison for the Institutes for Heideggerian Hermeneutical Studies. There we study with philosophers, read authors we seldom get to read in our daily lives, and savor the abilities of our colleagues and ourselves as scholars. We cherish these summertime oases for the connections they foster and the opportunities they provide to think and explore worlds too often left fallow in the exigencies of everyday. We thank Nancy Diekelmann for creating and nurturing this garden in the desert.

It is Nancy who believed in this book series enough to make it happen—and such achievements do not come easily. With Pam Ironside and the editorial board (David Allen, Michael Andrew, Patricia Benner, Karin Dahlberg, Daniel W. Jones, Kathryn Kavanagh, Fred Kersten, Birgit Negussie, and Thomas Sheehan), Nancy oversaw the two awesome volumes that precede this one. In addition to creating an admirable legacy, they forge a hard act to follow. We could only trust that others devoted to interpretive inquiry would come through for a volume on caring and culture—and indeed they did. This volume could not *be* without the talented scholars who submitted their best work. It could not have happened without an amazing cast of reviewers who responded to our call. We are exceedingly grateful for their timely and learned responses! Our sincerest thanks go to Cathy Andrews, Philip Darbyshire, Claire Draucker, Ann Harley, Diane Heliker, Joanne Hessmiller, Pam Ironside, Mary Johnson, Gail Lindsay, Sherry Sims, Becky Sloan,

Jeanne Sorrell, Betsy Stetson, Dianne Tapp, Cheryl Webb, Sharon Wyatt, and Tricia Young. And special thanks go to Christine Sorrell Dinkins, who could have been sitting under a palm tree in Florida when she edited this volume for us. Without these exceptionally able scholars, scattered as they are across three nations, *Many Voices* would not be heard.

Many Voices

An Introduction

Caring and Culture in Interpretation and Practice

Virginia Knowlden and Kathryn Hopkins Kavanagh

This volume of the *Interpretive Studies in Healthcare and the Human Sciences* book series brings together caring and culture. As a human experience, caring is crucial for the continued survival of the species as social and cultural, as well as biological beings. It is part of such diverse and basic human activities as parenting, counseling, befriending, and healing, all of which occur within sociocultural contexts. Socialized and enculturated as we are, we learn patterns of understanding and behaving in the world as we know it. Experiences of living contribute to new meanings and understandings. Amid new and always changing interpretations, caring remains both embedded in and reflective of culture. There are many ways to examine caring and culture, but because the book series emphasizes interpretive inquiry, caring and culture are explored in this volume through a variety of phenomenological, hermeneutic, and ethnographic approaches.

In this introductory chapter, we present a brief background on hermeneutical phenomenology and illustrate the applicability of the philosophical work of Martin Heidegger and Hans-Georg Gadamer in developing new understandings of care- and culture-centered, health-related phenomena. Caring and culture are classic examples of hermeneutic problems, for their meanings are often not apparent and require interpretation.

Martin Heidegger's work is particularly relevant to our discussion because of his thinking about Care and its structure. Gadamer informs us about culture, the key aspect of human adaptability (Kottak, 2000), through his ideas about understanding as "standing in history" in the sense that being in the world is manifested through tradition (Gadamer, 1975). Tradition is ontological in as much as it is through tradition that we understand the world and each other, learn culturally, and think symbolically. Culture, representing tradition, is neither passive nor deterministic but requires active appropriation, perpetuation, and transformation through human participation (Ulin, 2001). This involves active mediation between, for example, already-learned tradition (which includes the considerable authority of tradition) and the situation of the moment.

In this way, culture is operative in all acts of understanding and caring. It influences attitudes toward the world with prejudices (preconceived ideas or opinions that precede the facts) rooted in traditional learning and experience; indeed "[t]o have a 'world' means to have an attitude towards it" (Gadamer, 1975, p. 402). Knowing, anticipating, and understanding such attitudes or prejudgments ("prejudices" is the word Gadamer and his translators use, although it should be noted that prejudices are necessarily neither negative nor harmful but are essentially convictions, ideals, and preferences influenced by tradition) make possible the understanding of human actions based in culture. For instance, the ability to formulate a meaningful question depends upon some foreknowledge or anticipation of the situation. Likewise, it is these prejudgments that draw us into the always-implicit hermeneutic circle with its continual, dialectical movement of meaning and understanding of the relationship of the part to the whole. The value of this stance lies in its providing an alternative to ethnocentric scientism by allowing a "more comprehensive vision of human possibilities" (Ulin, 2001, p. 246). In contrast, "[a] person who does not accept that he is dominated by prejudices will fail to see what is shown by their light" (Gadamer, 1975, p. 324).

Culture is manifest through language, which includes all forms of communication, as well as through adaptation to and of environments. The primacy of language is consistent with the rule that "the limits of my language are the limits of my world" (Wittgenstein, 1961, p. 57). A variant of this understanding persists in the social sciences as the Sapir-Whorf hypothesis, which asserts that so close a relationship exists between culture and language that language in large part defines experiences for us by filtering a bombardment of sensations of all kinds, intensities, and durations to recognize and organize reality as we know it (Scupin, 2003). That sorting and codifying—that is, making sense of the world in which we live—reflects whatever language we have. If we have words for many variants of a situation, we apply them; if we have only a few, we recognize only a few possibilities in the situation. If we have none, we might miss the entire situation by neither attending to nor understanding it. In sum, we perceive that for which we have language and dimly perceive, at best, that for which we do not.

Although different languages (confounded as they are with different worldviews) craft differing ways of thinking and understanding (Kottak, 2000), language is also universal, even in the midst of language-contingent tradition. "[L]anguage speaks us" (Gadamer, 1975, p. 421) to the point that being can be understood only linguistically, but linguisticality permeates traditions and allows the "fusion of horizons" that Gadamer described as the engaging of differing traditions and the discourse that results through disclosure of those traditions.

While Gadamer contributed understandings of situation and context, Heidegger (whom Gadamer followed closely in his thinking) proposed Care as the Being of Dasein, human Being-in-the-world, the basic condition of existence known as Openness (Heidegger, 1962, 2001). The Being of Dasein shows up as our own being, that which matters to each one of us. Human Being-in-the-world has to do with the way that our being understands situations in a familiar, holistic sense, rather than in a fragmented way.

Following Heidegger, the essential matter is to understand "being." Although Dasein can be known only in its wholeness, Heidegger suggested that care is irreducibly composed of several *existentiale*, its fundamental characteristics (Boss, 1963; Heidegger, 1962). These *existentiale* indicate that we enter into various situations with a familiarity about the way we experience ourselves, immersed as we are in the surrounding world. We do this again even if the particular situation we find ourselves in is not one we have been in before. The *existentiale* include worldhood (the shared customs and language of people) or *Das Man*, Being-in (to be absorbed in the surrounding world), Being-with (to participate in another's world in a caring way), Being-there, Being-possible (to remain open to new ways of understanding ourselves and others), making room, states of mind, understanding as disclosedness, discourse, and truth (Heidegger, 1962). These *existentiale* composing care are briefly explicated in an interpretation and discussion of a healthcare-related situation later in this chapter.

All *existentiale* are encompassed by time, which "constitutes . . . the totality of the structure of Care" (Heidegger, 1962, H.328, p. 376). In Western culture, our ordinary understanding of time is that it is linear and consists of past, present, and future. Out of these arise Dasein's potentiality-for-Being. The past (having-been-ness), and the future (expectant-being, being-ahead-of-itself) are an integral part of the present (being-in-time, being-already-in), according to Heidegger. Yet, in actuality, it is the moment that matters, encompassing as it does past, present, and future. Experiencing our being as being-in-the-world in a temporal sense frees us to participate in another person's world in a caring way, for our being is not restrained by the past or the future. All of these are unified states of mind for Dasein (Heidegger, 1962, p. 377), and out of the *existentiale* arise Dasein's potentiality-for-Being.

Heidegger went on to define "Being-in-the-world as essentially care, Being-alongside the ready-to-hand . . . as *concern*, and Being with the *Dasein*-with of Others as we encounter it within-the-world . . . as *solicitude*" (Heidegger, 1962, p. 237). "Solicitude is guided by *considerateness* and *forbearance*" (p. 377). Heidegger distinguishes Caring for a being from Caring about a being. To care for someone or something means to take over, dominate, or displace a Being until the matter is resolved. It is in large part a matter of objectification and doing-for. There are events and situations in which this is imperative. Caring about a Being is to assist a being to care for oneself.

The art and science of human caring (Watson, 1979, 1999) as a fundamental concept and as a moral ideal has been developing over many years. In the health and human sciences, and specifically within nursing, perspectives on caring have been identified as falling into five basic conceptual areas: caring as a human trait, caring as a moral imperative or ideal, caring as an affect, caring as an interpersonal relationship, and caring as a therapeutic intervention (Morse, Solberg, Neander, Bottorff, & Johnson, 1990). However, with persistent lack of clarity, parsimony, and precision in descriptions and conceptualizations of caring, a clear and precise definition remains elusive. Instead, caring belongs to a family of meanings, all of which are contingent on diverse cultural orientations and change with time, so no fixed definition is possible. With their features shared, the meanings of "caring" become "a family affair among its senses" (Kaplan, 1964, p. 48). Nonetheless, all care and solicitude is for or about something (Gadamer, 1975; Heidegger, 1962).

Interpretation is as much a part of practice in healthcare as it is in inquiry. We use a brief story involving caring and culture to help illustrate their interpretation from the perspectives of Heidegger and Gadamer. The story was drawn from research focused on the understanding and practice of care and caring in a high-technology healthcare setting[1] (Knowlden, 1988, 1998).

Maria's Story

Maria is a young nurse with less than one year's experience in a Neonatal Intensive Care Unit (NICU), although she is experienced in work with normal newborns. In the Heideggerian sense she has been "thrown" into a new-to-her world of isolettes, lights, alarms, bells, and monitors. In response, she communicates considerable anxiety over her struggle to care for the babies and maintain her human connection in that environment. When asked to describe the roots of that dialectic in her work, Maria replied:

My first experience where I learned how to not nurse the machines but the patients was as a student in L&D [labor and delivery]. Nurses nursed the fetal monitors instead [of the mothers]. In class we learned not to do that—there's a patient at the end of the machines.

In the NICU, Maria observes a similar tendency for nurses to focus on the environment rather than on the patients:

I was absolutely overwhelmed. At first I was thrilled and excited that I can keep one of these [babies] alive. Then I couldn't stand it. I hated how others cared for the babies, their callousness, their attitudes. I felt they should still treat and give comfort. . . . [But] nurses nurse the . . . monitor instead of the baby. . . . I see machines as extremities requiring lots of care, lots of technical skills. You have to find a balance between [care of machines and care of babies], yet you can't ignore the alarms, the IV fluids.

People cover the isolettes with blankets, calling it minimal stimulation. But the babies don't necessarily calm down. You don't know how they're doing, and then the alarm goes off. Some babies are not powerful enough to get the heart rate at 200 so the alarm goes off. Sometimes [nurses] ignore the alarms, but the alarm means the baby needs something. Sometimes they put [the alarm] on three-minute hold. . . . They don't comfort the baby, or soothe, or check the leads.

It's been a very difficult nine months . . . [but] I feel I have the energy to comfort the babies, to give extra TLC [tender loving care] that some don't have. I get a lot out of seeing what comfort measures do for the babies. I express to others taking care of the baby what the baby likes. I like talking to parents about these comfort measures; that makes two of me there to hold the pacifier, the blanket. I've been able to extend myself into them, providing a bonding that they've been denied [by the baby being in the NICU]. . . . I started caring as I thought I should—making offerings of help to others who had burned out, so I felt better about the way a baby was being treated. Now I like it.

In addition to learning to be in the culture of the NICU, Maria found herself at odds with positions of the broader culture as those were reflected in medical and hospital policy. The first baby for whom Maria was the primary nurse, Cassie, had a condition that medical personnel decided required blood transfusions. The baby's parents objected to the treatment because they were Jehovah's Witnesses, who oppose on principle any use of blood or blood products (Andrews & Hanson, 2003). Maria found herself taking a stance: "I let the parents know that I was in a neutral position. I would be an advocate against aggressive treatment. I would respect their rights." Maria empathized with their concerns for the baby and her care. "Parents have enough problems. The last thing they need is to get the impression that nurses don't care." She was also concerned about bonding between the baby and the parents. "The father was not allowed to come in until after the lines are started, the baby intubated, and the ventilator on, and in the box." Sometimes there is no eye contact, and parents need encouragement and support to relate to this baby as their baby. "They're afraid to touch. I let them know they're doing something for the baby. It's really a part of the baby's care."

The Caring and Cultural Dialectic

The "Worldhood(s)" and Being-In

Maria finds herself in a busy NICU, a setting in which the tiny humans being cared for are dwarfed by the technology that sustains them. There she finds personal caring often preempted by mechanical demands and drifting into noncaring or perhaps "approximations of caring" (Watson, 1999, p. 34) that only indirectly affect the patient. In Maria's situation, other cultural dynamics further impinge on care. The physicians of the healthcare team deem it imperative to treat the infant with blood transfusions. As a result of parental objection, the case goes to court, and the parents lose their right to make decisions regarding their baby's treatment. Ordinarily, Maria depends on parents to help her stay connected to the babies, just as she tries to nurture connections between babies and the parents. In this case she finds herself facing a dialectic in which she feels the parents, as Jehovah's Witnesses, were more accepting of the baby's dying than of being given blood, while the medical personnel "could not let the baby die; [they] had to treat."

In the story, Maria is a Being fully present, standing with the humanness of the parents as she encounters them in the world. She is sensitive to who they are as people and to what they hold as values. She cares about the entire family and intends to be their advocate. But Maria is also a being involved in the common ethos of caring of the NICU, a setting that has its own traditions and expectations. As a result, Maria experiences anxiety and angst as her caring is thwarted by rules, regulations, and lack of agreement about how to best take care of this family. Gadamer (1996) points out that, just as care is always for or about something, "all anxiety is anxiety in the face of something or anxiety about something" (p. 157).

Jehovah's Witnesses are people of a religious faith with deep convictions against accepting blood and blood products into their bodies (Smith, 1986; Sugarman, Churchill, Moore, & Waugh, 1991). Although members of this religious group depend on conventional medical resources for healthcare, blood and any agent in which blood is an ingredient are not acceptable in treatment. As with any group, Jehovah's Witnesses want good medical care for their children but ask that healthcare professionals consider their convictions. Today, the issue around use of blood and blood products is increasingly avoided by use of effective, nonblood alternatives in most medical subspecialties (*No Blood*, 2001). However, situations such as that depicted in Maria's story continue to recur.

In requesting that intervention not contradict their beliefs, baby Cassie's parents are asking for care and treatment that is more inclusive than that afforded by an essentially science-based way of knowing and practicing. Orthodox biomedicine, with its highly scientific philosophy and culture, emphasizes curative medicine over (more holistic) healing (Baer, 2001; Hahn & Gaines, 1985; Loustaunau & Sobo, 1997; Payer, 1988). People who prioritize healing over cure also tend to value treatment of the entire person, a request that fits healthcare's stated protocols and standards (Dossey, Keegan, & Guzzetta, 2000).

Seekers of healthcare are increasingly diverse, oriented as they are to various combinations of cultural, social, and personal interest groups. We hear much about multiculturalism and community that allows and encourages change at whatever pace is comfortable for its participants (Goldberg, 1998; Willet, 1998). At the same time, in healthcare settings, the demands of complex technology increasingly challenge patient-centeredness in caring. Culture-specific care enables individuals and groups who may differ in background from healthcare providers to bridge the difference between clinicians' and consumers' life worlds (Leininger & McFarland, 2002). Cultural competence (the ability and process by which a care provider "continuously strives to work effectively within the cultural context of an individual, family, or community" [Andrews & Boyle, 1997, p. 16A]), like holistic care, is increasingly considered a standard of care (Andrews & Boyle, 2003; Engebretson & Headley, 2000). However, just as not all medical facilities and practitioners accommodate specialized blood-related requests in their medical treatment, not all care providers are sensitized to and educated in the need and ways to provide culturally congruent intervention strategies and care.

Also relevant to Maria's situation is American culture's emphasis on the individual (DeVita & Armstrong, 1993; Stewart & Bennett, 1991). It is the individual, not the family, that has rights and becomes the focus of medical attention. Biomedicine, like other institutions within the culture, is profoundly affected by the cultural continuities and changes shared with the rest of mainstream American society (Stein, 1990). This reflection of culture implies that the same prejudicial and discriminatory patterns around class, race, ethnicity, and gender that exist in broader society are likely to exist in medical practice (Baer, 2001; Kavanagh, 1991).

Medicine is powerful, enjoying as it does an authority bestowed with societal permission (Pfifferling, 1981). People do not carry with them the anxiety about health that they do about illness (Gadamer, 1996), thus when humans become ill, they tend to be more open to dependence on others. Like organized biomedicine, hospital bureaucracies are not merely powerful but have social control functions (O'Neill, 1986; Turner, 1987). That is, when the values and norms expectant of hospital administrators and practitioners clash with those of patients or their families, the archetypal institution exhorts its "corrective" (albeit culturally impositional and hegemonic) policies, which are typically reinforced by law as well as policy, as was the case with the Jehovah's Witnesses with whom Maria interacts.

Medical dominance (the authority held by the medical profession, and to some extent nursing and other healthcare disciplines [Gadow, 1980; Ladd, 1980]) serves in both the therapeutic encounter and in the broader public sphere to maintain a social distance between the physician and the patient (Lupton, 1994). It is not unusual for this gap to promulgate poor communication and failed empathy (Freund & McGuire, 1995). It is the opposite of the aforementioned "fusion of horizons" that facilitates communication and reveals the emancipatory potential of knowledge (Gadamer, 1975).

Being-With, Being-There, and Being-Possible

Maria discloses how solicitude in the sense of "Being with the Dasein-with of Others as we encounter it within-the-world" enables her to provide care to infants. "Disclose" is used advisedly here in the way that Heidegger used the term. Disclosedness can be understood as saying that "uncovering . . . [is] a way of Being" (Heidegger, 1962, p. 224). Disclosedness is understanding. Thus, understanding has its eye toward the future. Understanding uncovers our potential as human beings. Being-uncovering is a direct experience with the self for Maria, as well as a direct experience of her self with the baby's parents. Being-uncovering reveals how "I am" in this experience. It is Being-open to the possibilities in the process of discovery. Disclosedness as understanding is not a judgment or a way of behaving. Being uncovered is being human in the world. Disclosedness as uncovering reveals who we are. In Maria's eyes, Cassie's parents are as caring as any others might be. They are neither right nor wrong in their stance concerning the baby's medical treatment, but the "fusion of horizons" between them and Maria (that is, their co-participation in distinct traditions) allows conversation to develop dialectically. In this discourse, "[t]he unfolding of the totality of meaning towards which understanding is directed forces us to make conjectures and to take them back again" (Gadamer, 1975, p. 422). Maria desired to "be an advocate against aggressive treatment. I let the parents know that I was in a neutral position. I would respect their rights." Maria's position, then, is in direct contrast to that of the medical and other nursing staff, and to that of the court's decision to preempt parental rights and determine care for the baby. Maria experiences tension as she cares for this family—but she is trying to care for the family, not merely the individuals who compose it. It is the tension that reveals itself on every level of the dialectic between the part and the whole. In applied disciplines, interventionists constantly confront choices between respecting individual wishes and pressing for compliance. The same unresolved dialectic in other aspects of society (for example, teaching) means negotiating between recognition of and respect for differences that are meaningful to some but not the whole, and pushing for assimilation.

We uncover ourselves through our states of mind and emotions—whether we are anxious or content, happy or sad—and through all of our verbal and nonverbal communication. We reveal ourselves in the way we talk, listen, or are silent, what we look at, how we look, and what we miss in seeing. One's disclosedness uncovers our being. As we disclose, we uncover our self. Disclosedness and understanding show "what (one's) Being is capable of . . . Interpretation is the working out of possibilities projected in Understanding" (Heidegger, 1962, H.148, p. 188). Maria has come to understand how she wants to be with this family as she provides care, but she is left with a serious predicament. Her understanding does not provide a solution to the situation.

Maria demonstrates solicitude in her "Being with the Dasein-with of Others as we encounter it within-the-world" by becoming "like" or identifying with the parents. Maria is practicing by *projecting towards a potentiality-for-Being for the sake of which any Dasein exists*" (Heidegger, 1962, p. 385). Here Maria's understanding is not only disclosing and uncovering, but it is also understanding through acting, practicing for the baby's future, and for Maria's own potentiality-for-Being as well.

Maria in her understanding of the parents' worldview through observation, attentiveness, and conversation uncovers their Being. "The Being of that disclosedness is constituted by states-of-mind [in this instance, attentiveness, an essential part of Maria's caring], understanding, and discourse [or conversation]" (Heidegger, 1962, p. 224). Maria characterizes her attentiveness as "very, very sensitive," yet she is powerless to have the parents' desires upheld and can advocate only between them and the staff and between them and the baby, now changed in their view by the blood transfusion. Ideally, their voices would be heard in Maria's story. Advocacy does not imply paternalistically presuming that we understand what someone needs or wants, interpreting it our way and then behaving accordingly (Gadow, 1980). Instead, it means facilitating (inviting) their letting us know in some way so that we understand what *they* need or want—not what *we* think they need or want—and then facilitating their achieving that (Kavanagh, 1993). The healthcare provider does not define the interest or goals (Gadow, 1980). Such self-determination is being respected more often in healthcare, but in situations such as Maria's, other authoritative forces may prevail.

Our attention is directed toward the phenomena themselves, the facts and the events in a situation, so that they speak to us. Maria reveals herself through her own prejudgments and prejudices—Heidegger's forestructure or horizon (Heidegger, 1962, p. 365). Through Maria's openness to the facts that are presented to her, coupled with her forestructures, a "fusion of horizons" occurs that expands her understanding (Gadamer, 1975; Heidegger, 1962, p. 365; Reeder, 1988, p. 213). Thus, Maria does not set aside her own values in order to be an advocate, but she understands and supports the parents, making a future possible.

Discourse and Expertise

For Heidegger, discourse is what is expressed in language. We as humans have language awaiting our use. The words of a language are objects present-at-hand, able to be used. Discourse is what is heard, while keeping silent authentically implies one has something to say. Discourse that expresses itself is communication. Heidegger notes that discourse is more than idle talk and conversation. Maria has not limited her engagement to ordinary conversation with the baby's parents. Instead, clinical knowledge and practice are negotiated (Benner, Tanner, & Chesla, 1996). She has listened to them and heard *their* concerns about *their* baby. She has taken them seriously.

Maria has also listened to and heard the medical and hospital personnel in their solicitude in treating the baby. Maria has remained open to the dialogue from both sides. For Heidegger, "Listening to . . . is Dasein's existential way of Being-open as Being-with for Others" (Heidegger, 1962, p. 206). In her hearkening (p. 207), Maria heeds but is caught in overlapping conversations: her conversation with the baby's parents, the conversation between baby Cassie and her parents, and Maria's conversation with the NICU nursing and medical staff. Maria is the interpreter and facilitator of one to the other: parents to their baby, parents to the staff, staff to the parents, and staff to the baby. Despite being thrown into the world of the NICU, she has understood that the culture and the social norms that predominate do not need to shape her interpretation of what happens there; she sees other possibilities. From this discourse she has determined "the intelligibility of Being-in-the-world [as] articulated according to [what is significant]" (Heidegger, 1962, p. 206). Like understanding, the characteristics of discourse are "rooted in the state of Dasein's Being" (p. 206), and these characteristics are "what the discourse is about; what is said-in-the-talk, as such; the communication; and the making-known" (p. 206). Discourse is essential to disclosedness.

From what we know of her story, Maria is left in the classic situation of understanding a situation, and even becoming knowledgeable about it, without being able to intervene as effectively as she would like (Kavanagh & Kennedy, 1992). The dialectic between the part and the whole does not preclude a crucial movement from philosophical hermeneutics to a critical perspective with practical potential and intent. Making the shift from understanding to intervention begins with the movement from reflexivity to reflectivity and cultural self-assessment (Andrews, 2003). Competence must be accompanied by authority to practice, otherwise, in addition to leaving a gap between understanding and practice, understanding alone fails to expose forms of domination and to promote participatory or liberation strategies. As Ulin explains,

While self-reflection, effective historicity, and the cultural character of all interactions are indispensable ingredients of the process of totality that defines interpretation, they are not sufficient, at least as articulated in the hermeneutic tradition, to account for the complexity of interactions that are marked by social inequality. (Ulin, 2001, p. 140)

Maria is faced with complex realities. In becoming culturally competent, she is not only aware of differences in worldviews but also sensitive to their significance and meanings to those who hold them. In becoming knowledgeable about differences, she is open to learning individual situations and invites discourse. She also learns to be comfortable in encounters with people who come from backgrounds and worldviews other than her own and to incorporate culturally sensitive assessment, communication, and intervention strategies into her practice (Andrews & Boyle, 2003; Kavanagh, Absalom, Beil, & Schliessmann, 1999; Leininger & McFarland, 2002). However, even these practice issues do not ensure our in-depth understanding of Maria's story.

Being-Alongside

Through her solicitude Maria has been alongside the parents, as well as being-ahead of them in her concern for their relationship with their baby. She has enacted Care as the Being of Dasein. Heidegger states that concern is expressed toward things in the world, while solicitude is toward people, other Daseins. Caring is guided by tolerance, and Maria has demonstrated tolerance. She has expressed sympathy for beliefs and values different from her own. Maria in being-alongside has also made use of the ready-to-hand. "'Things' (are) . . . that which one has to do with in one's concernful dealings" (Heidegger, 1962, p. 97). In caring for the baby, Maria uses equipment, technology, and procedures that she takes for granted. These things have been useful in keeping the baby alive. They are ready-to-hand, "standing reserve" (Heidegger, 2001),

constitutive for the equipment we are employing at the time; . . . manipulable in the broadest sense and at our disposal. . . . Dealings with equipment subordinate themselves to the manifold assignments of the "in-order-to." And the sight with which they thus accommodate themselves is *circumspection*. (Heidegger, 1962, p. 98)

In practice, one looks around in order to see what is there and what is to be done. Notions of usefulness and activity are revealed as "Practical behaviors." Heidegger indicates that "in Practical behaviors one *acts*, and that action must employ theoretical cognition if it is not to remain blind" (Heidegger, 1962, p. 99). Maria strives to become expert in her practice; she begins by striving to "do no harm."

In being asked how she learned to handle these tiny babies, Maria replied, "I see machines as extremities requiring lots of care, lots of technical skills. You have to find a balance between [the baby and the equipment]." Clinical skill, clinical wisdom, and good judgment are all part of developing clinical expertise; experiential learning requires engagement in the situation and the possibility of "turning-around" preconceptions and interpretations (Benner, Hooper-Kyriakidis, & Stannard,

1999). Maria looks for a balance between caring for and caring about and in the tension caused between the mechanical, for the most part, objectification of care for Cassie's tiny body and the need for advocacy for the parents, the staff, and the baby. That advocacy includes considering ways in which meanings and expectations for Cassie may have been altered by the medical treatment given her.

Heidegger indicates that we are not concerned primarily with the tools. Maria knows that "science is necessary but not sufficient for becoming a wise clinician who communicates and works well with others to bring about the best outcomes for her patients" (Benner, Hooper-Kyriakidis, & Stannard, 1999, p. 438). The tools are there, waiting, as are Cassie, her parents, and the NICU staff. As a caring clinician, Maria engages in dialogue with all aspects of the situation (including Cassie's acuity, intellectual and emotional engagement in the interactive situation, and the needs of those involved). This working out (clinical reasoning) of knowledge, inquiry, relationships, and action in place (that is, praxis) and the ability to influence the situation (agency) (Benner, Hooper-Kyriakidis, & Stannard, 1999; Benner, Tanner, & Chesla, 1996) enable Maria to be caring in her management of the breakdown occurring in interaction between the baby's parents and the other NICU medical and nursing personnel, and possibly between the parents and their baby.

In the immediacy of everyday practice, Maria struggles with the balance between the requirements of the baby and those of the equipment amid the culture and expectations of the NICU setting. As Heidegger says,

Our concernful absorption in whatever work-world lies closest to us, has a function of discovering; and it is essential to this function that, depending upon the way in which we are absorbed, those entities within-the-world which are brought along in the work and with it [that is to say, in the assignments or references that are constitutive for it] remain discoverable in varying degrees of explicitness and with a varying circumspective penetration. . . .

Readiness-to-hand is the way in which entities as they are "in themselves" are defined. (Heidegger, 1962, p. 101)

In this way, Maria is creating a way to use the mechanics of the NICU in the form of *techne*, the knowledge that constitutes an ability to produce the practical work needed (Gadamer, 1996). One can balance knowing and caring for and about the human with the equipment, or focus on being technically expert in using the equipment. Healthcare providers have choices about how equipment is integrated with care, just as they do about inclusivity of worldviews or beliefs. Maria has an opportunity to develop a way of being-with the entire situation—cultural values, social norms, and instrumentation.

The world of the NICU is relatively new to Maria, and it differs greatly from the ordinary world in which she otherwise lives. The NICU calls for technical proficiency, but Maria's human capability is being called out as well. She has a stake in how others view her, not only the baby's parents and the NICU staff, but her family and friends, and, ultimately, how she views herself. Maria is more than an object delivering care. She struggles to maintain who she is in all her domains of living. In this one small story of the many that compose her life, Maria is bridging the gap between being-with the family and helping them to express caring, and caring for their baby with concern and considerateness. Through all this, she continues to disclose herself to herself and transcends what she was to what she has become.

Maria resists falling toward the "they" of the other nurses whose actions reflect greater experience with the tiny babies' needs than Maria's "novice" status (Benner, 1984). On the other hand, "they" may not demonstrate real expertise in the sense of focusing on the patient. As Heidegger (1962) notes, the "they" pulls every one toward "a leveling" and "averageness." Whether her assumption that some nurses are "burned-out" is accurate or merely a manifestation of their thrownness or Maria's into the NICU, there is no doubt that caring can be costly, for despite intensive care increasingly being a usual standard of care in the United States, caring for the critically ill is demanding and tense work (Kavanagh, 1988; Zalumas, 1995).

Others may or may not view Maria's compassion and involvement with this family as credible. Heidegger indicates that

one's own dasein and that of others is to be defined . . . in terms of certain ways in which one may be. In that with which we concern ourselves environmentally the Others are encountered as what they are; they are what they do.

In one's concern with what one has taken hold of, whether with, for, or against, the others, there is constant care as to the way one differs from them. (Heidegger, 1962, p. 163)

Maria strives to do this—to maintain herself without capitulation in the world into which she is thrown. It is "an era of shifting and emergent paradigms, of moving between worldviews and dualistic opposites; it is a time for openness, for exploration, a time of pragmatics, and heuristic means to move forward" (Watson, 2002, p. 5). It can be a rewarding and exciting time to care for and to care about others, and amid all the tensions of healthcare—splintered as it is by narrow, linear approaches—it is a time in which it is essential to care for and nurture the self as well.

Conclusion

This introductory essay has explicated Heidegger's and Gadamer's ideas about caring and culture as viewed philosophically, interpretively, and in a nurse's practice. It is our hope that the readers of this volume will relate these and other aspects of caring and culture to the excellent chapters that follow.

Note

1. Maria's story comes from an interview concerning communication of caring in nursing practice in community and high-tech health care situations (Knowlden, 1988, 1998). The study was funded by the Charles A. and Anne Morrow Lindbergh Foundation.

References

Andrews, M. M. (2003). Culturally competent nursing care. In M. M. Andrews & J. S. Boyle (Eds.), *Transcultural concepts in nursing care* (4th ed., pp. 15–35). Philadelphia: Lippincott.

Andrews, M. M., & Boyle, J. S. (1997). Competence in transcultural nursing care. *American Journal of Nursing, 98*(8), 16A–D.

Andrews, M. M., & Boyle, J. S. (Eds.). (2003). *Transcultural concepts in nursing care* (4th ed.). Philadelphia: Lippincott.

Andrews, M. M., & Hanson, P. A. (2003). Religion, culture, and nursing. In M. M. Andrews & J. S. Boyle (Eds.), *Transcultural concepts in nursing care* (4th ed., pp. 432–502). Philadelphia: Lippincott.

Baer, H. A. (2001). *Biomedicine and alternative healing systems in America: Issues of class, race, ethnicity, and gender.* Madison: University of Wisconsin Press.

Benner, P. (1984). *From novice to expert: Excellence and power in clinical nursing practice.* Menlo Park, CA: Addison-Wesley.

Benner, P., Hooper-Kyriakidis, P., & Stannard, D. (1999). *Clinical wisdom and intervention in critical care: A thinking-in-action approach.* Philadelphia: W. B. Saunders.

Benner, P., Tanner, C. A., & Chesla, C. A. (1996). *Expertise in nursing practice: Caring, clinical judgment, and ethics.* New York: Springer.

Boss, M. (1963). *Psychoanalysis and daseinsanalysis* (L. B. LeFebre, Trans.). New York: Basic Books.

DeVita, P. R., & Armstrong, J. D. (1993). *Distant mirrors: America as a foreign culture.* Belmont, CA: Wadsworth.

Dossey, B. M., Keegan, L., & Guzzetta, C. E. (2000). *Holistic nursing: A handbook for practice* (3rd ed.). Gaithersburg, MD: Aspen.

Engebretson, J. C., & Headley, J. A. (2000). Cultural diversity and care. In B. M. Dossey, L. Keegan, & C. E. Guzzetta (Eds.), *Holistic nursing: A handbook for practice* (3rd ed., pp. 283–310). Gaithersburg, MD: Aspen.

Freund, P. E. S., & McGuire, M. B. (1995). *Health, illness, and the social body: A critical sociology* (2nd ed.). Englewood Cliffs, NJ: Prentice Hall.

Gadamer, H-G. (1975). *Truth and method* (G. Barden & J. Cumming, Trans.). New York: Seabury Press.

Gadamer, H-G. (1996). *The enigma of health: The art of healing in a scientific age* (J. Gaiger & N. Walker, Trans.). Stanford, CA: Stanford University Press.

Gadow, S. (1980). Existential advocacy: Philosophical advocacy: Philosophical foundation of nursing. In S. F. Spicker & S. Gadow (Eds.), *Nursing: Images and ideals—Opening dialogue with the humanities* (pp. 79–101). New York: Springer.

Goldberg, D. T. (Ed.). (1998). *Multiculturalism: A critical reader.* Malden, MA: Blackwell.

Hahn, R. A., & Gaines, A. D. (Eds.). (1985). *Physicians of Western medicine: Anthropological approaches to theory and practice.* Dordrecht, The Netherlands: D. Reidel.

Heidegger, M. (1962). *Being and time* (J. Macquarrie & E. Robinson, Trans.). New York: Harper & Row. (Original work published 1927)

Heidegger, M. (2001). *Zollikon seminars: Protocols—Conversations—Letters* (F. Mayr & R. Askay, Trans.). Evanston, IL: Northwestern University Press.

Kaplan, A. (1964). *The conduct of inquiry.* New York: Harper & Row.

Kavanagh, K. H. (1988). The cost of caring: Nursing on a psychiatric intensive care unit. *Human Organization, 47*(3), 242–251.

Kavanagh, K. H. (1991). Invisibility and selective avoidance: Gender and ethnicity in psychiatry staff interaction. *Culture, Medicine, and Psychiatry, 15*(2), 245–274.

Kavanagh, K. H. (1993). Transcultural nursing: Facing the challenges of advocacy and diversity/Universality. *Journal of Transcultural Nursing, 5*(1), 4–13.

Kavanagh, K. H., Absalom, K., Beil, W., & Schliessmann, L. (1999). Connecting and becoming culturally competent: A Lakota example. *Advances in Nursing Science, 21*(3), 9–31.

Kavanagh, K. H., & Kennedy, P. H. (1992). *Promoting cultural diversity: Strategies for health care professionals.* Newbury Park, CA: Sage.

Knowlden, V. (1988). Is caring surviving in high-tech nursing practice? Unpublished interview data from the research grant supported by the Charles A. and Anne Morrow Lindbergh Foundation, Minneapolis.

Knowlden, V. (1998). *The communication of caring in nursing.* Indianapolis, IN: Sigma Theta Tau International, Center Press.

Kottak, C. P. (2000). *Anthropology: The exploration of human diversity.* New York: McGraw-Hill.

Ladd, J. (1980). Some reflections on authority and the nurse. In S. F. Spicker & S.

Gadow (Eds.), *Nursing: Images and ideals—Opening dialogue with the humanities* (pp. 160–175). New York: Springer.

Leininger, M., & McFarland, M. R. (2002). *Transcultural nursing: Concepts, theories, research and practice* (3rd ed.). New York: McGraw-Hill.

Loustaunau, M. O., & Sobo, E. J. (1997). *The cultural context of health, illness and medicine.* Westport, CT: Bergin & Garvey.

Lupton, D. (1994). *Medicine as culture: Illness, disease and the body in Western societies.* London: Sage.

Morse, J. M., Solberg, S., Neander, W. L., Bottorff, J., & Johnson, J. (1990). Concepts of caring and caring as a concept. *Advances in Nursing Science, 13*(1), 1–14.

No blood—Medicine meets the challenge. (2001). Videotape produced for Watch Tower Bible and Tract Society of Pennsylvania. Brooklyn, NY: Watchtower Bible and Tract Society of New York.

O'Neill, J. (1986). The disciplinary society. *British Journal of Sociology, 47*(1), 42–60.

Payer, L. (1988). *Medicine and culture: Varieties of treatment in the United States, England, West Germany, and France.* New York: Penguin Books.

Pfifferling, J-H. (1981). A cultural prescription for medicocentrism. In L. Eisenberg & A. Kleinman (Eds.), *The relevance of social science for medicine* (pp. 197–222). Dordrecht, The Netherlands: D. Reidel.

Reeder, F. (1988). Hermeneutics. In B. Sarter (Ed.), *Paths to nursing knowledge* (pp. 193–238). New York: National League for Nursing Press.

Scupin, R. (2003). *Cultural anthropology: A global perspective.* Upper Saddle River, NJ: Prentice Hall.

Smith, E. B. (1986). Surgery in Jehovah's Witnesses. *Journal of National Medical Association, 78*(7), 668–669.

Stein, H. F. (1990). *American medicine as culture.* Boulder, CO: Westview Press.

Stewart, E. C., & Bennett, M. J. (1991). *American cultural patterns: A cross-cultural perspective* (Rev. ed.). Yarmouth, ME: Intercultural Press.

Sugarman, J., Churchill, L. R., Moore, J. K., & Waugh, R. A. (1991). Medical, ethical, and legal issues regarding thrombolytic therapy in Jehovah's Witnesses. *American Journal of Cardiology, 68*(15), 1,525–1,529.

Turner, B. S. (1987). *Medical power and social knowledge.* London: Sage.

Ulin, R. C. (2001). *Understanding cultures: Perspectives in anthropology and social theory* (2nd ed.). Malden, MA: Blackwell.

Watson, J. (1979). *Nursing: The philosophy and science of caring.* Boston: Little, Brown.

Watson, J. (1999). *Nursing: Human science and human care: A theory of nursing.* Boston: Jones & Bartlett for National League for Nursing.

Watson, J. (2002). *Assessing and measuring caring in nursing and health science.* New York: Springer.

Willett, C. (Ed.). (1998). *Theorizing multiculturalism: A guide to the current debate.* Malden, MA: Blackwell.

Wittgenstein, L. (1961). *Tractus logico-philosophicus.* London: Routledge & Kegan Paul.

Zalumas, J. (1995). *Caring in crisis: An oral history of critical care nursing.* Philadelphia: University of Pennsylvania Press.

1

Difference, Dialogue, Dialectics
A Study of Caring and Self-Harm

Andrew Estefan, Margaret McAllister,
and Jennifer Rowe

Overview

Healthcare practitioners are regularly confronted with a range of complex client issues. In practice, clinicians respond to individual needs, yet their responses are shaped and constrained by significant social discourses. When clinicians are not aware of the interaction between practice and those discourses that influence practice, there is a tendency to homogenize people, to routinize, and to reproduce the status quo. Thus, difference is not fully appreciated, dialogue tends not to occur, and dialectics within practice are overlooked. Critical reflection on these factors may reveal possibilities for changing the nature of caring practice.

In this chapter the nexus of practice, discourse, and education is investigated in the context of nursing people who self-harm. The discussion is contextualized by drawing on the findings of a study that examined nurses' practice within specific in-patient workplaces. The findings identify dominant discourses as they shape and constrain nursing care. Tensions that impact on a clinician's ability to care and lead to a tendency to struggle with difference are discussed. Based on the findings, an alternative approach to educating health professionals and encouraging critical reflection on practice is proposed.

Introduction

Skillful caring practice in mental health nursing has been shown to be a powerful influence on client recovery. Through therapeutic management, clients learn to understand problems, develop strengths and social connections, feel more satisfied with services, and become more likely to continue therapeutic work (Dingman, Williams, Fosbinder, & Warnick, 1999; Kelly, 1998).

Skillful nursing care takes into account psychological and social contexts and consequences of health problems, as well as specific details of disease (Reed & Ground, 1997). Within specific contexts, there is constant interaction between individual practice and collective discourse that shapes and constrains what nurses say and do. For example, a nurse may understand the holistic needs of a client but be constrained from providing those needs by a hospital's agenda, which might be to prioritize standard procedures and fiscal outcomes. Thus, rather than view caring work as a dyadic encounter, it may be more accurate to see it as interplay between three things: client, clinician, and context. Given that this interplay is complex and involves competing discourses, caring practice is not always predictable and stable. If we are to advance care for clients who self-harm, then these layers of complexity need to be revealed and deconstructed. In this way we facilitate the emergence of a caring practice that is cautious and considerate of clients with unique issues and needs.

This chapter explores from a post-structural perspective the caring work of nurses engaged in helping clients who self-harm. The chapter begins by providing an overview of the issue of self-harm and proceeds to discuss findings from a discourse analysis that investigated the practices of a small number of Australian mental health nurses, working with self-harming clients in in-patient healthcare services. Finally, we suggest ways that education and practice can be revised in order to understand nursing practice contexts as dialectical rather than dichotomous and so embrace difference and act on the tensions of day-to-day caring work. While the issue under focus is the practice of responding to individuals who self-harm, many of the insights may resonate as meaningful for clinicians aspiring to the challenges of providing individualized care to clients in other contemporary healthcare contexts.

Self-Harm Issues

Deliberate self-harm is a common and distressing behavior for the individuals engaging in it and for their families and significant others, and it frequently requires professional healthcare. Broadly defined, self-harm is any behavior that results in injury to the individual who enacts it. In order to focus discussions, the term is used here to refer to acts such as cutting, burning, or otherwise injuring the body. It excludes reckless behavior, clear suicidality, psychotic phenomena, or stereotypical behaviors seen in some learning disabilities and organic diseases (Vaughan, 1995).

Self-harm is distressing and costly to the individual, to the healthcare provider, to society, and to the culture within which it occurs. Briere (1996) estimates the prevalence of self-harm to be 4% of the population and up to 13% in clinical populations. Self-harm remains a social taboo, and despite the myth that self-harm is a form of attention seeking, it is frequently completed in private (Vivekananda, 2000). Very few incidents of self-harm come to public attention. Even when the client is in therapy, she or he may not reveal the behavior. A study by Van der Kolk, Perry, and Herman (1991) revealed that up to 18% of therapists did not know their client was self-harming.

Self-harm has been the subject of much scholarly discussion since the early 1930s, yet there is no one theory that completely explains the phenomenon, and no single treatment approach to ameliorate it (Shaw, 2002). Psychodynamic theories see self-harm variously as a form of anger turned inward, a way of showing psychic distress without talking about it, a mechanism of repressed guilt in relation to sexual conflict, or a form of catharsis for emotional extremes (Calof, 1997; Favazza, 1996; Menninger, 1938).

Behavioral theories focus on the ways self-harming behavior becomes self-reinforcing. An act of self-harm leads to a biochemical surge of endorphins that produces an immense calming effect, and the individual may learn to use self-harm as a way of self-soothing. Furthermore, operant conditioning focuses on the ways self-harm may be a learned behavior, modeled by parents and peers as a way of dealing with conflict or managing emotions (Bennun, 1984; Fennig, Carlson, & Fennig, 1995).

Although these theories are dominant in understanding self-harm, two more marginal discourses are also relevant—discourses of trauma and feminism. Trauma studies began to proliferate in the 1980s when Post-Traumatic Stress Disorder (PTSD) was named as a condition seen in Vietnam veterans along with those who had survived catastrophes and severe childhood abuse and neglect. Trauma theory sees self-harm as a coping strategy to manage feelings of anxiety, powerlessness, dissociation, intrusive memories, and compulsions to reenact the trauma and punish the body (Miller, 1994; Van der Kolk, 1989).

Feminist discourses of self-harm attempt to explain why this behavior is seen predominantly in girls' and women's development and why it emerges in adolescence. Incidents of self-harm are three to four times more common in women than men and more common in younger than older adults (Mental Health Foundation, 1997). The incidence may be higher in women for many reasons. Women may be socialized to deal with emotional pain in emotional ways, whereas men may deal with emotional upset in physical ways. Women may act on themselves, and men on others. Women may experience more abuse as a child and as adults than men, and women remain more vulnerable to abuse as adults.

Despite this gender imbalance, Favazza (1996) contends that self-harm is becoming more common in males, perhaps because more males are self-identifying experiences of childhood abuse; males are becoming socialized to be emotionally literate; and society is becoming less tolerant of acting out behaviors, such as verbal and physical abuse. The issue of self-harm may have more to do with power and resistance than it does with gender.

Nevertheless, feminist discourses such as relational psychology (Machoian, 1998; Rogers, 1996) are enlightening because they extend the psychoanalytic understanding and the contexts of relationship and environment. When self-harm is associated with loss, abandonment, or abuse, it may be seen as a kind of protest against destructive, disempowering, or unsatisfying relationships—a sign of being silenced or trapped. Self-harm may then be seen as an extreme form of self-expression, when the person's voice is not otherwise heard (Shaw, 2002).

The focus for thinking about self-harm is shifted from individual pathology to a symptom of a larger relational crisis. Relationships are clearly important in providing emotional sustenance and in facilitating healthy, happy lives. Feminist therapeutic approaches strongly assert that positive relationships need to be developed and false or ineffective relationships need to be exposed (Gilligan, Rogers, & Tolman, 1991). Feminist discourse also led the way in theorizing differently about self-harm. Self-harm began to be thought of as qualitatively different from suicide, even though the two may at times coexist (McAllister & Estefan,

2002). Self-harm also began to be thought of as a way of using the body to communicate and to claim power (Crowe, 1996; Foucault, 1980).

Corporeality understands the body as the site where cultural experiences are inscribed (Curry, 1993). The body is an object that is always socially influenced. It is marked and shaped, and yet it is also experienced as unique to the individual, the seat of one's subjectivity and sense of self (Caillois, 1984; Crowe, 1996). This paradox is something that people learn when they struggle with the idea that they can both act and be acted upon. People can be subjects and objects at the same time. Corporeality sees the body as a battleground where the person acts out this struggle with the self—a self who is unique, personal, and subjective, and a self who is a social subject, molded and constrained by beliefs and practices that have been embedded by society. For example, when a woman cuts herself, she is the subject of her bodily experience, not simply the object of others' experiences of it. She is also acting as the self who is personal and who wants to express her internal pain, and the self who is a social product who is frustrated with being treated as an object.

Beyond the relational view, self-harm is also currently being theorized as a biosocial and a cultural disorder. The biosocial theory sees disorder biologically in that there tend to be characteristic signs in many individuals: heightened sensitivity to emotion, increased emotional intensity, and a slow return to emotional baseline. Socially, the problem lies in the way coping mechanisms for this emotional dysregulation are invalidated (Everett & Gallop, 2000; Linehan, 1993). When the person acts in self-harming ways, that behavior is invalidated, a cycle of guilt–self-harm–invalidation–guilt is established, and self-harm recurs.

Favazza (1996) suggests that self-harm is neither purely biological, psychological, or social but rather involves a combination of these factors as they operate within the web of culture. Favazza examined various religious practices across a number of cultures in which self-mutilation is sanctioned. In a religious and cultural context, self-mutilation acts as a rite of passage by providing a stepping-stone to wisdom and self-knowledge, aiding the development of healing oneself and others, and restoring a sense of power and control. This view of self-injury moves it beyond the realm of individual psychopathology and provides it with significant social purpose and cultural meaning.

As a result, self-harm has different meanings for different individuals and groups and therefore requires knowledgeable, skilled, and flexible responses from healthcare workers. According to Osuch, Noll, and Putnam (2000), self-harm can be categorized into six subscales: as a way to regulate affect, reduce feeling desolate, punish/please others, influence others, assert magical control, or self-stimulate. Such diverse motivations are rarely appreciated by nursing staff because most receive no formal training about the nature of self-harm and are vulnerable to prevailing public attitudes, which tend to be negative or based on myths (Hemmings, 1999).

In sum, self-harm is a complex human behavior that has meaning at individual, social, and cultural levels. For the individual, self-harm is a bodily medium through which people may express and reveal their psychological distress. At social and cultural levels, self-harm reflects women's experiences of distress in a given situation and reveals how the behavior is socially and culturally embedded.

The Culture of Care

According to cultural theorists such as Foucault (1980), culture can be reproduced or transformed within social relationships. Cultural practices tend to be reproduced when hegemonic forces are in place and when people comply with the prevailing order largely because it has been taken for granted and accepted. The dominant cultural group's agenda goes ahead unchallenged and even unnoticed. Yet culture can also be transformed when peoples' consciousness is raised, and they begin to notice hegemony, to realize how dominant groups have a tendency to silence differences of opinion, and to marginalize groups that do not conform to mainstream ideas. In this view, power is a resource that is accessible to all people within society, not just those in authority, and it can be used to challenge and perhaps transform everyday cultural practices.

In the healthcare culture, particularly within the Australian psychiatric healthcare context in which this study is located, certain preferred practices continue to be supported, perhaps unconsciously, by the majority. Those practices include reliance on the medical model for diagnosis and treatment and on behavior modification for shaping clients' social behaviors to help them become more socially competent or, indeed, more socially acceptable (Johnstone, 1997). At times, these practices are ill fitting, producing limited outcomes, perhaps even delaying progress in clients. Health workers' therapeutic repertoire is limited because dominant practices are so all pervading.

McAllister (2001), for example, described self-harm in a hospital setting as a scenario wherein many people, not just the client, get caught up in harm's way. The client who hurts herself and then shows her wounds to a busy nurse may be labeled medically or behaviorally as either a "personality disorder who is acting out," "attention seeking," or simply "making trouble." None of these labels prompts effective treatment, and yet they continue to be officially sanctioned and institutionalized within care plans and protocols. When the healthcare system makes unrealistic demands for consistency and controlled caring, health workers will typically struggle with standard rules and perhaps fail in their duty to care.

The client who self-harms presents significant challenges to nurses and health agencies that are not always equipped to respond effectively. Being ill equipped to respond to self-harm poses risks to both clients and nurses. For the client, there is the risk of invalidating, insensitive, and painful treatment that can be re-traumatizing and perpetuate self-harm (Linehan, 1993). For the nurse, there is the risk of frustration, burnout, and vicarious traumatization from being exposed to a perplexing and confronting behavior (Alston & Robinson, 1992; Hartman, 1995). Yet clients continue to seek help and want to tell their stories (Ahuja, 2000), and nurses continue to want to help clients recover (McAllister, Creedy, Moyle, & Farrugia, 2002). Given that clients do articulate their experiences and nurses seek to assist the client toward recovery, the question remains why practice or care continues to be problematic for nurses and clients.

Having set the scene by describing characteristics of self-harm and issues concerning this phenomenon, we briefly discuss significant discourses represented in the literature. This discussion assists the reader in understanding the practice context and issues that potentially influence nursing care for people who self-harm.

Significant Discourses

Discourse refers to a way of thinking, talking, or writing about reality (Cherryholmes, 1988). Discourses act as forms of containment of knowledge, setting parameters and limiting the ways in which a practice can be thought or spoken about and consequently experienced. Knowledge in mental health is shaped, constrained, and sustained through an interaction between talk in the clinical area (Horsfall & Cleary, 2000), and policy and practice directives that impact on the work of nurses in mental health. Therefore, mental health nursing is a discursive practice—a practice that is subject to and constitutive of discourse. Everyday individual and collective interactions shape discourses and, in turn, practices, so that some assume dominance while others are marginalized. Discourses of risk, management, outcomes, efficiency, professionalism, and care dominate the literature relating to self-harm and nursing.

The Discourse of Risk

The terms *risk* and *risk management* are not new concepts in mental health care but have become increasingly formalized into policy and practice directives in acute inpatient services (Doyle, 1998; Hazleton, 1999; Sherman et al., 2001). These concepts have traditionally shaped nursing practice and have been found to be important in nurses' perceptions and talk. For example, Hazelton (1999) found that nurses return to themes of safety and risk and believe that issues concerning safety and the management of a "difficult clientele" largely structure their work (p. 226). Risk and risk management are important health discourses in the way health problems are conceived and responded to in contemporary society (Peterson & Lupton, 1996). Risks are estimated and managed as part of a problem-solving approach characteristic of late modernity. Risk identification and management resonate particularly in mental health in order to construct and manage pathology and abnormal behavior.

Examining media representations of this discourse illustrates how it operates in the broader community. The media make significant contribution to the widespread perception that those with mental health problems pose a risk to communities (Munro, 2000), and media reporting continues to stigmatize mental illness by using negative or outdated language. Recently, for example, the television program *Providence* (Masius, 2002) portrayed a person disturbed by auditory hallucinations and suffering schizophrenia as wild, uncontrollable, and bent on homicide and fire lighting. There is also evidence to suggest considerable prejudice in the community against the mentally ill (Heald, 1999). Common public attitudes toward people who self-harm range from fear to horror, disgust, and avoidance (Johnstone, 2002). This combination of prejudice and media distortion has the potential to be self-perpetuating, reproducing the status quo both in public attitudes and nursing practices.

The prominent media message suggests that those with mental health problems pose risks that require control. Subsequently, nurses are under social pressure to prioritize their practice according to clients who pose the greatest risk (Bowers, 1997). This is, however, a one-sided view of a multidimensional picture. In this polarized, dichotomous perspective, the client is constructed as a risk to society, situating the nurse in a surveillance role—protecting society from the client. The nurse must be (however erroneously) perceived as the one who is risk-free and the provider of safety. The client is then perceived in the opposite manner. Risk and risk management constructed from this perspective is a discourse that maintains a status quo of dichotomy, whereby the nurse is seen as the provider of care and safety and the client as vulnerable and in need.

On the other hand, a dialectical reading of risk situates the client as being both *of risk* (a danger) and *at risk* (vulnerable) (Hazleton, 1999). From this perspective, tension exists between the public moral discourse, in which the client is positioned as always potentially dangerous, and the caring discourse, which recognizes the inherent vulnerability within the potentially dangerous client (Hazleton, 1999). There also exists a dialectical relationship between security and danger, and between trust and risk (Mercer, Mason, & Richman, 2001). Simply stated, public perceptions of dangerousness require increased security of and for clients. Control more than care remains prioritized, and the nurse is engaged mainly as a "social policeman" (Hazleton, 1999).

Risk and Management

There appear to be three ways in which management can be construed. The first is in the workplace, where the care environment is controlled in a top-down fashion. This form of management values procedure and serves to maintain a functioning workplace. It involves management processes such as staffing and resource allocation. The second form of management involves the management of workers to perform tasks within time and cost-containment frameworks. This kind of management melds the clinical environment and clinician through devices such as clinical paths, policies, and standardized procedures. These policies, procedures, and clinical pathways inform and shape the care provided and thus impact the client. The third form of management extends worker and environment management to encapsulate the client. It involves managing the client in order that symptoms and risk are contained (Busfield, 2000). Such approaches clearly have the potential to constrain care, yet they can also positively influence treatment approaches.

Management discourse has the potential to streamline work and structure the clinical environment, contributing to the therapeutic milieu and maintenance of therapeutic boundaries. It can also, however, alter nurses' focus toward workload rather than client (Muir-Cochrane, 2001). Although management discourse can be helpful, it may constrain nurses' views of their practice, whereby it becomes difficult to recognize a nursing role in the absence of risk or symptom exacerbation.

Efficiency and Outcomes

Efficiency, indicated in economic and outcome measures, is strongly embedded in current risk-management discourse. There is increasing governmental expectation that limited public resources are expended on the basis of evidence of efficiency. Economic management and rationalization of health services are afforded priority (Bonner, 2001). Health providers have come to rely upon, value, and take for granted the naturalness of outcomes-focused services. Discourses on risk-management efficiency intersect at workplace and work-practice levels and exert pressure on nurses to act in ways that efficiently minimize risk, manage clients, and contain costs—all outcome measures. When this effective, efficient, management-focused, and outcomes-oriented work is done, we argue that nurses (and others) tend to consider the nurse's role to be complete. Traditional practices of nurturance, comfort, education, motivation, and support go undervalued and unnoticed and ultimately may not be provided.

Within this context nurses are "managed" in order to improve efficiency, effectiveness, outcomes, and cost containment. This in turn influences their practice. In relation to self-harm, a survey of mental health nurses caring for clients illustrates that nurses frequently failed to request additional supervision for clients even though they had been identified as at risk (Childs, Thomas, & Tibbles, 1994). Concerns for efficient or cost-contained management was a primary consideration.

Embedded in these approaches is tension between maintaining the order of things and attending to individual clients. Nurses are pressured to conform to economic and organizational agendas. Practice is constructed within a role in which nurses need to respond to the unexpected yet, at the same time, follow a path of maximum predictability toward certain outcomes. This demand has consequences that manifest not only in nurses' responses to clients but also in nurses' intrapersonal responses to their work, that is, how they manage themselves, a further aspect of the risk-management discourse that pervades nursing care.

The Managed Self

Self-management is central to effective caring in that the ability to attend and to be proactive and responsive to the needs of others intersects with the ability to know and manage self. The managed self has been the topic of theorizing in contemporary literature. Staden (1998) refers to the work of Hochschild (1983) and states that nurses need to manage themselves in order to appear caring. Describing this as the "managed heart," these authors suggest that nurses are required to manage both their conduct and their emotional responses to clients. Clearly then, the management discourse has implications for the nurse as person, as well as professional.

The self-harm literature also reflects this notion. Hartman (1995), for example, warns of the potential for vicarious traumatization in nurses who do not attend to their own needs when they care for clients who self-harm. It may be hypothesized that if nurses are convinced that their role is to manage order and contain risk, they may deny the consequences to themselves of their interactions with people who self-harm or their ability to appropriately manage their own responses.

What is described above is a form of role ambiguity that may increase work-related stress—a situation that in turn makes it more likely that clinicians will take a managed approach to practice. Work-related stress is on the rise (Dallender, Nolan, Soares, Thomsen, & Arnetz, 1999), and several studies have linked the increasing burnout of nurses to changes in the delivery of healthcare (Brown, Bartlett, Leary, & Carson, 1995; Clinton & Hazleton, 2000; Stordheur, D'hoore, & Vandenberghe, 2001). Burnout can be defined as the loss of physical, emotional, and mental energy (Musick, 1997) and is characterized by emotional detachment (Brown, Bartlett, Leary, & Carson, 1995), high levels of stress (Clinton & Hazleton, 2000), and the use of detachment tactics and dissociation (Crowe, 2000).

Detachment may be seen in the ways nurses distance themselves from clients. Niven (1994) reports that increased stress can lead to cynicism toward clients who may then be held responsible for the workplace stress that nurses experience. In this case, it is not surprising that some nursing practices are grounded in an orientation that objectifies the client and invalidates their needs (Brown, Bartlett, Leary, & Carson, 1995). Such practices may be skillful in that they have a good fit with the dominant managing frameworks, and yet they are patently not responsive or therapeutic. The picture is further complicated when the concept of caring, central to the language and ideology of nursing, is overlaid.

Caring Discourse in Nursing Practice

Caring discourse is multilayered. On one level, caring discourse directs nurses to respond to clients in certain ways, and these directions may at times pull nurses in different directions. For example, caring is frequently discussed in terms of being human and valuing ordinariness (Taylor, 1994), but it also involves using expert professional ethics (Barker, 2000) and developing an identity separate from the self through a new professional identity (Roach, 1992).

Caring discourse also contains conflicting philosophies, such as the phenomenological lens of Benner and Wrubel (1989) and the postmodern lens of Watson (1995). Many nursing authors and theorists have proposed that caring is central to understanding the nature and practice of nurses (Benner & Wrubel, 1989; Buller & Butterworth, 2001; Leininger, 1978; Watson, 1995). Yet others have argued that caring cannot be nursing's exclusive realm since other professions also claim a caring agenda (Barker & Reynolds, 1994).

Whether central or associative, caring is steeped in nursing ideology, professional constructs, and broader cultural and social discourses. The notion of caring is affective for it evokes images of kindness, compassion, and patience. These behaviors are embedded in practice ideology and normalized in professional nursing models. What is less clear is how caring ideology intersects with practice realities and how it might be influenced by imperatives of the managerial health service environment that typify the current context of mental health nursing. This leads to speculation about how care, thus embedded, may serve to reproduce the status quo and constrain both the purpose and actions of nursing practice. Skillful practice as care cannot, it seems, be taken for granted.

One writer has suggested that an alternative way of defining and understanding the central purpose of nursing may be to think and speak of it as *being with* the client (Wilkin, 2001). Wilkin argued that being with a client requires acknowledgment of the contingent and particular of the client situation, a basis upon which nurses can define their practice roles and skills. It could be that in this alternate discourse, both nurses and clients may be well situated to discover areas of strength, resilience, and need as a basis for therapeutic practice. This perspective has, in common with humanistic constructions of holism, an interest in context. It is, however, different in that it is not a totalizing approach wherein the central agenda is of managing the client. Rather, it is one in which contingency and concern for the particular become the work for clinician and client.

Whatever the perspective, caring in some form is embodied in the day-to-day acts of nursing practice, and the dynamics of skillful practice continue to be debated. Further, when placed in the broader picture of discourses that shape and constrain practice in any specific context, tensions and challenges become apparent. Discourses serve many functions, not least of which is to shape, establish, and sustain the status quo. Yet often unheralded are specific actions and behaviors that move against the tide and provide a view of possibilities for skillful practice. The context of nursing practice with clients who self-harm is one such practice field.

It is apparent that there is much to be investigated, understood, and challenged in order to better situate the self-harming client and the nursing practice that responds to this complex health experience. In this practice context there is strong evidence that there are many deficiencies in nursing approaches, and that these deficiencies seem to be continuing unabated (Johnstone, 1997; Perego, 1999; Shaw, 2002). Examining this practice context from a post-structural perspective is one (as yet underutilized but potentially helpful) critical approach to use. It may uncover taken-for-granted practices, reveal discourses that subtly shape actions and reproduce the status quo, and promote understanding of constraints, tensions, and possibilities for change. The next section of this chapter reports such a study.

The Study

The study set out to explore the following questions:

1. What are the dominant discourses that shape and constrain nurses' practice with clients who self-harm?
2. What power mechanisms operate in these discourses to enable or constrain effective nursing care of people who self-harm?
3. What knowledge do nurses value to inform their practice with clients who self-harm?

A Foucauldian approach to discourse analysis was used to investigate the research questions. The strength of this approach is that wider influences on practice can be made visible, while at the same time the impact of these discourses on everyday nursing responses to clients can also be evoked and illustrated. Discourse as it is applied to this study is defined as "a patterned system of texts, which may be found in communications or social structures" (Lupton, 1992, p. 145). In the context of discourse analysis, texts are any communicative event and are the object of analysis (Ballinger & Payne, 2000).

Foucault (1980) theorized the role and function of discourses in the social world. For Foucault, discourses create "epistemes" or, put more simply, "the order of things" (Danaher, Schirato, & Webb, 2000). This "order of things" makes certain things sayable, some things possible, and other things impossible. Through a process of classification and allocation of meaning and value, sense is made of things, and what can be known and spoken about is shaped. Epistemes are unconscious and not thought about, but they are influential, as they are things upon which meanings and practice are constructed.

Foucault (1980) further argued that power exists among people and that analysis of it should focus not on its essential nature, but on the point of application. This is reflected in Foucault's (1977) genealogical approach to discourse analysis. Genealogy begins by problemizing an issue, examining its historical and political emergence, and producing a critical picture of the phenomenon under investigation (Howarth, 2000). As applied to the current study, the literature review revealed that the discourses of risk, management, outcomes, and efficiency are politically and socially situated to drive current health agendas and to shape and constrain nursing practice. The texts for the discourse analysis were generated from the practice of five nurses who worked in in-patient mental health services.

Conducting the Study

Prior to conducting the study, ethical clearance was obtained from the University Ethics Committee. Interview data from five practicing registered nurses, all relatively new to mental health nursing, formed the primary text for discourse analysis. The nurses were self-selected in a purposive, convenience-sampling process (Morse, 1991). Each nurse participated in one individual semi-structured, audio tape-recorded interview that lasted approximately 45–60 minutes. This approach to data collection enabled participants to discuss in a safe, confidential space their experience of practice with the client who self-harms. As the participants were master's degree students undertaking the same course, individual interviews were chosen so that the nurses would not be open to peer scrutiny. The notion that the fear of judgment or the need to appear to be a good person (or nurse) may produce idealized or conforming responses (Polit & Hungler, 1995) also informed the data collection method. Therefore, individual interviews were selected for contributing to rigor and to ethical research conduct. In the interviews, an *aide-mémoire* was used to ask all participants the same broad questions, such as "Tell me about a time you have worked with a client who self-harms," and "Who else was there and what did they do?" These questions prompted participants to talk about aspects of practice they found significant in ways that were evocative. They discussed their own experiences and their understandings of other nursing practice occurring in their workplaces. A funneling approach (Minichiello, Aroni, Timewell, & Alexander, 1995) was then used to explore specific aspects of these nurses' practice, producing text.

Data were transcribed verbatim, and each participant text was labeled with a letter: *A* through *E*. Texts were read and reread in order that the data could be engaged with as a whole. At this preliminary stage of data analysis, operational discourses emerged, and the data were scrutinized for significant statements that reflected the perceived naturalness of the clinical environment and nursing responses. In other words, this process uncovered how Foucault's "order of things" was represented (Foucault, 1980; Danaher, Schirato, & Webb, 2000).

The next step taken in the study was to consider how everyday practice is constructed by and within the context and culture of the in-patient mental health environment. Once a broad picture of the discourse/practice of each of the participants had been gained, transcripts were reread to isolate key points of the text. Critical questions such as "What influences how practice is spoken about?" "What is not being said?" and "What is in the margins of the text?" helped the researchers make visible the ways that power was being enacted and resisted. Returning to the whole transcript and considering the parts in relation to the whole facilitated theorizing how discourses exist, how they are supported and maintained, and how they influence practice for these nurses in their individual clinical environments.

To maintain consistent analysis, the process of reading and rereading, noting the whole, the parts, and the parts in relation to the whole, was repeated for each transcript. Once this process was completed for each participant, common themes were sought in all texts. These shared aspects of practice then formed the basis for discussing and theorizing about the prominent discourses that operated for these nurses (Minichiello, Aroni, Timewell, & Alexander, 1995). Eliciting shared aspects of practice also served to assist in examining practice possibilities that were marginal within the more prominent and accepted, "common sense," or normalized discourse/practice.

Study Limitations

The understandings generated by discourse analysis are bound by context. Post-structural approaches to inquiry are grounded in the notion that truth, rather than an objective reality, is local, multiple, and intersubjective (Gitlin, 1989). This study aims to evoke aspects of context-specific practice in what is certainly a partial yet also sustainable view. Therefore, the findings of this study, conducted in Brisbane, Australia, in 2002 with a small number of nurses working with clients who self-harm, are not generalizable. Furthermore, the participants in this study were undertaking further education at the time of their participation, shaping the lens through which they experience and report their care. Their interpretations of practice are likely to be affected over time.

Participant Backgrounds in or with Self-Harm

Participants' knowledge and education in self-harm were various. One participant reported receiving no education regarding self-harm in his undergraduate education. This led him to "hit the books" as a means of developing a theoretical understanding of self-harm. Another participant stated that her initial education regarding self-harm happened on the ward when she was a newly registered nurse, through a process of mentorship with a more experienced practitioner. Two of the remaining three participants reported receiving a broad overview of the issue in their undergraduate education.

One nurse had received greater theoretical input regarding self-harm. This participant was able to recount a comprehensive level of instruction regarding self-harm. She identified having learned that self-harming clients may be attempting to cope and wanting not to die: "I was taught that it was a way of coping, but in our particular society it was not an accepted way of coping" *(E)*. This participant went on to explain how these aspects of self-harm were contextualized for her by saying:

In other societies and cultures it is [seen as a way of coping]—even in the Aboriginal culture. What we term self-harm is part of their culture in dealing with grieving and other aspects . . . so we learned about the physiology, too, of what self-harm does. And that gave it more of a context because some people drink, some people over-eat, some people have other risk behaviors that have that same physiological effect on the body, but they're not as shunned by society as [are those who] self-harm. So it gave a context to what self-harm was for the first time and that helps to not just see the self-harm when you're with someone who does self-harm. *(E)*

Participant *E* referred to her education as giving her the ability to look past the behavior of self-harm and be aware that it may occur for many reasons. This is an important component of practice (McAllister & Estefan, 2002), because behaviors alone are not diagnostic.

What was common among the participants was that, despite practicing in mental health services, none had been taught skills to respond to a person who self-harms. The only participant who recalled any content relating to practice skills spoke generically of being present for and observing the client: "Just being supportive and understanding—showing empathy. Just the basics. Just those basic fundamentals at a beginning level just to be supportive. If I remember rightly—what were the warning signs. Just the warning signs in people" *(D)*.

These participants had little if any formal knowledge on which to draw as a foundation for their practice with people who self-harm, and yet they did work with this client group as part of their mental health nursing practice and recounted and reflected upon their experiences. In their accounts it became clear that the participating nurses experienced tensions in their work. Embedded in these tensions were interactions between discourse and practice. Three primary tensions were identified:

management and nursing practice, psychiatry and nursing responses, and experience and nursing practice. They are described below and illustrated with extracts from the participants' accounts.

Interpretation

Management and Nursing Practice

Management, as workplace and work-practice organizer, was seen to be an overarching, significant discourse that influenced nursing practice in positive and negative ways. Management may promote efficiency and standardized procedures by regulating practice, making it more reliable and more accountable, thus minimizing chaos and disorder. On the other hand, management may constrain nursing work by reducing the role to measurable tasks, encouraging conformity over creativity, focusing on compliance with rules, and ensuring that workers conform to procedures. In this view, there may be tension when the needs of the workplace compete or contrast with the needs of the client. Being task focused rather than client focused is one consequence.

Nurses in this study commented upon ward cultures that were driven by hierarchy and a top-down decision-making model. This created tension for the work they wanted to perform:

Nurses feel very frustrated with management. From the very top down, there are shifts and changes. At the moment from the very top down there is a very belligerent medical model approach. . . . there's not a team feel that comes down. It's still very much hierarchical management and by the time it gets down to the bottom nursing staff are down here. *(E)*

This dynamic led participant *E* to comment that the nurses "feel unheard. They feel frustrated. They are wanting to do things on the ward that they don't feel supported in. So all of this transmutes into caring for the patient, because the patient is the last one in the line."

Frustrated nurses experienced difficulty in practicing effectively with the client because their autonomy was being constrained. This promoted a sense of powerlessness in these nurses, although there were clear sites of resistance. Participant *E* described how some nurses responded to this workplace culture and attempted to assert control over their practice:

And there are times, I know there are times when staff are ventilating and it may be simply, "Okay, the kitchen is locked between this time and this time and I'm not opening it." And that's—there are reasons for that because we have people who just walk in off the street and help themselves to liters of milk and handfuls of food out of the patient kitchen. So it does have a reason for being locked, but I have seen it where the total intolerance of opening the kitchen at any other time is perhaps a ventilation of frustration that staff member is feeling, because they're not getting heard and there's that uncertainty in their mind. *(E)*

In this scenario, nurses appear to be demonstrating resistance to the control that is exerted over their practice, but it has negative consequences because clients' freedoms and quality of life are being overlooked. In this case, nurses, feeling exposed to rigid arbitrary decisions about their practice environments, adopted the same inflexible characteristics toward their clients, as evidenced in their interactions. Freire (1972) suggested that oppressed people tend to adopt the characteristics of their oppressors as a means to assert themselves.

The management–nursing practice tension is also evident in nurses' responses to clients. Management discourse shapes nursing practices by preferring behavioral techniques to humanistic understanding. This preference required chastising the client for behaviors that disrupted the environment: "Well probably some sort of punitive measures I guess, brought upon her in the sense that, you know, telling her off—telling her that she's done the wrong thing" *(A)*.

The management discourse also involved seclusion in response to an act of self-harm. For participant *D*, this approach was unsatisfactory and created additional concerns, such as legal issues, apprehension about the emotional effect on other clients, and the dignity of the secluded client:

People who self-harm are removed from that, from that particular area of self-harm and usually placed in seclusion or placed in a locked area [where] they can be observed. Obviously to protect the nurses and anyone else from any further action or suing. Probably to take the stress away from other co-patients that might witness the self-harming and to keep an eye on the person for the damage that they might do. . . . That if that person has self-harmed or is intending to self-harm, remove them from that environment and lock them in a place where they can't self-harm. Strip them and medicate them. *(D)*

Such extreme interventions were not uncommon in participants' accounts of their practice. Participants revealed that they either ignored the self-harm, based on the assumption that to ignore the behavior is not to reinforce it, or overreacted, in which case the client was forcefully contained. Both polemic responses seem to be shaped by the management discourse whereby behavioral strategies manage both client and environment. Ignoring self-harm enabled nurses to continue to manage the ward and clients' behaviors. Secluding clients enabled crises to be contained and those clients nursed with a minimum of disruption to the environment.

These responses were common features of practice yet frequently engendered other difficulties for nurses. Management discourse in the form of standardized and rule-bound routines and protocols appeared so firmly embedded in nurses' conceptions of their practice that to think about responding differently was not easy. This occurred despite participants' ability to recognize that these practices sometimes failed. A participant reflected on a time when a client had been secluded following an episode of self-harming. This client was placed into seclusion ostensibly for her own safety and to reduce outside stimuli to enable her to settle down.

She'd been medicated, we had stripped her of absolutely everything. She had no jewelry, nothing. She was in a hospital nightie. I mean all of these procedures are demoralizing but at that point it was to keep her safe. She was in a quiet room under cameras and fifteen-minute observations and each time I'd go in to see how she was going, she had self-harmed. She was progressively bleeding all over the place and I could not work out what she was doing. And I would sit with her and talk and that was one time when I didn't feel that I was in any way therapeutic other than keeping this person safe and I wasn't being successful in that. I wasn't keeping her safe. And it eventuated that she was peeling her toenails off. Because I looked at her fingernails and they were down to the quick and she was peeling her toenails off and using her toenails to lacerate herself. And she almost, um, her arm became so hugely infected that she had compartment syndrome and almost had to go to theater. She did quite severe damage. (E)

What this powerful account demonstrates is how well-intentioned—but rigidly and unreflectively executed—interventions can be damaging to the client and counterproductive to the ward environment. Placing the client in seclusion was a considered response to self-harm, in that nurses were seeking to prevent further injury to the client, and a discursively shaped practice in that it was accepted as the most effective means of containing the self-harm. Nurses did not question the appropriateness of this standardized response. Their behavior was constrained by a discourse so powerful that it narrowed vision and failed both nurses and clients. This failure was also evident in another account of this type of response:

She tried to put instruments in her shoes. She'd break plastic knives and forks and—um, put them anywhere she could. She'd even been secluded on one particular time, apart from her shoes and still managed to get an item out and start cutting her arms with it. *(D)*

What nurses appeared not to recognize in these episodes of care was the invalidating nature of the intervention. The client self-harmed, and this communicative act was met with an injunction. That is, the client was punished for communicating his or her distress. Such invalidation has the potential to cause further self-injury (Linehan, 1993). Furthermore, the notion that seclusion is a low-stimulus environment for a person who self-harms is questionable. It may be argued that the need to self-harm is produced by considerable interpersonal distress (Crowe, 1996). Thus, confining the client to an isolated environment fails to address the intrapersonal distress and avoids relational practice. Such an intervention reveals that the physical body is privileged in nursing interventions. The physical body is amenable to management via protocols and environmental control, and so the crisis can be contained. Secluding the client may not reduce the intrapersonal crisis, however, and practices such as seclusion illustrate how the multidimensional aspects of the person may be invisible to nurses. Therefore, a dialectical practice of caring for the vulnerable body by accessing, interpreting, and validating the intrapersonal was unattainable for these nurses. The ability to practice within the dialectic was further complicated by the tension between the psychiatric discourse and the nursing responses to the client.

Psychiatry and Nursing Responses

For nurses in this study, the psychiatric discourse pathologized self-harm and rendered the meaning and motivation for the act invisible. Psychiatry is a powerful discourse in the shaping and constraint of nursing, because, when practicing by this discourse, nurses may perceive that they have few therapeutic practice options (Horsfall & Stuhlmiller,

2001). This perception was clear in many accounts, where nurses described feeling impotent to respond to the self-harming client. The psychiatric discourse correlates self-harm with Borderline Personality Disorder (BPD). Those diagnosed with BPD are commonly believed to be manipulative and attention seeking (Dear, 2000), and therapeutic intervention is often directed toward behavioral approaches to ameliorate these behaviors. When practice is shaped in this way, two-way communication between nurse and client is effectively shut down, and the client's attempts to communicate are ignored or misread. The notion that self-harm is an attention-seeking behavior permeated participants' accounts of practice.

I think it's just—they're just seeing an attention seeker—ignore. I think it's just to ignore them sort of, yeah. Yeah, maybe just to be ignored. I don't think it serves any function . . . I think perhaps the nurses don't know how to deal with it. (B)

With this statement, participant B was making visible the effect of being taught to ignore self-harm as an attention-seeking behavior. The practice is grounded in the notion that if the behavior is responded to, it will be reinforced and thus will be more likely to occur. While physical injuries were attended to, the client's distress was not. Psychiatric discourse, thus constructed, embeds an irony, wherein the body is responded to, and the intrapersonal dimensions of the person are marginalized and rendered invisible. In describing how this occurred in practice, Participant C explained: "You don't make a big deal out of it. You just clean them up and get the doctor to it to look at it and you play it down. Make sure they are physically all right and maybe talk to them about it later."

For another participant it was important to attend to the emotional dimension of the client, although she felt her practice being constrained by how she was expected to respond. This feeling demonstrates a tension between the psychiatric discourse and caring discourse characterized by seeking to *be with* the client:

I suppose not to make too much fuss about the cut itself. To be fairly casual . . . not to nurture that behavior. But be empathetic and like on the ward, we got the doctor to come in and I assisted the doctor to stitch this patient up . . . and uh, maybe then sit down with her later on but not too much fuss over it. (B)

A further response that indicated nurses' caution toward reinforcing clients' perceived manipulation and desire for attention came from participant A:

The nurses are always aware of, um, I guess patients that are manipulating in behavior. It's the, um, I guess no-one likes to be taken for a ride. And, um, they're always very conscious of that fact and perhaps too much so to the extent of maybe being detrimental to some of the patients. And it's too easy sometimes to perceive someone as, um, manipulating you where in fact this could be just a normal part of their disease process.

The power of the psychiatric discourse can be seen in how it constrained the ways nurses thought about their clients as "manipulative attention seekers" who exhibited behaviors that are pathological. Nurses then relied on a behavioral model that sought to minimize the likelihood of rewarding and increasing these negatively valued behaviors. Ironically, the psychiatric discourse silenced the client's intrapersonal distress and rendered their attempts at communication invisible. What nurses saw instead were clients who were two-dimensional characters—a body and a behavior, seemingly devoid of emotion, reason, and motivation.

Psychiatric and management discourses were thus significant in shaping nurses' responses to clients who self-harm. The study participants, however, offered evidence of sites of resistance in practice, of the inherent power of these discourses. There were negative dynamics that reflected resistance but also positive dynamics. Data analysis revealed accounts of inspiring practice with the client who self-harms. Participants were able to richly describe episodes of care, where relationships with clients had been strengthened, and therapeutic progress had been made. One participant recalled an interaction whereby talking to the client gave her a helpful insight into the client's motivation for self-harm:

She was awfully anxious. I remember she was quite shaky and anxious. And . . . she was taken back to the ward and she's actually the same person I mentioned before when we sort of stitched her up and cleaned her up and also I had a talk to her and she's the one that said it let the bad out. *(B)*

The insight gained for this nurse was that the client's reason for self-harm was unrelated to manipulation or attention seeking. Thus, the nurse was able to access the client's subjective experience. Talking with

the client in this way went against the dominant discourses of management and psychiatry and became an act of resistance. This response
constituted an opportunity for new ways of practicing and opened a
channel of communication between nurse and client. This experience
prompted the nurse to continue to engage with the client and allowed
further insights to develop: "She said she had to do it, she had to do it.
She was in a like a panic. She had to do—I mean there was no way, if
I use those words—'attention seeking'—there was much deeper—she
had, she had to do it to get herself to feel better again" (B). Other nurses
described similar experiences during which engaging with the client
opened up spaces for therapeutic encounters to occur. One participant
told of a helpful encounter she had with a client, despite encouragement
from other nurses not to engage the client in this way: "I just spoke to
them like they were a person. I sort of let them—which I was told wasn't
really the right way to handle them—but I sort of let them control our
discussions in some ways" (C).

Nurse C talked of her experience of seeing beyond the behavior
and appreciating the need to engage with the client as a person. Her
motivations were grounded in a deep concern for the client's well-being:
"To me it was better to help her straight away and get her out of the
system, than to ignore her, send her out and have her come back—
what is it—recidivism or whatever it is?"

In working toward this outcome nurse C engaged with the client
and made space for rapport to develop that engendered trust and mutual
respect. Within the space, the nurse was able to work with the client
toward experimenting with alternative ways of being and coping. She
powerfully illustrated this point:

I just put my point of view and once I got to know her . . . I was pretty up front
with her. Like, I pointed a few things out to her that she didn't like a couple
of times. She lost her temper with me a couple of times, but I think that actually
helped because she actually voiced how she felt instead of . . . she didn't actually
go off and cut. . . . And then I do actually remember saying that to her "Oh,
you've lost your temper" and she looked, stopped and looked at me, and sort
of thought, "Oh, I have," and she cried. She told me she never cried and I got
her to cry. Just things like that. I don't know. I prayed to God I was doing the
right thing the whole time, because like I said, I really didn't know.

Traditional psychiatric discourse emphasizes objectivity and favors
distance between the professional and the client (Wilkin, 2001). Engag-

ing with the client enabled the nurse to recognize the client's humanity, and thus the interaction became a site of resistance to dominant perspectives of practice. This participant reflected later in the story on how working with this client had both moved her as a human being and energized her as a nurse. Seeing the client in this way enabled a more satisfying outcome for both nurse and client—one in which recognition of the client's experience created spaces for therapeutic interpersonal contact to occur.

Acknowledging the client as unique and requiring involvement and engagement does not come without risks to the nurse, however. As one participant indicated, being in an environment where self-harm is perhaps poorly understood can render nurses vulnerable to the traumas the client experiences and the client's expressions of this trauma:

But it was hard when other people . . . because she did go into seclusion . . . there was a few times when I wasn't about or I would come back from a lunch break or have wandered out and then found her locked in seclusion. It was quite hard seeing her in seclusion after spending such a long time with her and she'd tried to self-harm. *(D)*

An approach that was seen as helpful in practice to both client and nurse was the acknowledgment of the function that self-harm serves for the client. One participant talked about how she approached a client who had self-harmed:

When I was dressing her wounds, I was talking with her about self-harm and the theory behind self-harm and telling her that I recognized that it was not an attempt to kill herself and compared it with other things that other people might do to relieve anxiety and discussed that with her and while I was dressing the wounds and we just talked about it . . . and she was responsive to that. *(E)*

Participant *E* demonstrated understanding the function of self-harm to the client, as well as allowing herself to appreciate that an act of self-harm is not necessarily a defeat for the therapeutic endeavors of the nurse. Engaging with the client in this way is a resisting practice, an ironic one, effectively turning away from the psychiatric focus on the physical and behavioral and toward new ways of *being with* the client that acknowledge and act upon subjectivity. Such practices provided nurses with glimpses of the potential intersubjective benefits of engaging with clients. Sites of resistance to psychiatric discourse have the potential, then, to open up new practices for nurses. These sites are marginal and require further consideration and dialogue.

Experience and Nursing Practice

A beginning mental health nurse *(E)* gave the previous account of practice. Her account demonstrates intuitive knowing-in-practice, one that was a regular feature in all of the accounts provided by participants in this study. This fact reveals a surprising aspect of the practices of neophyte mental health nurses. It has been suggested that the use of intuition is a component of expert practice derived from the integration of theoretical understanding with practice exposures (Benner, 1984). Further, it has been suggested that caring requires a high degree of competence (Sourial, 1997). Participants' accounts of practice in this study demonstrated high levels of intuitive practice in those who would, in Benner's approach, be termed novice practitioners. Further, these accounts demonstrate features of interpersonal and clinical competence.

This intuitive feature of neophyte practice may be a potential source of rejuvenation for nurses who work with clients who self-harm. These new mental health nurses discovered spaces in which engaging with the client was developmental for both nurse and client. The continued development of this naive practice may be at risk, however, from experienced practice that is predominantly shaped by more managerial discourses.

Dominant rationalist discourses value what is known as the "authority of experience" (hooks, 1994), but experience is only one source of knowledge. Nurses tend to value experience over other ways of knowing, yet experience does not equate with critical knowledge, as it may be based on ritual, tradition, or routine. Nurses in this study engaged with and responded to clients intuitively, forming a site of resistance to the discourse of experience. Carper (1978) refers to personal knowing, ways of knowing that are related to the personal rather than the professional. Nurses in this study vividly articulated practices that reflected personal ways of knowing.

Participants in the study reported that their attempts to engage with clients in this way were, at times, criticized or questioned by more experienced nurses who offered them mentorship and guidance. The new nurses were exposed to the authority of experience that has the potential to shape and constrain their practice. The data gained from this study suggest that the potential for development of these sites of caring practice is already under threat from exposure to dominant discourse. Participant *A* recalled a practice episode during which he was unsure of his response to a client who self-harmed; he subsequently discussed his approach with a more experienced registered nurse:

I realized it wasn't exactly the right thing to do, but I could understand why the patient did it. And so, that's why I sort of, um, let her have that leniency. . . . He [the registered nurse] was shocked that she didn't come to him for starters and then more so shocked that I didn't sort of defer to him and said 'Well, that's what you're supposed to do in the future. She's not really your . . . patient to take care of and 'cause it is a fairly serious matter and needed to be dealt with in a certain way and you're a beginning practitioner. It would have been best if I'd have handled it.' And I said, 'Yeah, yeah, fair enough.' I just took it all on board, um, because I'm still learning.

Participant *A* then went on throughout the interview to discuss the care of this client and to refer back to his status as a beginning practitioner. His accounts of interactions with the more experienced registered nurse showed how that nurse reinforced the notion that, as an inexperienced mental health nurse, participant *A* lacked the skills and knowledge to effectively respond.

Another participant was cautioned for spending too much time with her client: "I didn't think I'd spent any more time with her than I did with any of my other patients. But they seemed to think—it's a bit like, you know, they're a PD [personality disorder], you get 'em in and you get 'em out" *(C)*. Recognizing her role as a learner, nurse *C* sought guidance about how to respond effectively to this client. She recalled another registered nurse offering to coach her through an effective interaction: "And one of the other nurses sort of said 'Oh, well, we'll play good cop, bad cop. You know—I'll be the arsehole and you can be the . . . the nice nurse.'" This approach seemed inappropriate to the participant. Intuitively she was aware that this was not an acceptable interaction. Her work with the client had been helpful, and in a reflective session with a different registered nurse, the participant reported that she was encouraged to go with her instincts, leading her to reject the idea that there was value in playing games with clients. This participant demonstrates how it is possible for beginning nurses to resist dominant but unreflective approaches. The excerpt also reveals that drawing upon the authority of experience is not always a helpful practice. Put simply, experience has limits and naïveté has possibilities.

Another participant was actively encouraged to practice according to her instincts by a supportive preceptor. The participant described the mentorship she received, and yet she was also aware that her practice was open to the wider influence of the ward. In discussing her understandings of why people self-harm, she referred back to some on-the-job learning and coaching that had helped her to form the opinion that attention seeking was a primary motivator for self-harm. "Maybe it's the attitude of the ward sort of, what rubbed off on me. . . . I think the nurses, most of them, or the doctors don't seem to understand self-harming" (B). This participant had previously reported that a client had told her that self-harm helped her to "let the bad out" (B). Yet, even with this new understanding and supported practice, her ideas of and practices with the client who self-harms were being constrained by the wider authoritative discourses of psychiatry and management.

Neophyte mental health nurses possess an as-yet unrestrained intuition that enables them to respond effectively and developmentally to the client who self-harms. The texts evoke a view of new nurses, less restrained by prevailing discourse, being able to access their intuition and to use this in their encounters with clients. Engaging with the client, a practice in contrast to the tenets of traditional psychiatric discourse, can be seen as a site of resistance. Participants valued spending time with clients and in doing so discovered ways to respond that validated both the client and the nurse's role as a health caregiver. In these ways being a novice appears to offer certain freedoms, illuminating fresh or creative ways of being with clients that sit outside the norms. These freedoms may be mediated over time by the more dominant imperatives of managing and containing risk.

A second site of resistance was found in participant A's refusal to accept established protocols for referring clients to their nurses. Participant A was aware this would not be likely to meet the client's needs and chose to respond in a client-focused rather than a system-focused way. This choice was beneficial to the client. Broadly interpreted, this resistance involved not going along with the accepted ways of doing things and was, in that regard, a feature of many participants' accounts of their practice.

Participants in this study, by nature of their newness to mental health nursing, questioned events occurring in the clinical environment. Yet experience within the workplace culture was more highly favored than naïveté. As a result, participants were sometimes led to doubt their knowledge and desire to care for the self-harming client. The participating nurses experienced tension in the discourse between experience and naïveté.

It would seem that there are benefits to being inexperienced. Nurses new to mental health are engaging intersubjectively with clients to create fluid and contingent spaces for caring to occur, and in these ways the nurses challenge and subvert predominant ways of knowing about and doing nursing that objectify clients and oversimplify their motivations. The practices and ideals embedded in the accounts of the nurses in this study represent an encouraging site of resistance to the culture of managed ward environments, enabling these new mental health nurses to trace paths toward self-awareness and improved outcomes for clients.

The study, while limited in size, is rich in insights about the discourse practice interface it reveals. We argue that preparation for practice may assist clinicians to acknowledge and negotiate the obvious tensions and hegemonic discourse constructs inherent in the workplace and engage in responsive practice. Education is an important transformative site. The final section of this chapter discusses educational possibilities that may prepare clinicians for practice cultures such as the one illustrated in the reported study.

Building Caring Literacy Through Critical Education

As this study revealed, many clinicians deliver care intuitively, automatically, or reactively. For the neophyte nurse, intuition created therapeutic spaces for engagement. In more experienced nurses, their automatic care was often unhelpful. Because many clinicians are not formally trained in specific client issues such as deliberate self-harm, they may have no other resources to draw upon. Therefore, the beginning nurse can only access the wisdom of others, which may be heavily socialized by dominant discourse. Alternatively, nurses may only have access to their own personal, perhaps unarticulated, caring values (McAllister & Walsh, 2003). Similarly, the experienced nurse who may not have access to a supportive or helpful peer may have to depend on herself. Either is vulnerable to the powerful yet hidden forces of dominant discourses that may not always contribute to clients' well-being.

As long as practices that occur with self-harming clients remain hidden, they cannot be publicly scrutinized, evaluated, or systematically improved. In this way, many clinicians, despite the formal imperatives of practice, have little "caring literacy." Education and practice training in the context of deliberate self-injury is a means of addressing this issue and can focus on building a caring literacy in clinicians and consumers. Education can be approached from a variety of standpoints, including critical pedagogical principles (hooks, 1994).

Preparing to Teach Transformatively

In preparing to engage students, teachers need to consider a number of curriculum development principles. Teachers who attempt to reveal the dominant paradigm open it up to scrutiny, debate, and perhaps revision. On the issue of self-harm, this may mean exploring standard practices, reflecting on common language used to speak about issues, and identifying issues and experiences currently at the margins of clinical practice. See Table 1 for a suggested program for teaching therapeutic responses to self-harm to health care givers.

Another step is to make an effort to subvert taken-for-granted aspects about the clinical world. The provision of case studies that illustrate helpful and unhelpful practices is an example of how this may be achieved. Further, the use of case studies enables students to appreciate the importance of subjective experience in caring relationships.

Classroom activities that aim to expose false dichotomies in the experience may also be illuminating. In self-harm, those dichotomies include thinking of either suicide or self-harm (when both may be occurring), thinking of past issues as irrelevant to the present (many psychological theories value either one or the other), and valuing actions rather than inaction (when the best practice may be to wait, to accept the moment, to be with the client throughout his or her distress rather than jumping to action). Thinking deeply about these dichotomies may help students generate more inclusive and helpful ways of thinking about issues and of embodying the practice value of engagement.

In planning content it is important to be cautious of what are known as "totalizing" or "essential" discourses (hooks, 1994), which tend to assume that there is something essential, stable, or universal about people

Table 1. Self-harm Education Program

Affective and Cognitive Attributes	Theories and Practices
Empathic	— Patterns and biopsychosocialcultural theories of self-harm (Braun, 1987; Favazza, 1996; Heron, 1990; Linehan, 1993; Van der Kolk, 1989)
Sensitive	
Intersubjective	
Efficient	
Effective	— The nature of self-harm (using various testimonials)
Ethical	— Clinical practices
Informed	— Psychosocial needs, strengths, and risk assessment (Antonovsky, 1987; Rapp, 1989)
Assertive	
Culturally sensitive	— Therapeutic framework
Empowering	— Long-term therapies: group therapy, individual therapies, dialectical behavior therapy (Calof, 1997; Linehan, 1993; Yalom, 1995)
Enabling	
Using critical thinking	
Using lateral thinking	— Therapeutic communication
Using creative reasoning	— Engagement: compassion, empathy, active listening, intersubjectivity
	— Containment and safety: emergency care, space, contracts, contingency plans
	— Awareness raising: Zen, dialectic critique, reflection
	— Resilience building: making social connections, developing resources, working on strengths, reframing problems
	— Legal issues
	— Innovations: clinical pathways for self-harm, emergency contact card consultation liaison, clinical supervision

and situations when what is more accurate and helpful is to see differences and specific needs. Examples include diagnostic categories for people who self-harm that are stigmatizing, sexist, or ostracizing; practices that exclude or dissuade people of minority cultures from using the health service; and paternalistic practices that patronize the client, making her or him feel stupid or inferior.

One way of foregrounding difference is to introduce specialized topics, such as self-harm, within undergraduate preparation programs. This idea is, however, both novel and unsettling. It is unsettling in that curriculum changes are often met defensively by dedicated teachers who are committed to claiming their piece of the calendar year for an important learning topic. However, it may be possible to both allay teachers' fears and encourage embracing this novel idea by taking content from topic areas already dense with information, which may be impeding that subject's ability to operate effectively. In this way, topics such as "Communication" or "Interpersonal Skills" or even "Nursing Practices" that must cover broad areas are given meaning, context, and consequently life by placing them in a specific context such as the study of self-harm. As a result, students may be more likely to understand the significance, relevance, and application of communication and caring skills.

The difference with teaching specifically to a client issue such as self-harm, rather than teaching generally to theoretical concepts, is that the students' learning is situated in ideas and skills that are directly relevant to practice. It is our experience that students then learn for themselves how to apply specific skills learned in a self-harm topic to other situations with clients. For example, engagement and resilience-building skills are relevant to other clinical situations but come to life when they are taught within discrete contexts. Another advantage in teaching this way is that students can graduate with expertise in specialized areas and thus move beyond being a jack-of-all-trades but master of none. Finally, it is a way of working with difference, rather than marginalizing and overlooking unique clinical populations and needs.

Giving Voice to Consumers and to Clinicians

Personal stories present a means of revealing the problems of everyday practice in an embodied and memorable way, rather than presenting lecture material taken from textbooks. While a valuable learning aid, the textbook can be daunting and impersonal. Taking words from a page can teach many important things but may do little to engender in students an appreciation of the subjective realities of clients. Personal stories bring both the practicing nurse and the consumer to life and situate the subjective experience as readily accessible to the student in the educational arena. They provide text in which discourses are embedded and so serve as a means of examining tensions between discourse and practice. This can offer a complimentary subjective and social approach to the objective viewpoint of both text and teacher.

This approach is particularly helpful in an area such as self-harm, for those who self-harm are a marginalized group. Silence is one of the keys to marginalized groups' maintaining their position. In contrast, storytelling is a means of vocalizing issues and perceptions that then become open to interpretation and understanding of the subjective. The storytelling approach serves to both create and value dialogue. Dialogue makes private thoughts and reflections public, opening ideas up to scrutiny, challenge, and revision. Dialogue disseminates insights, helping others to gain from access to multiple perspectives. By teachers' valuing dialogue in the classroom, students are challenged to find ways of introducing dialogue in the clinical setting. A further benefit to dialogue is revealed as it opens up power issues to scrutiny and enables power to be reconceptualized as a means of working with others and as a means of engagement.

Using Power Differently

Attempting to establish an equal relationship between teacher and student superficially subverts the criticism that power relationships between teacher and student are exploitative. But equality is an illusion since teachers and students are not the same. They have different agendas, different needs, different desires, different rewards, different skills, and different knowledge of nursing. A powerful lesson for students to learn within the classroom is that differences can exist; indeed, they are enriching. Students can be encouraged to apply this insight to clients with whom they work.

It is useful to look at ways students can moderate hierarchy in client–clinician activities and to discuss the nature and basis of power and authority. The idea is not to do away with power, but to trace its sources and effects and to learn how to use authority and influence differently (Sinclair, 1998). Power and leadership are not always about demonstrating control, using force, dominating, or coercing, but also refer to acting in a position of authority.

To work in a participatory way with clients is to be conscious of power—not to fear or avoid it, not to assume that clients do not have power, or that power should rest only with those who are providers, but to harness authority and distribute it more equitably. In the case of self-harm, it may be important to notice actions as acts of power that can be harnessed and used to build strength rather than exacerbate distress.

Silence in a client who acts by self-harming is still a form of communication. The challenge in the clinician–client context is to work toward the client's learning to use her or his voice for self-expression. When a client shows her or his wounds to a clinician, the client is sending a powerful message as well as claiming and using authority. The situation in turn requires a response from nurses. This is a time to reflect on the idea that communication takes many forms. Power is a resource available to both client and clinician; it can be worked with to find therapeutic ways of changing. Rather than assume that reasons for self-harm are known and common to all clients, it is important to put dogma aside and search for meaning with the client. This shared approach to power is characteristic of the skilled practice of engagement.

A further helpful insight may be to see self-harm as a powerful action and not as evidence that the clinician always needs to limit or control the risky and at-risk client. According to Van der Kolk (1989), deliberate self-harm may reveal paradoxically the person's will to survive. All of these readings uncover strength in spirit that may not otherwise be noticed. Rather than a signifier of failure, self-harm may point to victories. Encouraging students to engage with clients by sharing these views with the client opens up the possibility that he or she may look at the self differently, to notice strengths as well as needs.

Rather than aiming to do work on the client, in skilled caring practice one can aim to work *with* and *for* the client (Wilkin, 2001). Since the hospital system has long encouraged nurses and others to deliver care to patients, to be the expert, active, and managing partner, this shift in standpoint requires some practice and can be challenging. But by the nurse's working alongside the client and negotiating care with her or him, the client is more likely to feel understood, more likely to feel cared for, and more likely to feel motivated to begin the work involved in changing habits.

People who self-harm, like all other healthcare consumers, have unique and different needs that clinicians need to understand, accept, and respect, as well as to help motivate the client to change. Yet, the healthcare environment focused on risk, management, and outcomes, despite the good intentions of many, continues to be problem centered. Further, the notion that clients constitute a risk to be managed engenders paternalism in health services (Johnstone, 1997). Power and control are taken away from clients, and opportunities to share expertise and build partnerships are effectively denied. Within the learning experience, it is useful to encourage a different view of power and to offer an alternative to problem-centeredness.

Moving Beyond a Problem Orientation

As McAllister (in press) has argued, the problem-orientation may be useful in helping to isolate problems, target areas of change, and apply interventions dispassionately and rationally, but these actions are not always appropriate. The discourses of risk and associated management, for example, isolate and focus on problems. Care practices involve risk management, while engaging with the client is pushed to the margins. Furthermore, constantly searching for problems may prevent the nurse from appreciating things that are going right for a person. It may also be that some problems may never be resolved completely, and the focus on the negative is inherently pessimistic.

Problem-centeredness has also been roundly criticized by postmodern theorists as no longer relevant in a posthumanist age (Welton, 1995). Problem-centeredness is a totalizing discourse that tends to assume that problems are at the center of human existence, rather than incidental. Problems and difficulties become peoples' main concern, rather than feats and achievements. Problems are seen as something to be overcome rather than tolerated and perhaps integrated.

An alternative approach takes a solution orientation to the client (Antonovsky, 1987; Jackson & McKergow, 2002; Rapp, 1989). Unlike a problem orientation, a solution orientation does not simply identify and reveal difficulties; it also does not place the problem at the center of the nurse–client interaction. A solution orientation acknowledges problem solving as part of the nurse–client work but foregrounds the presence of both problems and strengths. Like the problem-solving approach, it is a form of clinical reasoning. But a solution orientation involves logic and creativity, deductive and inductive thinking, imagination and reason, problem solving and solution searching. A solution orientation also works with what is going right with an individual or group and seeks to maximize those potentials through engagement in order to build on strengths, achievements, and capacity. See Table 2 for a summary of contrasts between orientations to problems and orientations to solutions.

When instructors include discussion of solutions, students may be able to see the limits of dominant discourses such as the psychiatric discourse or the illness model and to employ strategies that are wellness oriented (Antonovsky, 1987). Searching for solutions also requires more

Table 2.   Problem and Solution Orientations

Problem orientation	Solution orientation
— Asks what is wrong and why?	— Asks what he or she wants to change and how?
— Explores historical causes and present difficulties in order to find a remedy	— Explores present and focuses on exceptions to expose hidden strengths and resources
— Searches for underlying issues, i.e., the "real" problem	— Invites client to clarify main issues and priorities for health service
— Assumes client is deficient, resistant, misguided, or naïve	— Assumes client is competent, resilient, and resourceful

imagination and creativity than the conventional problem orientation, which tends to privilege logic and reason. Classroom activities can include lateral thinking and imaginative exercises that help students to rethink the familiar and to think about the strange in novel ways. While these strategies are discussed specifically in relation to a course on self-harm, the critical pedagogy outlined can be used in other courses that aim to extend skillful caring practices. Such approaches help to question the everyday and to uncover discourses that shape and constrain caring practices.

Conclusion

This chapter has described and illustrated some of the dominant discourses that influence skillful caring within the context of the relationship between nurses and clients who self-harm. It has used the findings of a discourse analysis of nursing practice to illustrate these discourses. The chapter reveals that clinicians who approach their practice unconsciously and without adequate preparation are at risk of applying discourses that fail the client. Dominant discourses have a tendency to be totalizing and to homogenize difference. Dominant discourses also tend to produce negative power relations and support the status quo. All these issues are at odds with the caring rhetoric, which values mutual relationships, an optimistic view of change, and respect for the unique qualities of individuals and groups.

We suggest that education is a powerful means of prompting new thinking in caring practices. In order to shift thinking about caring practice, it is necessary to reflect on practice, uncover hidden dogma and ideals, challenge and replace taken-for-granted practices, and adopt approaches that are consciously and cautiously used to help clinicians respond to unique needs of diverse clients. Our suggestion is to use the principles of critical pedagogy to sensitize students to how discourses influence practice, to help them see the ways that difference in society is marginalized and contained, and to teach them how to use power differently.

References

Ahuja, A. (2000, February 22). Self-harm: The secret agony. *London Times*.

Alston, M., & Robinson, R. (1992). Nurses' attitudes towards suicide. *Omega, 25*(3), 205–215.

Antonovsky, A. (1987). *Unraveling the mystery of health: How people manage stress and stay well*. San Francisco: Jossey-Bass.

Ballinger, C., & Payne, S. (2000). Discourse analysis: Principles, application and critique. *British Journal of Occupational Therapy, 63*(12), 566–572.

Barker, P. (2000). Reflections on caring as a virtue ethic in an evidence-based culture. *International Journal of Nursing Studies, 37*, 329–336.

Barker, P., & Reynolds, B. (1994). A critique: Watson's caring ideology, the proper focus of psychiatric nursing? *Journal of Psychosocial Nursing and Mental Health Services, 32*(5), 17–22.

Benner, P. (1984). *From novice to expert: Excellence and power in clinical practice*. Menlo Park, CA: Addison-Wesley.

Benner, P., & Wrubel, J. (1989). *The primacy of caring: Stress and coping in health and illness*. Menlo Park, CA: Addison-Wesley.

Bennun, I. (1984). Psychological models of self-mutilation. *Suicide and Life Threatening Behavior, 14*(3), 166–186.

Bonner, G. (2001). Decision making for health care professionals: Use of decision trees within the community mental health setting. *Journal of Advanced Nursing, 35*, 349–356.

Bowers, L. (1997). Community psychiatric nurse caseloads and the "worried well": Misspent time or vital work? *Journal of Advanced Nursing, 26*, 930–936.

Braun, B. (1987). Treatment of Multiple Personality Disorder. American Psychiatric Press, Washington, DC.

Briere, J. (1996). A self trauma model for treating adult survivors of severe abuse. In J. Briere, L. Berliner, J. Bulkley, C. Jenny, & T. Reid (Eds.), *The APSAC Handbook on Child Maltreatment* (pp. 140–157). London: Sage.

Brown. D., Bartlett, H., Leary, J., & Carson, J. (1995). The Claybury community psychiatric stress survey. *Journal of Advanced Nursing, 22*, 347–358.

Buller, S., & Butterworth, T. (2001). Skilled nursing practice—A qualitative study of the elements of nursing. *International Journal of Nursing Studies, 38*, 405–417.

Busfield, J. (2000). Introduction: Re-thinking the sociology of mental health. *Sociology of Health and Illness, 22*(5), 543–558.

Caillois, R. (1984, Winter). Mimicry and legendary psychasthenia. *October, 31,* 17–32.

Calof, D. (1997, January–February). Chronic self-injury in adult survivors of childhood abuse: Developmental processes of anger in relation to self-injury (Part II). *Treating Abuse Today, 6*(1), 61–68.

Carper, B. A. (1978). Fundamental patterns of knowing in nursing. *Advances in Nursing Science, 1,* 13–23.

Cherryholmes, C. (1988). *Power and criticism: Poststructural investigations in education* (Issues in contemporary educational thought, Vol. 2). New York: Teacher's College Press.

Childs, A., Thomas, B., & Tibbles, P. (1994). Specialist needs. *Nursing Times, 90*(3), 32–33.

Clinton, M., & Hazleton, M. (2000). Scoping the prospects of Australian mental health nursing. *Australian and New Zealand Journal of Mental Health Nursing, 9,* 159–165.

Crowe, M. (1996). Cutting up: Signifying the unspeakable. *Australian and New Zealand Journal of Mental Health Nursing, 5,* 103–111.

Crowe, M. (2000). The nurse-patient relationship: A consideration of its discursive context. *Journal of Advanced Nursing, 31,* 962–967.

Curry, D. (1993, Spring). Decorating the body politic. *New Formations: A Journal of Culture/Theory/Politics, 19,* 69–82.

Dallender, J., Nolan, P., Soares, J., Thomsen, S., & Arnetz, B. (1999). A comparative study of British mental health nurses and psychiatrists of their work environment. *Journal of Advanced Nursing, 29,* 36–43.·

Danaher, G., Schirato, T., & Webb, J. (2000). *Understanding Foucault.* London: Sage.

Dear, G. (2000). Self harm in prison: Manipulators can also be suicide attempters. *Criminal Justice Behavior, 27*(2), 160–175.

Dingman, S., Williams, M., Fosbinder, D., & Warnick, M. (1999). Implementing a caring model to improve patient satisfaction. *Journal of Nursing Administration, 29*(12), 30–37.

Doyle, M. (1998). Clinical risk assessment for mental health nurses. *Nursing Times, 94*(17), 47–49.

Everett, B., & Gallop, R. (2000). *The link between childhood trauma and mental illness.* Thousand Oaks, CA: Sage.

Favazza, A. (1996). *Bodies under siege: Self-mutilation and body modification in culture and psychiatry* (2nd ed.). Baltimore: Johns Hopkins University Press.

Fennig, S., Carlson, G., & Fennig, S. (1995). Contagious self-mutilation. *Journal of the American Academy of Child and Adolescent Psychiatry, 34*(4): 402–403.

Foucault, M. (1977). *Language, counter-memory, practice: Selected essays and interviews.* Ithaca, NY: Cornell University Press.

Foucault, M. (1980). Truth and power. In C. Gordon (Ed.), *Power/knowledge: Selected interviews and other writings* (pp. 109–133). New York: Pantheon.

Freire, P. (1972). *Pedagogy of the oppressed* (M. B. Ramos, Trans.). Harmondsworth, UK: Penguin.

Gilligan, C., Rogers, A., & Tolman, D. (1991). *Women, girls and psychotherapy: Reframing resistance.* Binghamton, NY: Harrington Park Press.

Gitlin, T. (1989). Postmodernism: Roots and politics. In I. Angus & S. Gally (Eds.), *Cultural politics in contemporary America.* London: Routledge.

Hartman, C. (1995). The nurse–patient relationship and victims of violence. *Scholarly Inquiry for Nursing Practice, 9*(2), 175–192.

Hazleton, M. (1999). Psychiatric personnel, risk management and the new institutionalism. *Nursing Inquiry, 6,* 224–230.

Heald, M. (1999). Speaking out . . . A TV debate reveals the extent of public prejudice against people with mental illness. *Nursing Times, 95*(24), 19.

Hemmings, A. (1999). Attitude to deliberate self harm among staff in an accident and emergency team. *Mental Health Care, 2,* 300–302.

Heron, J. (1990). *Helping the client: A creative practical guide.* Sage, London.

Hochschild, A. R. (1983). *The managed heart: Commercialization of human feeling.* Berkeley: University of California Press.

hooks, b. (1994). *Teaching to transgress: Education as the practice of freedom.* New York: Routledge.

Horsfall, J., & Cleary, M. (2000). Discourse analysis of an "observation levels" policy. *Journal of Advanced Nursing, 32,* 1291–1297.

Horsfall, J., & Stuhlmiller, C. (2001). *Interpersonal nursing for mental health.* New York: Springer.

Howarth, D. (2000). *Discourse.* Buckingham, UK: Open University Press.

Jackson, P., & McKergow, M. (2002). *The solutions focus: The simple way to positive change.* Yarmouth, ME: Nicholas Brealey.

Johnstone, L. (1997). Self-injury and the psychiatric response. *Feminism and Psychology, 7*(3), 421–426.

Johnstone, M. (2002, December). Self-injury as meaning. *Auseinetter, No. 3,* Issue 16, 7–9.

Kelly, D. (1998). Caring and cancer nursing: Framing the reality using selected social science theory. *Journal of Advanced Nursing, 28,* 728–736.

Leininger, M. M. (1978). *Transcultural nursing: Concepts, theories and practices.* New York: Wiley.

Linehan, M. (1993). *Cognitive-behavioral treatment of borderline personality disorder.* New York: Guilford Press.

Lupton, D. (1992). Discourse analysis: A new methodology for understanding the ideologies of health and illness. *Australian Journal of Public Health, 16,* 145–150.

Machoian, L. (1998). *The possibility of love: A psychological study of adolescent girls' suicidal acts and self-mutilation.* Unpublished doctoral dissertation, Harvard University Graduate School of Education, Cambridge, MA.

Masius, J. (Director). (2002). *Providence.* NBC Television. Produced by T. Kring.

McAllister, M. (2001). In harm's way: Hidden aspects of deliberate self harm. *Journal of Psychiatric and Mental Health Nursing, 8*(5), 391–398.

McAllister, M. (in press). Doing practice differently: Solution focused nursing. *Journal of Advanced Nursing, 41,* 528–535.

McAllister, M., Creedy, D., Moyle, W., & Farrugia, C. (2002). A study of Queensland emergency department nurses' actions and formal and informal procedures for clients who self-harm. *International Journal of Nursing Practice, 8*(4), 184–190.

McAllister, M., & Estefan, A. (2002). Principles and strategies for teaching therapeutic responses to self harm. *Journal of Psychiatric and Mental Health Nursing, 9,* 573–583.

McAllister, M., & Walsh, K. (2003). C.A.R.E.: A framework for mental health. *Journal of Psychiatric and Mental Health Nursing, 10*(1), 39–48.

Menninger, K. (1938). *Man against himself.* New York: Harcourt Brace & World.

Mental Health Foundation. (1997). *Suicide and deliberate self-harm: The fundamental facts.* Mental Health Foundation. Retrieved [3 July 2002], from *http://www.mentalhealth.org.uk/page.cfm?pagecode=PBBZ0101.*

Mercer, D., Mason, T., & Richman, J. (2001). Professional convergence in forensic practice. *Australian and New Zealand Journal of Mental Health Nursing, 10,* 105–115.

Miller, D. (1994). *Women who hurt themselves.* New York: Basic Books.

Minichiello, V., Aroni, R., Timewell, E., & Alexander, L. (1995). *In-depth interviewing: Principles, techniques, analysis.* Sydney, Australia: Longman.

Morse, J. M. (1991). Strategies for sampling. In J. M. Morse (Ed.), *Qualitative nursing research: A contemporary dialogue.* Newbury Park, CA: Sage.

Muir-Cochrane, E. (2001). The case management practices of community mental health nurses: "Doing the best we can." *Australian and New Zealand Journal of Mental Health Nursing, 10,* 210–220.

Munro, R. (2000). "Psycho" headlines add to mental illness misery. *Nursing Times, 96*(7), 12.

Musick, J. L. (1997). How close are you to burnout? Learn how to control stress before stress controls you. The American Association of Family Physicians. Retrieved 14 May 2002 from www.aafp.org/fpm/970400fm/lead.html

Niven, N. (1994). *Health psychology: An introduction for nurses and other health care professionals.* Edinburgh, Scotland: Churchill Livingstone.

Osuch, E. A., Noll, J. G., & Putnam, F. W. (2000). The motivations for self-injury in psychiatric inpatients. *Psychiatry, 62,* 334–346.

Perego, M. (1999). Why A and E nurses feel inadequate in managing patients who deliberately self harm. *Emergency Nurse, 6*(9), 24–27.

Peterson, A., & Lupton, D. (1996). *The new public health: Health and self in the age of risk.* London: Sage.

Polit, D. F., & Hungler, B. P. (1995). *Nursing research principles and methods.* Philadelphia: Lippincott.

Rapp, C. (1989). The strengths model of case management: Results from twelve demonstrations. *Psychosocial Rehabilitation Journal, 13*(1), 23–31.

Reed, J., & Ground, I. (1997). *Philosophy for nursing.* London: Arnold.

Roach, M. S. (1992). The aims of philosophical inquiry in nursing: Unity or diversity of thought? In J. F. Kikuchi & H. Simmons (Eds.), *Philosophical inquiry in nursing.* (pp. 38–44). Newbury Park, CA: Sage.

Rogers, A. (1996, 3 February). *Writing on their bodies, I: Understanding self-mutilation with adolescent girls through creative writing in psychotherapy.* Paper presented at Harvard Medical School Conference titled *Child and Adolescent Self-Destruction,* Boston.

Shaw, N. (2002). Shifting conversations on girls' and women's self-injury: An analysis of the clinical literature in historical context. *Feminism and Psychology, 12*(2), 191–219.

Sherman, M. E., Burns, K., Ignelzi, J., Raia, J., Lofton, V., Toland, D., Stinson, B., Tilley, J. L., & Coon, T. (2001). Firearms risk management in psychiatric care. *Psychiatric Services, 52*(8), 1057–1061.

Sinclair, A. (1998). *Doing leadership differently: Gender, power and sexuality in a changing business culture.* Carlton South, Australia: Melbourne University Press.

Sourial, S. (1997). An analysis of caring. *Journal of Advanced Nursing, 26,* 1189–1192.

Staden, H. (1998). Alertness to the needs of others: A study of the emotional labor of caring. *Journal of Advanced Nursing, 27,* 147–156.

Stordheur, S., D'hoore, W., & Vandenberghe, C. (2001). Leadership, organizational stress and emotional exhaustion among hospital nursing staff. *Journal of Advanced Nursing, 35,* 533–542.

Taylor, B. (1994). *Being human: Ordinariness in nursing.* London: Churchill Livingstone.

Van der Kolk, B. (1989). The compulsion to repeat the trauma: Re-enactment, revictimization, and masochism. *Psychiatric Clinics of North America, 12*(2), 389–411.

Van der Kolk, B., Perry, C., & Herman, J. (1991). Childhood origin of self destructive behavior. *American Journal of Psychiatry, 148*(12), 1665–1671.

Vaughan, P. (1995). *Suicide prevention.* Birmingham, UK: PEPAR Publications.

Vivekananda, K. (2000). Integrating models for understanding self-injury. *Psychotherapy in Australia, 7*(1), 18–25.

Watson, J. (1995). Postmodern nursing and knowledge development in nursing. *Nursing Science Quarterly, 8*(2), 60–64.

Welton, M. (1995). *In defense of the lifeworld: Critical perspectives on adult learning.* Albany: State University of New York Press.

Wilkin, P. (2001). The other side. *Mental Health Nursing, 21*(5), 28. Retrieved 11 February 2002 from *http://proquest.umi.com/pqdlink.*

Yalom, I. (1995). *The theory and practice of group psychotherapy.* New York: Basic Books.

2

"These Are the Children We Hold Dear"

Jacqui Kess-Gardner

Introduction and Conclusion by Kathryn Hopkins Kavanagh

On Writing the Self: An Introduction

This story began nearly twenty years ago. It has taken that long for it to be lived and written. During that time, it has also become increasingly accepted that writing is a method of inquiry (Becker, 1992; Morrison, 1992; St. Pierre, 1997). Stories like this one lack precedents and prototypes. They are born of fits and starts. As time goes on and reflection deepens and meanings become clear, the story becomes both a creation of its author's heart and "an experience with language" (Heidegger, 1971, p. 57). How does one relate the pain and pleasure of transformation—unanticipated and unrelenting as they, and it, may be—as experiences revealing themselves over time? "I am borne into personal existence by a time which I do not constitute" (Merleau-Ponty, 1962, p. 347). According to Heidegger (1962), our sense of how we are faring discloses "one's being-in-the-world as a whole" (p. 137). Experience matters, for it molds by wrenching us personally into the mediating world in desperate ways concurrently shaped by history and biography and invented on the spot.

The personal story has been described as "an existential struggle for honesty and expansion in an uncertain world" (Ellis & Bochner, 2000, p. 749). Central to the construction and interpretation of narrative is "the essential sway" of its grounding, self-sheltering and concealing as that may be (Heidegger, 1999). That grounding in space and time allows emptiness, clearing, and "be-ing"— the resonance of enowning (Heidegger, 1999)—that births the multiple "I's" of the writer who understands and explains her life through featured stories, plots, characters, and the empathic stance of hermeneutics (Hones, 1998; Josselson, 1995). The image of the self is never a simple reflection of experience but always strives for explanation (Hankiss, 1981). It is writing the experience that exposes both what matters mean and what *really* matters. There are always issues that culture tries to shroud in non-engagement (Chávez & O'Donnell, 1998), things that are not spoken about. Disability and giving birth to an other than "perfect child" are two of those.

Narrative is a story of events and experiences placed within the context of particular life histories (Brody, 1987; Stuhlmiller & Thorsen, 1997), but experience differs greatly from observation. Autobiography naturally takes on the form and content of its author—she who lives the story. Feminist autobiography draws women out of obscurity and places them in history by validating their experience (Etter-Lewis, 1991; Reinharz, 1992)—experience that is shaped both by individuality and by culture with its gathering of the dynamic tensions of history. Any woman engaged in interpretive inquiry in this transpersonal, transhistorical (Levin, 1989) world learns about herself. However, not everyone is a storyteller.

There are tell-all ethnographic diaries (Malinowski, 1967; Tedlock, 2000) and first-person field accounts (Behar, 1996; Cesara, 1982). The literature is replete with narratives of the self (Richardson, 1994), personal experience narratives (Denzin, 1989), personal essays (Krieger, 1991), personal ethnography (Crawford, 1996), autobiographical ethnography (Reed-Danahay, 1997), ethnographic autobiography (Brandes, 1982), ethnographic memoir (Tedlock, 1991), cultural biography (Frank, 2000), and "confessional tales" (Van Maanen, 1988). Whatever the genre, interpretive inquiry's plea is for "kinder" (in lieu of cold and analytical) writing (Childress, 1998). In all of these, the inquirer is both observer and observed, participant and pawn, as emotional and behavioral experiences and memories unfold. When it is herself she reflects upon and studies in the struggle toward finding coherence (Linde, 1993), the encounter becomes tangible and unavoidable. She must trust herself to know her own mind and recount it faithfully. And she must also trust the reader to respect her story. Writing is therapeutic (Ben-Ari, 1995; Jourard, 1971) by reclaiming the self (Etter-Lewis, 1991), but sharing intimate experiences with non-intimates requires a different mettle. Sharing newly revealed realities means exposing one's soul. There is always that risk of ridicule or rejection.

Autobiography that displays multiple layers of consciousness and engagement connects the personal to the cultural genre of personal narrative not bracketed in the realm of science but accessible and readable as story (Ellis & Bochner, 2000; Jago, 1996; Kolker, 1996; Ronai, 1995; Tillmann-Healy, 1996). In "These Are the Children We Hold Dear," the reader experiences the struggle for meaning and control in the connecting text of the Gardner family and kin. The gaze shifts, backward and forward, dialectically revealing emotions, faith, self-consciousness, embodiment, and the channeling of human potential. At all times, the truth is inescapable: "we are nowhere but in the present" (Behar, 1996, p. 176). These connections invite readers to "live their way into the experience" (Denzin, 1994, p. 511), embedded as it is in everyday expediencies and caring in historically, socially, and culturally contextualized lives.

Despite acceptance of writing as a form of inquiry, there is always that hint of common wisdom in Hurston's claim that "women forget all the things they don't want to remember, and remember all the things they don't want to forget. The dream is the truth. Then they act and do things accordingly" (Hurston, 1978, p. 9). The blurring of diverse representations of everyday life—and of its disruptions great and small—and the democratization of knowledge have given voice and new critical awareness that allow the beliefs and behaviors of the inquirer to inhabit the historical moment of the subjects of inquiry (Tedlock, 2000). Narratives of women's lives register the tensions between conventional roles and unconventional expectations thrust by chance upon the unsuspecting. Meanings and boundaries are unsettled as potential tragedy instigates self-doubt and marginalization. The inquirer views herself as the phenomenon; there is no "other," no subjectifying or objectifying (Laing, 1968; Levin, 1989), only mindfulness of an intertwining of subject and object in other aspects of the self. It is what is said to be the way of the Buddha's sensing: "Just as it is, in its as-it-is-ness, whatever you see or whatever you hear is for ever blessed. It is neither one nor two" (Shibayama, 1974, p. 223).

The authenticity of narrative and knowing is shown up by meaning, the raison d'être of interpretive inquiry. Meaning is grasped through the search for understanding by uncovering the values, beliefs, and assumptions (Polkinghorne, 1983) intrinsic to and generally taken for granted in everyday living. Addressing the issue of the narrative's ontological authenticity validates the reflexivity, coherence, and potency of interpretive inquiry. There is a hearkening, that is, openness to hearing with releasement, achieved by the virtue of retrieval of the experience informed by its *pre-understandings* (Fink & Heidegger, 1979; Levin, 1989).

In Jacqui's story, which follows this introduction, the transformation is neither gentle nor docile as she searches for herself among the instability of unanticipated caring needs and expectations. In this loving family inclined toward music, it is sound that takes on meanings of "letting, freely, spontaneously, joyfully yielding" (Levin, 1989, p. 224) and echoing with "the vibration of the sound with my whole sensory being" (Merleau-Ponty, 1962, p. 234). But the physical reality with which Jacqui and her family live threatens both silence and implosion, as in "Beethoven ventilating, with a sound he cannot hear, the cave-in of recurring rage" (from "Beethoven, Opus III," Clampitt, 1999, p. 50). Fortuitously, it is an extended family with intuitive faith and spiritual practices that enable a belonging to the wholeness of Being and a commitment to appropriate self-formative practices (Levin, 1989). For Jacqui, religious faith tempers the unconcealment that allows the ontological difference between Being and being. In this family's culture, it is caring faith that counts—that makes existence "this botched, cumbersome, much-mended, not unsatisfactory thing" (from "A Hermit Thrush," Clampitt, 1999, p. 274).

In lives richly studded with strengths, challenges, and convictions, survivors emerge phoenix-like and triumphant from the detritus of enormous odds. The human face is a fragile thing. Human societies are quick to label people unattractive or render them unacceptable based on physical difference and disfigurement (Banner, 1983; Macgregor, 1979). "In the sphere of social integration, anomie emerges" (Benhabib, 1986, p. 250). Heidegger speaks of thrownness "in the distress of the abandonment of being and in the necessity of decision" (Heidegger, 1999, p. 169). Jacqui's story is one of a fundamental estrangement with Being as she previously knew it, for it seemed no longer adequate. But even in suffering, hearkening, listening, and learning to let go and let be (Levin, 1989), this story speaks to gathering the time "that embraces or holds-around the moving and the resting things" (Heidegger, 1982, p. 252). Others have put it more simply: "Sometimes you just have to take the leap, and build your wings on the way down" (Yamada, 1997). According to a Harris (1986) poll, half the people in the United States who are disabled (based on definitions involving limitations in performing major life activities) do not consider themselves disabled (Frank, 2000; Harris et al., 1986). Jacqui's story resonates with caring that enables. It vindicates with anxious clarity that objectification and medicalization of human experience cannot touch the details of real and embodied circumstances (Gadamer, 1996; Kleinman, 1995). It is, in large part, simple faith that saves the day and heals, embedded as it is in Jacqui's lifeworld—"present-at-hand" (Heidegger, 1962, p. 42) and subject to being played as if a thing between art and spirit.

Jacqui's Story: In the Beginning

"Don't smear my make-up," joked Jacqui as she waved a carefully manicured hand at her husband, James, as he tried to wipe the perspiration from her brow. Any moment now Jacqui would deliver their second baby. "Leave her alone, James," said the physician warmly. "Let her keep her makeup on if she wants. You know how vain she is." James laughed with the doctor as the obstetric team readied for the birth. Jacqui was happy and labor had been a breeze. Nothing could have prepared this couple for what would happen next.

Mine was a normal pregnancy. I was as healthy as a horse. James did not wine me, but he dined me well on the Chinese food I loved and craved. Unlike my first pregnancy, we were both more mature and ready for this baby. My marriage was secure, I was madly in love with James, and Jamaal, our son, was a true delight and a gift from God. Life was good. I was blessed with a husband I adored and a son who was articulate, well-mannered, and talented. Already studying piano at the Peabody Institute at the age of four, Jamaal awed audiences during Sunday concerts at the Conservatory. My husband really wanted a second child, and so did I, after some seductive and gentle persuasion. I was hoping for another boy because I have this thing about being queen of the house. I wanted another boy because I marveled at the idea of another son who looked like James. Jamaal looked like a miniature version of my husband. Yes, another boy would be perfect.

"Push now!" shouted the doctor—at least it seemed like he shouted. Within seconds, the baby's head emerged. Everyone squealed with delight, and I beamed with pride. I had given birth to another boy. The cord was cut, and Jermaine was whisked away to be weighed and checked.

Suddenly the room filled with tension so thick it was tangible. A reluctant red-haired nurse came over to us and said, "Mr. and Mrs. Gardner, we think something is wrong with your baby. We can't get his eyes open and his face is disfigured." A moment hours-long went by. I began laughing hysterically at this silly nurse. Surely, she was joking. I quickly looked around the cold delivery room. The faces I saw convinced me that this was no joke. The piercing pain I felt was unbelievable, all the worse for getting such news in this vulnerable and compromised position—on my back, legs agape, feet still in stirrups, getting my episiotomy stitched up.

There were tears in my doctor's eyes as he tried to calm me, which frightened me because he is always in control of all situations and certainly in control of his emotions. This was *reality*. "No!" I thought. I blinked and shook myself. This was a bizarre dream, and I would awaken any moment with my perfect baby in my arms. But, no, reality just got worse. James and I were taken solemnly to the recovery area. I would rather have been a corpse headed for the morgue.

My new son had the most beautiful head of black, curly hair I have ever seen. From the neck down, he appeared perfect. But his hairline came down his forehead in a "V" over each eye, or where the eye belonged, giving him an evil look. His facial features were monstrous. He looked like an alien. I wanted to die. One of his eyes had never formed and was sealed shut. The other eye was damaged; the "white" was yellow and about the size of a raisin. The damaged eyelid could not close. He had no eyelashes or eyebrows. His disfigured nose had nostrils that flared out, exposing the inside. His ears seemed unusually small, and he was not very active. Ironically, his complexion was beautiful, and he had the most perfect rosebud mouth. It was excruciating to look at him, and I refused to look again.

In the not-so-private recovery room, James and I rocked in each other's arms and cried. We tried to relive this pregnancy to see what went wrong. I didn't drink, smoke, or use any type of drugs. I ate healthy foods, exercised daily, and slept whenever I was tired. Heck, I was the healthiest I had ever been, so why did this happen? Did I work too hard, too long? I was a hairstylist on my feet most of the day. Fluorocarbons in the hairspray? I was so sure it was my fault! Was I too casual about my niece recently being diagnosed "mildly retarded," so God was going to fix me with a disaster of my own? Or . . . just maybe I loved Jamaal too much, and God had to put me in my place. "Damn God!" I screamed. "What did I do to deserve this?"

I come from a very religious upbringing, but there was no consoling me at this point. I hated God with a capital *H* and did not trust him any more. James was going through his own hell. He wept like a child in my arms and kept saying, "Baby, I'm so sorry. I insisted we have another child and look what happened." James blamed himself, and I blamed myself. We even discussed having incompatible genes and genetic counseling, after the fact and after Jamaal! When one gives birth to a child with a handicapping condition, one actually mourns the death of the perfect child that was expected. You go through the grieving process—denying, being angry, bargaining, being depressed, accepting. At the moment, I was pissed off with God for this one! I was raised in a Christian household with both parents and six siblings. I didn't stop praying; I was afraid to. But I didn't trust God anymore.

The doctor came in after getting cleaned up and hugged me tight. We wept. He apologized again, as if that was either relevant or helpful, and told us it was no one's fault. Whatever happened to Jermaine's eyes happened during the first trimester. He promised to have more tests run so we could understand *why*. The *why* seemed the question of importance, for some odd reason. It was as if, once we knew the *why*, we could then undo what was done. The doctor announced that he was not performing the planned tubal ligation as I might want to become pregnant again. I prayed silently that Jermaine would not make it through the crucial first twenty-four hours. But I knew already that I would *never* attempt another pregnancy. Never!

A Newly Created World

My physician arranged for a private room, not wanting me to share a room with another mother. He then said he would see me in the morning and left. I dialed my mother's house, and the phone was picked up on the first ring. I gasped for air. "Hello, Priscilla," I whispered, trying to gain control and sound sane. Priscilla is my mother; we have always called her by her first name. "Hi, Jacqui. Well, how are you?" All hell broke loose in me. "The baby looks like a monster and he's blind and he's ugly and I'm not bringing him home and I'm not coming home either and I'm going to tell everyone he died and what am I going to do?" I said at breathless, lightening speed.

My wise mother paused a few seconds. "Oh, my God," she said, "I'm so sorry." Then, without ever losing it, she said in firm and measured phrases: "These are the children we hold dear. We don't give *our* children away. We bring them home, and we nurture them. If a mother can't love her child who has a problem, what makes you think a stranger would? Get yourself together, bring him home, and love him. We will love him, too. It will be hard, but you can do it." Priscilla's words were soothing, as well as firm. In a typical Black American family, when the mother says, "Jump!" you ask only "How high?" I took some time to hear what she said. She waited in silence, but I could hear her crying. I said, "But why me, Priscilla?" And she said, "But why not you, love?"

I knew she was right. Feeling somewhat better, I called my oldest and closest sister, Cookie. My mother had already called her while I was trying to compose myself after our conversation, so she knew about Jermaine. Nevertheless, we wept like there had been a death in the family. It felt that way. We cried like insane women and spent the first ten minutes crying in each other's ear and blowing our noses. We do that sort of thing. We are as close as two sisters can possibly be and genuinely feel each other's pain. We refer to ourselves as "The Presidents" in our family because we like to think that all major decisions come by us. We consider ourselves equals. Cookie said she did not know how we would get through this, but she would make calls to my friends and customers (I owned a hair salon) so that I could be spared the "Oh you poor dear" routine. We sobbed and joked about Jermaine becoming the next Stevie Wonder.

I felt stronger after these two conversations and determined to hold "my baby." I had not referred to him as "my baby" since he'd entered this cruel world. I had to make up to him for the love that I felt I had selfishly deprived him of while I was hosting my own pity party. He needed me, I realized, and I was much ashamed of the fact that I had turned my back on him. I wanted him to die in his sleep so I did not have to deal with explaining him to anyone. I didn't want my friends to know I was capable of such a "freak accident." I knew I was vain and dead wrong, but there it was. I called my mother-in-law, Gladys, who by then had heard about Jermaine from James. She was taking the news badly but assured me we would "stick together" and would make sure that Jermaine had everything he needed. I was so blessed to have a family so supportive! And I would soon enough learn that not everyone is so kind.

With the phone calls behind me, I knew what I had to do. Still apprehensive, I told the nurse I wanted to see and hold my baby. She asked whether I thought I could handle it and if I wanted her to accompany me. I told her this was something I had to do alone and thanked her for her concern. I told the nurse I wanted to fix my makeup before I remet my son. True, he would never see my face or the makeup I insisted on applying. I painted my lips with my brightest lipstick and combed my hair so it bounced when I walked. I selected a kelly green satin robe with a matching belt and gold metallic slippers with two-inch heels. The nurse asked if the heels weren't a little high. I assured her I felt fine. I had only given birth, which no longer felt like a big deal to me, compared to the hand I had just been dealt. I sprayed cologne on my neck and wrists. I began my journey.

That walk to the nursery where the "different" babies were placed to shield the moms from the pain of having to interact with the mothers of "perfect" babies was the longest I've ever taken. It was not because of just having delivered a baby, for I was numb of physical pain. My heels clicked along the corridor, resonating with my heartbeat. Thoughts crowded my mind. I could not sort them out. How would I raise this child? My mother's voice echoed in my mind. I walked faster, knowing I had so much to do, and I had wasted precious hours like an unfit mother. I wished James was there, but it was the middle of the night.

Besides, wishing had not helped much yet, so alone I strode. The hospital was quiet at nearly two in the morning and smelled medicinal. I thought about Jermaine, my son whose name I had not yet called, and what he looked like—still hoping this was some cruel joke and he would reveal himself to be any other newborn. The nurse knew who I was when I entered the dimly lit nursery, even before I introduced myself. I guess the "powers that be" had called ahead to put the nursery nurses on the lookout for a psychotic mother. The nurse used a gentle tone one might take with a completely irrational mental patient. She assured me she'd be in the next room and then took me to Jermaine. She placed him in my arms and left us alone.

Hot tears flowed down my face. This was *not* a dream. This baby was *mine*. The nurse came back within minutes to see if I had slit Jermaine's wrists or my own (bad joke), and I asked her if I could attempt to nurse him. I was led to a cozy area with a wonderful mahogany rocking chair and sat down with my Jermaine. He looked so helpless and so hungry for love; so alone, so pitiful, and so different from any child I had ever seen. Jermaine was small. I still did not know his birth weight; that tidbit was lost way down on the priority list. I shot a glimpse at him, thinking that a quick look would make the situation a little better. I then stared at him a long time. I quickly put my hand over my mouth to muffle my gasps. I examined the rest of his body to see that he was intact. He was, and I was relieved. His forehead protruded and his eyes were widely spaced. The child had only one visible eye. While one had never formed, the other was a milky mass of blue-white slime. He had no bridge for his nose and the nose was grossly crooked. My tears fell on his unusual face, and I kissed his beautiful rosebud mouth. I hugged him and squeezed him like there was no tomorrow. What a pleasant thought—no tomorrow. I'm a real talker, always have been, and began a dialogue with my new son.

Hello, Jermaine. I'm your mommy, and I love you very much. I am so sorry for acting so horrible after your birth and being a terrible mother so far. Please forgive me for not being there for you and know it will never happen again. I will make it up to you and give you the best life that I can. I will read to you, talk to you, and play beautiful music for you. I will make sure that you are the smartest, most positive, and most loved, and best-adjusted blind kid in the world. Please don't hate me. And please don't hold this against me.

I kissed him again and thought he seemed to respond. I will never forget that kiss, because I feel like he was aware of the bond that would forever connect us. Our bonding began at that moment. I then began to breastfeed him, and he latched on immediately. Unlike his older brother, who had taken his good sweet time, Jermaine nursed like a champ, and I genuinely loved him. I was in *love*. We were one. I was obsessed with making his life great. I knew at this point that I would die for him if I had to. I knew I had a lot of work to do. I sang to him as he nursed and told him about the wonderful family he was going to come home to, about his tall handsome daddy and his articulate big brother. The nurse came in to take Jermaine back to the nursery. I could tell from her face that she knew the reunion had gone well. We smiled at each other, and she patted my shoulder, telling me I was going to be okay. I knew she was right. I felt safe at the hospital.

It was now 3:30, and I had not called James. I wanted to tell him about Jermaine. He informed me that he had just gotten back from attempting to commit suicide. He meant to drive himself off the express-way but decided he could not leave me alone to face the music. I cried. He was a total wreck. I consoled him the best I could, which wasn't well at all. I told him about my reunion with Jermaine. James was re-lieved when I told him I loved Jermaine. He said that made it easier for him. He told me he loved me and I was "one hell of a woman." We said goodnight.

The Roller Coaster of Hope

I walked back to my room with long strides and an air of new confi-dence. I was going to be fine. The nurse told me that three of my sisters and my brother, parents, and mother-in-law were trying to reach me. At that ungodly hour, I called each one back. Then I tried to sleep. I tossed and turned, had nightmares, dreamed of a baby with two perfect eyes, and woke up in tears. This was going to be rough. I wasn't fine, not in the least was I okay. Soon after, I heard clattering breakfast trays and delighted moms and dads discussing the births of their "perfect" babies. The hurt started all over again. I started to cry, and James came in and consoled me.

James and I decided it was time to call Jamaal. Karen, my baby sister, put him on the phone, and I hesitatingly said, "Hi, babe. You have a new brother." Jamaal squealed with delight. I then told him that Jamaal had a disfigured face, what I meant by *disfigured*, and that he was blind.

Our angel said, "Is that all? Bring him home, and we'll be his eyes." I was too full of emotion to do anything but hand the phone to James. Jamaal repeated what he had said, and James cried, too. How could this child have parents who were such wimps?

A nurse came in to say that Jermaine's pediatrician had come to examine him and wanted to see us in the nursery. Again I fell to pieces. It seemed this was becoming a way of life for me. The doctor hugged me as I decorated his starched white jacket with my navy-blue eyeliner, much to my embarrassment. He shook hands with James. He said he could not imagine what went wrong with Jermaine. He told us that an ophthalmologist was waiting to tell us his findings. We went over to where Jermaine was in the incubator to see the tall, expressionless doctor who didn't even give us the time to exhale before he began to spew poison in his blunt monotone. "Dr. Doom" said, "Your baby's blind, but has light perception in the good eye." Hell, I thought, there was a "good" eye? On he went. "He will need a cornea transplant, but it probably won't restore sight. The left socket has no globe at all but just a cyst with garbage in it. I wouldn't get my hopes up, if I were you, because it does not look good, and I don't think that he will ever see. Here are the numbers of the doctors where they'll do the surgery." I was too stunned to be angered by this doctor's attitude. We were speechless. He left without a compassionate word or gesture. James and I were totally bewildered. Jermaine would *never* see.

We rushed back to my room to lick our wounds in peace, only to find a social worker there. He was a chipper little guy with a big magnetic personality. He headed a support group for parents of handicapped children. We liked him instantly. He spoke to us at length, putting us in touch with our true feelings about Jermaine and letting us know how normal it was to feel shock, hate, denial, blame, and on and on. We really needed to hear this. He gave us information about the group we would eventually join. When he left an hour later, I felt like he cared about how we felt and how we would deal with our situation. I'd told him how I had wanted Jermaine to die and how I was as mad as hell about this new problem that would not go away. He nodded appropriately, while James and I expressed our sorrow and pain. James didn't talk that much, but I *had* to talk. It was the only way that I could get a grip on things—as it was, I was losing my grip fast. He told us our feelings were normal and how talking with parents with similar plights would help us to work through this madness. The social worker gave us hope when no one else had given us any so far. We needed what he offered: support and understanding. Later a woman came in to give us literature about stimulating blind infants and explain that it would be a whole new ball game. My education about blindness began here.

Five days after Jermaine was born, we were admitted to one of the most famous hospitals in the country so that Jermaine could undergo his first cornea transplant surgery. I had no chance to go home to see Jamaal, or to collect myself. Things were happening much too fast. Jermaine was to have a cornea transplant in the morning. Time was of the essence. The doctors would also try to repair his eyelid so it might close. We answered the same gazillion questions over and over again for different people, had blood work done, and were on display for the many students who frolicked through gawking as if we were from another planet. I prayed for a miracle. Yes, I was still praying, although I was mad as hell at the creator. My life would never be the same again.

We were housed in a huge room separated by dirty and stained cloth curtains that had seen more than their share of grimy hands. The curtains formed cubicles. I hated it. This place was the pits—this huge place of international fame. I guess we didn't have enough money to merit a decent and clean room. Hell, I had General Motors Blue Cross and Blue Shield, so why were we in a dump like this? Well, lucky for them, I didn't have time to ponder over accommodations. We, of course, were the center of attention. No one had ever seen a child who looked like Jermaine—mothers included, so I constantly got visits from other mothers and anyone else who took a notion to ask, "What's wrong with your baby?" This was going to be some life.

We met the new doctors. One resembled Santa Claus without the beard. He was kind and careful not to give false hope. He spoke with a thick German accent about cornea transplants and then asked if there were questions. Was the man mad? Of course I had questions! "Will Jermaine see? Will he live? Can this nightmare be over *now*?" He tried his best and turned us over to the other doctor, a handsome young African American man who would repair the eyelid. His air of confidence convinced me all would go well. I asked if he was concerned about Jermaine's skin keloiding once it was cut or pierced. He said he felt that Jermaine would not keloid, which proved to be wrong. "Dr. Confidence" should have said he didn't know if he would keloid or not. By the time these doctors left, James and I secretly thought Jermaine might see.

Next, we had an appointment with a plastic surgeon. This suave guy had no mercy on us. He was so bold as to tell us that there was absolutely and positively, mind you, *nothing* that could be done to correct the facial deformity of Jermaine's face until he was about fifteen years old. Great! During the most important years of his life, he would be dealing with a disfigured face in this beauty-oriented society. Could things get any worse? Little did I know that this doctor from this world-renowned institution didn't know what he was talking about, but he went on to make his prediction—the way we found most doctors tend to do. He said, feebly, that he was sorry and left James and me with our mouths wide open. Suicide was looking better and better with each encounter with these professionals.

I didn't sleep at all that night because I couldn't get used to being in a cubicle with no door and people coming in and out at will. I was also worried about the surgery. During the night, Jermaine was put under an ultraviolet lamp because he had become jaundiced. Morning came, and he was taken to surgery, which went well, according to the experts. The new cornea looked clear. Jermaine's eyelid was puffy and sore and looked like he'd fought fifteen rounds and lost. I dared to hope that with a clear cornea, Jermaine's chances of seeing would be much increased. I thanked God. Stitches were everywhere, and it gave me goose bumps to look at the wounds. To make matters worse, I had to give Jermaine three doses of ointment and drops four times a day, which were painful for my little warrior. The nurses would gladly have applied the medications to Jermaine's eyes, but I insisted on doing it myself. Not only did I want to make sure it was definitely done, but I was his mother, and that is what mothers do.

A week later we went home, leaving the cocoon of the hospital. It felt real good. I had already lived through my family's supportive but pained faces as they looked at Jermaine for the first time. It was time to face the real world. I missed Jamaal so much, and I was neglecting him by spending so much time with Jermaine. Before I went to the hospital to give birth to Jermaine, Jamaal was the first person I thought about in the morning and the last one I thought about at night. I had no idea what this whole Jermaine business would do to him but prayed he would not become too affected by it. Thank goodness Jamaal was so in love with Aunt Cookie that he really barely knew I existed. This was convenient, given the amount of time I was spending chasing corneas. Jamaal was also intrigued by his new brother and did not seem bothered by his different looks. He was elated, boasted proudly to his friends, and wanted to hold Jermaine, constantly. What a neat kid Jamaal was!

After being home a couple of hours, I called the Board of Education's Special Education Department. I explained that I had a ten-day-old blind child and was concerned about his education. The woman chuckled and asked me if I didn't think this was a little premature. I took offense at her comment and told her that the child would be forever blind, and I needed her help now. She made an appointment for me to have Jermaine evaluated for placement in the city's Parent-Infant Stimulation Program. I would be contacted as soon as they could do the paperwork. I was also told about a Kennedy Institute family support group that offers parents a shoulder to lean on, as well as the services of an occupational therapist, physical therapist, and a social worker. I looked into these resources immediately, and within weeks Jermaine was having sessions with an occupational therapist twice a week. Jermaine's cornea, by this time, had clouded, which meant his body was rejecting it. Sadly, we were back on the transplant list again. I felt I would be chasing ambulances forever, in search of the perfect cornea, each one being someone else's tragedy as well as my own.

Beyond this, I was not ready for the reception that I would receive in the outside world. Well-wishers came to see my child and looked in horror as they tried to maintain their calm. Even some family members avoided me like the plague. We got invited to fewer and fewer affairs until we eventually began living in seclusion with just each other and our families to lean on. Going to the store became a nightmare as people followed us around to gawk at our "different" baby. One woman I'd never seen before asked, "What in the world did you do to that baby's face?" By this time I was fed up and said, sweetly seeping venom, "I banged him in the face with a bat." It sent her scurrying, mumbling about "you young mothers."

Jermaine's home lessons were coming along nicely, and so was he. I had good days and bad ones. I noticed that he never smiled, although he was already several months old. The director of the Maryland School for the Blind gave me a list of books to invest in to become an expert on teaching my blind child. She also told me that if vision were Jermaine's only problem, the school for the blind was probably not where we would want him to attend since students there tended to be multiply handicapped. From the books I learned that blind children, lacking the luxury of visual cues, smile later than their sighted counterparts. Boy, did I have a lot to learn. Something as small as a smile means a lot when you are not privy to one. That priceless moment of a mom's smiling into her baby's eyes and she or he returning that smile. . . . I sang or read to Jermaine, looked into his expressionless face, and prayed he would smile. I tried teaching him to smile by moving his mouth up at the corners, but it didn't work.

James and I took turns carrying him around in a harness so he would not experience being lonely. I liked having him with me, and I could sing to him and, being the talker I am, talked him half to death. That may explain why he grew up to be a child of very few words. We never left him alone unless he was sleeping. We also played classical and contemporary music, along with some Stevie Wonder and Lionel Ritchie, nonstop. Our house was never quiet as I was praying for a miracle of music for him, but not expecting one.

Everyday without fail, my sister Keetie, who was more faithful to God than the rest of us, would call to have prayers with me and to tell me that God had a plan for Jermaine and me. She emphasized that God gave Jermaine to me for a good reason. I did not want to hear that crap. I was never rude to her because she is such a sweet sister, but I politely told her that she could spare me the preaching and scriptures because a good God would not leave me hanging like this. She always had a comeback, no matter how belligerent I became. She continued to call and to tell me that God was in control and would, in his own time, amazingly work wonders in our lives. I told her that I'd like to see how faithful she'd be if this were her life. She assured me that God does not make mistakes, and it was up to me to ask for guidance and to let go and let God. I realized this girl was not going to go away but would badger me until I asked God for forgiveness and guidance. I did exactly that.

The Flood Waters Part, the Mountain Reveals Itself

I kept increasing my resources, contacting the National Federation of the Blind, for example, and trying to get a handle on raising and advocating for a blind child. We were back on the waiting list for yet another cornea, so I kept a bag packed and stayed near the phone. This time the surgery did not go well, and neither did the hospital stay. The doctors had to put a breathing tube down Jermaine's throat, and he ran into serious complications. He came back from surgery on a respirator, moaning as if it were his last breath. Strange as it may seem, I no longer wanted to lose him. I was in for the long haul, ready to go to war for my little prince. "Dear God, let him live," I begged. "We have work to do."

While in the hospital, I took the liberty of reading Jermaine's records because I had read in my mountains of literature that, as a parent, it was my right to see what was written about him. Much to my surprise there were all kinds of rubbish in there that I was not aware of. According to doctors' reports, Jermaine was deaf in his left ear. "Damn," I thought, "all that singing and talking and music appreciation in vain!" Next the report noted that one kidney was larger than the other, possible retardation, abnormalities of the face (of course), abnormal genitals (Give me a break!), unusually small ears, and the list went on. I wanted to prove these jerks wrong, and where did they get their flawless reputation anyway? They had labeled him, and I was pissed. How in hell could they make such a call without extensive testing, and I didn't remember authorizing such tests. They were now dealing with an informed and irritated Black woman. I gave the very next intern who came into our cubical hell for not disclosing to me what was in Jermaine's records. I told him it was my parental right to know everything that was written about me or my child and that the secrecy would end here and now. He was conspicuously undone. I told him that I received no public assistance and "don't even think about treating me as a charity case." I also told the now-flushed young man that although this was a teaching hospital, I wanted no one who was not involved directly with Jermaine's case to question me or to pry into his records. I added that my warning included the hoards of young medical students that marched through daily. I asked if I had made myself clear; he annoyingly and sheepishly said, "Yes." From that point on, I was treated with new respect and as Jermaine's official advocate.

Jermaine's therapy continued. I ignored completely the "possible retardation" diagnosis because these so-called professionals didn't know squat about my child. I read up on retardation, and Jermaine didn't fit the profile. I was not buying into it. I was sure it was confusing to measure growth and milestones on a blind child who is delayed in all those areas that have to do with vision—hand-eye coordination, tracking objects, playing peek-a-boo. Jermaine was the teacher for all of us as we learned to relate to our blind child.

At home we functioned in our very own little "safe haven." We did not have a lot of visitors as people had begun to stray away from us. After all, what do you say to the parents when you look at their child and are completely shocked by his appearance? When James, Jamaal, Jermaine, and I went public, people said the cruelest things imaginable. We tried to keep Jermaine's face covered when we went out, but people are attracted to babies and want "a quick peek." They would get the shock of their lives and ask what we had done to his face. This happened more than I care to mention. We went to the Washington zoo. James had Jermaine in the harness facing him as we felt that with Jermaine strapped to his front, we could let Jamaal enjoy the zoo without people commenting on Jermaine. Wrong. People went out of their way to see what the baby looked like, and we spent the entire day trying to explain Jermaine's condition.

On one occasion we were shopping at a supermarket, and a woman followed us around trying to get a peek at Jermaine. Finally Jamaal turned to her and said, "You are being rude, and you're hurting my brother's feelings." From that day on, I took my cue from Jamaal and refused to let people make me uncomfortable. We took turns going to the store or left Jermaine with a family member when we went shopping. What cowards we were! Then Jamaal had a party at his Montessori school and asked if I could go with him. I said, "Sure, let me get a sitter for Jermaine." He said, "Let's take him with us. The other kids are bringing their siblings." My sister Cookie said, "Girl, it's time to stop hiding." She was right.

Jermaine was becoming more of a social being at home and doing a remarkable job with the occupational therapist. James and I, on the other hand, needed help, and we needed it now. James walked around trying not to look upset and doing a horrible job of it. Whenever our eyes met, they filled with tears. We didn't go out anymore, and we avoided friends. Friends didn't know what to say, so they avoided us. They wanted to think we were fine, so we acted fine. James had a hard time masking his emotions because he wears them on his sleeve. I, on the other hand, deserved an academy award for my portrayal of "The Happy Woman." Friends wanted to think I was my usual bounce-back-from-anything self. It let everybody off the hook to say "I knew you'd be able to handle this," "You're special," and "I couldn't do it, but I knew you could." Preposterous! How could they possibly think I was okay? I should have let them know how badly I felt, but it was not my way to do that. Actually, I'm not sure I knew how I wanted people to react, but in retrospect, I wanted them to say, "I know you're in pain, and I don't know what to do or what to say to you, but please don't shut me out. Let me know what you're feeling." I guess you have to be really savvy to pull that one off.

I ached because Jermaine would never see my face or enjoy my favorite time of year in autumnal russets and golds. I was depressed because he would miss the magic of Christmas decorations. I was darn mad at Jamaal for wanting to be blind so he could "get all the neat attention that Jermaine gets." I was furious at James because he was the father of my baby, and I often wondered, if I had married someone else, could I have delivered such a child? I was mad at everyone and needed professional help . . . fast!

The Kennedy Institute sent us a social worker to help us deal with some issues we were avoiding. She looked like Rapunzel but was not the least bit mushy, which was good because the last thing I needed at this point was a weeping willow therapist. She came every week for an hour or more and got to know us, and we told her things we had not told a living soul. She was the medicine we needed: she didn't judge, listened well, and responded appropriately. She never looked shocked at anything I said, which shocked me.

One day I had an unusually hard time dealing with my feelings. I hated my life, and I hated not going to work. I hated everyone, and it just didn't seem fair that we were so sad all the time. Jamaal was out of school, and James would be home soon. I planned to turn on the gas in the kitchen, gather my children and my husband (who felt the same way), and do away with the whole mess. It was a very comforting thought, and I had gone over the scenario in my mind for an entire day. We'd all be together, and this entire hurt would be over. I should have called the social worker, but I didn't. I went about straightening the house and getting things in order to leave for Cookie. I did not want the house to be a mess when they removed our bodies. After the house was cleaned, I told Jamaal how much I loved him and gathered Jermaine in my arms, telling him I did not blame him for the sadness and loved him deeply. I called Cookie for idle chitchat, giving her no clue this was the last time she would speak with me. We had once discussed how either of our deaths would send the survivor over the edge. We even joked about doing the makeup of the one who went first. But this was real. I was about to commit the murder of my loved ones and kill myself as well. I said good-bye casually to Cooks and hung up.

Then I began thinking about Daddy, who would be devastated by my death. I knew it would wipe him out. He would wonder where he'd gone wrong in his religious teaching, which preaches against suicide and murder. He would wonder why I had not come to him if I was in so much pain. He still treated us like we were his little girls and would do things like call my house to say he's bought some eggs and milk and to stop down and get them. He would call and ask me to "play a piece on the piano" for him, or to hear Jamaal play, and he'd tell me how proud he was of how I was raising Jamaal. When I was thirty, Daddy was still sneaking me an allowance. He was a clown and delighted in saying extra long prayers at Thanksgiving dinner when he knew we were starving, and he would open one eye to watch "The Presidents" giggle. I couldn't do this to him. Daddy saved my life. I never told him that. I told the social worker, and she told me my feelings were normal, even the thoughts of suicide, in situations like mine. She said I was in recovery because I could talk about the way I felt rather than suppressing it. She made me promise to give her a call if I ever felt like harming myself or my family again. I promised.

I threw myself into prayer and my two boys. Jamaal was doing really well with his piano lessons. I would strap Jermaine into his adaptive highchair and let him strike the keys, which he seemed to enjoy. I met an amazing woman during one of our hospital stays. She and I exchanged horror stories and had "bitching sessions." She bought Jermaine the most unique gifts, such as twin vision books that were in Braille and print so I could read them to him. She never forgot about Jamaal, which meant a lot to me. She had given birth in somewhat similar circumstances, so I never had to fake it with her when I was hurting. We were the best therapy for each other, and I owe my sanity to her.

Notes over the Pain

One evening after Jamaal had finished his lesson, I put Jermaine up to the piano in his high chair, and James and I went downstairs with Jamaal. Shortly, we heard the piano and the song, "Lightly Row," which

Jamaal had just finished playing. James and I looked at each other, and we looked at Jamaal. If Jamaal was with us, who was playing the piano? We sneaked back upstairs and saw my Jermaine playing the piano like he had been doing it all his life. And he was smiling. I uttered, "Thank you, Jesus!" and then I screamed. Jermaine was so startled that he too screamed and would not play the piano again for two weeks. The child could play the piano! We called our parents, who didn't believe it, and we couldn't prove it because Jermaine wouldn't do it again. But we knew he had done it; we were there. James thought it was a fluke, and Jermaine would never do it again. He was wrong. Jermaine was not quite nine months old.

After a while our sessions with the social worker became shorter; we were healing. I had something else in Jermaine I could nurture, his music. We were asked to speak at a seminar for professionals and parents of handicapped children, all expenses paid. We had never left Jermaine overnight before, but my mother agreed to baby-sit. James backed out from speaking but went along with me for support. I went on to speak at several healthcare seminars. These helped me talk from the heart and to heal. It also gave other mothers the opportunity to say how they really felt once the "presenter" admitted that she hated her child when she first found out he was so different. Many said that I helped them, but they helped me by allowing me to help them.

A year passed, and it was indeed a rough one. Writing a poem was what I felt was needed at this time. Actually, it was a song, but since my singing leaves a lot to be desired, I called it a poem when reciting it in public after my presentations. In private, I would sing this song to Jermaine and mean it from the bottom of my heart:

You are my world, although you cannot see.
I'll be your eyes for you and you be the sun for me.
You make up my world, you made me realize,
Though eyes are important, without them you *can* survive.
One year ago today, life seemed uncertain
But God let me take a look behind life's stage curtain.
And now I'm on top of things and you're so much higher.
I'll teach you to love and learn;
We'll set this old world on fire.
'Cause you are my world, you are my inspiration.
Though you cannot see with your eyes,

I know you'll survive.
Your name is *Jermaine*
And I do love you so.
There is no more pain.
Just thought you should know.

Jermaine was walking at almost a year and could now pull himself up to the piano and play to his heart's content. He spent most of his free time there and laughed while playing. He was so obsessed with the piano and his music that I would feed him there. He refused to do anything else, which included using the potty. I pried him off the piano bench for a midday break, and he fell asleep at the piano every night. We introduced him to new music weekly. He leaned toward difficult songs and classical pieces, pronouncing other music "junk." He's had wonderful piano teachers, including a man I met after seeing a television show on teaching blind children to play piano. I felt he was the teacher I was looking for, so I called him the next day. I told him Jermaine was two and half years old, and he said, "I think that's a bit young for formal lessons." Then pausing, he said, "Incidentally, who is that playing in the background?" I poked out my flat chest and proudly answered, "My two and half year old." He gasped and said, "Oh my gosh! Bring him right over!" I did.

As time went on, Jermaine was in the papers and magazines. He was interviewed, appreciated, exploited, and invited to play at the White House and with Stevie Wonder. He was on national television, made international debuts—and learned to demand any number of things, such as that no one clap during his performances, or he would stop or threaten to play "baby songs." He could not stand to hear his own music played back, because he was his own worst critic, and he hated applause. And he would play and play and play, not stopping when he was expected to. We would have to pry him off the bench, screaming at the top of his lungs. I would bribe him to keep still in concerts. What next?

I was concerned about the plastic surgeon's notion of waiting for reconstructive surgery until Jermaine was fifteen. The truth of the matter is that I simply had no faith in his opinion. Marcy Slayer, president of the International Craniofacial Foundation and wife of Kenneth Slayer, a well-known reconstructive surgeon, had seen Jermaine on TV. She said the plastic surgeons from that nonprofit organization could rebuild Jermaine's face in a way that would make him presentable. "Praise the

Lord," I said. "This is too good to be true." We would fly to Texas for a team evaluation—fifteen specialists, including surgeons, a psychologist, social worker, anthropologist, and speech therapist. We were told the surgery should be done as soon as possible and that the plastic surgeon who said to wait for fifteen years needed to have his own head reconstructed. The organization would pay for the family's flight to Dallas, put us up, provide food, and provide a semi-professional football player to keep Jamaal occupied while James and I dealt with Jermaine's evaluation. Could life be sweeter? We set the date and walked around on a cloud until James and I got scared. "What if it doesn't work? What if Jermaine dies? What if this is a terrible joke?" The deal included an ABC camera crew. Family reactions were split on our decision, some in favor and some with lists of "what ifs." We went.

Jermaine by now, at four, had developed quite an interesting personality and had loads of imaginary friends. He took on different personalities, all of them named for composers or movements of music. The psychologist worried about which one would be undergoing the surgery and whether the others would mind. On the morning of the evaluation, Jermaine was "Rondo." I knew what the team was thinking. James and I laughed, not the least bit concerned about Jermaine having multiple personalities, but these professionals were taking this seriously. We pulled Jermaine to the side and told him to "get his act together" before they pulled the plug on the surgery idea. He did. Temporarily.

We saw doctor after doctor. Jermaine had pictures taken of his skull and face from every angle, cat scans, face measurements, nose measurements, socket measurements, each specialist doing what he or she did best. We finally met Dr. Slayer, who would do the major portion of the surgery. He looked like a runway model with such confidence that I thought anyone this arrogant has to be good! He explained about facial clefting syndrome, hypertelorism frontal nasal dysplasia. I tried to look like I had a clue, but I asked him to explain. He looked a tad annoyed that we did not share the magic of medical jargon but began describing Jermaine's condition in lay terms. The cameras rolled as he described the surgery: moving Jermaine's eye sockets closer together, taking a bone from his skull to make a bridge for his nose, using gristle from his ears to make a tip for his nose, and possibly making eyebrows. He could also move Jermaine's face up. He would stretch the skin and make and reshape it, holding the stretched skin in place with bone grafts. Another specialist was on hand if we decided to have a prosthesis made for Jermaine's eye socket. Appearance is important, even to blind people, and I planned to do everything I could to make Jermaine appear as normal as possible.

The team met to compare its various findings. We were taken around, interviewed, and finely dined, while charming Jamaal wrapped rich ladies around his little finger with his precocious conversation. Jermaine was another story. I never knew what he would say or do. He had wowed people at the fancy club we'd been taken to by performing on the black lacquered piano for twenty minutes before dinner with two news stations present—the reporters were tickled when I had to get down on my hands and knees to work the pedals for most of his songs, since his four-year-old legs could not reach them. Marcy and her friends ordered extra cherries for Jermaine's coke, and one blond southern belle ordered Jermaine fries ("cut potatoes" in this ritzy restaurant), a burger (from ground steak), and lots of ketchup. She drawled into Jermaine's ear as she fed him the fries, "Let's dip 'em in the ketchup," sending him into hysterical laughter. It was a fun evening and wonderful to see how the other half lives.

Around this time Jermaine began labeling everyone he met with a number, symbol, or direction. Eggie and Uggie were twins who lived in the Technodrome, which happened to be located under our baby grand piano. Jermaine changed voices in his conversations with his imaginary friends. One night he, Eggie, Uggie, Timer, and Sonata were upstairs playing in his room. I was talking with Cookie on the phone when she asked who was talking in the background. I told her it was Jermaine and "the friends." "Making all that noise?" she asked. I said, "Yes." "Girl, go to his room and see if anyone else is in there." I refused. "Go ahead, Girl, remember those Alfred Hitchcock movies? What if there are little people in there?" she whispered, laughing her wicked witch laugh. We both laughed. Just then Jermaine said, "Mommie, come here and see what we're doing." I told him I hoped they were having fun. I was not about to crash that party!

During his own concerts, I sat next to Jermaine while he played. He would lean over to ask me how his music sounded. I would tell him that he played beautifully or that he needed more dynamics or that he should play more softly, and so on. He could be manipulative if he didn't get what he wanted when he was at the piano. I followed Jermaine's lead, while James paced and sweated through concerts. Jermaine could not be afforded the luxury of warming up prior to playing. Once he touched the piano, he would play an entire concert. When he heard songs on a tape, he would play them in that order, all six, or ten of them, never deviating from the original. I would pretend he was playing what we'd planned, but he might change songs midstream, and I'd be as stunned as the next person. I never provided lists for his performances and looked forward to his getting older and getting some structure in his playing.

The night before the surgery we ate dinner in our room because I really felt the need to hold my man and my children close to me. I felt a little weird as time neared for us to check into the hospital. James pulled me close, and I love when he does that. We had come a long way and fought this battle together. We had been through hell these past four years, and anything else would be piece of cake. The admitting procedure went smoothly. Jermaine had a private room because the media would be in and out, and if he had a roommate it would violate the roommate's privacy. The big room had a pullout chair that I would use later. I put Jermaine in his pajamas and said his prayers with him. I prayed to God that night like I never prayed before, asking him to spare Jermaine's life and bring him through the surgery safely. Life is strange that way. Only four years earlier, I'd prayed for God to take his life because I did not think I could deal with this. Now I was begging for the life of this child who meant so much to me. I simply could not imagine how I could have been happy without Jermaine in my life. He had taught me to love and fight, and I'd become damned good at both of those.

The nurses came in to chat and were very nice. The hospital was buzzing with excitement, aware that Jermaine had come with a camera crew. All were on their best behavior. I wanted to befriend the nurses who would be taking care of Jermaine after the surgery. I would have to depend on them.

Jermaine went to sleep immediately, and I called Cookie, who was waiting for my call. I began to cry and told her I was scared. She did what she did best, saying all the right things. We cried on the phone just as we did when Jermaine was born, but this was different. This was going to be the answer to a different prayer, and it was up to me to get myself together and rise to the occasion. We stayed on the phone for over an hour. I told her not to spoil Nikki, our Rottweiler (who never had table scraps except when Cookie was around). Cookie said it was a good thing Nikki could not talk because "the Cook" had given her steak and crab cakes. Cookie and I said goodnight and hung up.

Morning came quickly, and I awoke to sounds of the crew in the hall setting up for when Jermaine would leave his room. I went into the bathroom to metamorphose through waking up and looking human at this awful hour. Jermaine slept. I chose a red and white long polo shirt and white pants and flat white shoes. I put on my makeup and a pair of red schoolboy glasses. I woke Jermaine, washed him, and dressed him. We played a learning game until the crew was ready for us. "Who painted 'The three musicians'?" I asked. "That was Picasso," said Jermaine in his raspy voice. "Good, who invented the piano?" Jermaine answered without hesitation, "Bartolomeo Cristofori." What a kid! I was so proud of him, and he was so brave! What a lump in my throat!

We walked down the halls with the camera running, and reporters told people who came into the hallway to take their children back into their rooms if they did not want them on film. Many chose to stand and watch the media circus. A Black orderly told us he really wanted to wheel Jermaine to surgery and that he wanted Jermaine's autograph afterward. I went with the stretcher as far as the staff would allow me. Jermaine said goodbye as if he'd be back in ten minutes. I smiled.

I saw the neurosurgeon, who must have been reading my mind. "Mrs. Gardner, I met you when you were here for the evaluation. I'm the one who is going to protect the music center in Jermaine's brain." I thanked God, hugged the doctor, went back to Jermaine's room, threw myself on his bed, and wept until James and Jamaal appeared. It upsets Jamaal to see me cry, and he assured me that Jermaine would be all right. "You believe in God, Mommy?" I told him yes. "Then you don't have to worry about Jermaine." I smiled. Switching gears, Jamaal went on to tell me about the Southern Methodist University football star Marcy had set him up with so that James and I could concentrate on what was about to take place with Jermaine. The operation would take six to eight hours. James and I went back to the hotel, had a big breakfast, and fell on our knees to thank God for bringing us to Dallas and to beg him to spare Jermaine's life and grant us a successful surgery. We knew there was nothing we could do. Jermaine's fate was now and always has been in God's willing and loving hands.

Eventually we were called and told that Jermaine was out of surgery.

The cameras rolled as we were ushered to the recovery room. "Please God," I prayed, "Let this not be a disaster." I held back the tears as I ran to Jermaine, who was in a nurse's arms moaning, hoarsely, and calling for me. The nurse whispered a very southern "It's OK . . . Mama's comin'."

The sight of Jermaine was frightening. I could see in James's face that he felt the same way. Jermaine's entire head was wrapped in a huge bandage that was saturated with blood. His face was triple the size it was earlier. His eyes were swollen and he looked as if his face had been used for a punching bag. I swept him up in my arms and hugged him tight, thankful to God that he was alive. I told him that I loved him. I would deal later with how horrible he looked. The old Negro gospel song "I Don't Believe He Brought Me This Far to Leave Me" echoed in my mind as I silently asked God to calm me. Just then the nurse came over and explained to me that Jermaine's swelling was normal after such traumatic surgery and that in a few days Jermaine would be running down these halls as if he never had surgery. "Pacify me," I thought. "There is no way he will run down the halls in a few days." I was dead wrong and loved it! True, the first 48 hours were crucial. Jermaine was watched constantly. Jamaal cried when he saw him and asked why I had let them do this to his brother. I told him that I had prayed about it and that everything would be fine. But I was having a hard time believing that one myself.

The staff at the Humana Institutes in Dallas was phenomenal. We were put in a luxurious room in the hospital, complete with designer sheets. We were only a minute away from being with Jermaine. Whenever we needed to—and we needed to often—we could reassure ourselves of his uneventful recovery. Jermaine was on a morphine drip for pain and was, basically, out of it most of this risky time. I was relieved because never did I want him to experience pain from a surgery we had elected him to have. James and I kept constant watch over Jermaine, as did the very competent staff.

I was especially impressed with the nurses who cared for Jermaine. They were extremely caring and seemed to know their stuff. There was one nurse, in particular, who really caught my attention—an African American nurse who took a special liking to Jermaine. She was articulate and knew a lot. Although I admired her knowledge, I also felt jealous of her. She was so caring, and she knew how to care for Jermaine when I didn't. I wished I were a nurse; they were so respected at Humana

Institutes and so sure of themselves. They were crazy about Jermaine, and I wondered whether they really liked him or they enjoyed being the nurse to a somewhat celebrity.

The nurses on the unit that Jermaine was assigned to went out of their way to explain everything they were doing to Jermaine and why. They answered the many questions that I had and never seemed to tire of my having to know the "whys" of everything they did. I couldn't tell if it was just Texan hospitality that made these nurses unique or whether nursing schools there were turning out such conscientious, compassionate nurses. Whatever the reason, I felt fortunate that Jermaine was being cared for by these nurses. With the exception of the neurosurgeon who promised me before surgery that he would protect the music center in Jermaine's brain, a lot of the doctors—even in friendly Texas—left a lot to be desired in terms of seeming compassionate.

Some of the staff came in to visit Jermaine on their days off. Wonderful volunteers kept Jermaine and Jamaal entertained. Two of the operating room technicians invited us to dinner when Jermaine was released from the hospital. We had our first-ever fried catfish dinner, complete with homemade corn bread. The kindness of the staff at Humana and the people of Texas caught me totally off guard.

Marcy Slayer was a real gem, too. She made sure that we were comfortable and had everything that we needed. One day, after she went to the toy store to buy toys for Jermaine for his recovery, she suggested that James and I go out to get away for a couple of hours. I protested. I did not want to leave Jermaine's side. "I'll sit with Jermaine, Jacqui. You go out and spend some time with your husband." I was deeply touched by the love and care she displayed. This was the wife of a world-renowned plastic surgeon who spent her evening rocking my Black, blind child in her arms. Tears streamed down my face as I marveled at God's greatness and that of this white woman who looked at Jermaine with love—a woman whose foundation had assisted with the finances that enabled Jermaine to undergo this extremely costly surgery.

The day we left the hospital, Jermaine said he could not wait to play the piano. He had not played in over a week. His wanting to play the piano was a good sign, I thought. We decided that he could play for the doctors, nurses, and staff as a "thank-you" for their support, care, time, and talent. Marcy made arrangements to have a grand piano brought to the atrium of the hospital, and a concert date was set for four days after Jermaine's surgery. We went back to the hotel and located a piano in the ballroom for Jermaine to practice on.

James and Jamaal relaxed in our donated suite while Jermaine and I went to the ballroom. Jermaine was bouncing down the hall—bandages gone, but with staples across the top of his head. His swelling had gone down, and he was looking a whole lot better in the face area. He had a new nose that gave him a rather impish look, and he was cute, finally. He kept saying to all he met, "Do you like my new nose?" I thanked God as I walked into the ballroom for the caring hotel people who allowed our family to reside in a huge suite for three weeks and who treated us like royalty. I thanked God for the surgeon's gifted hands. I thanked him for all of the genuinely caring and very rich people of Dallas who had adopted our family.

I began to feel eerie as we approached the piano. I was holding Jermaine's hand and he seemed eager to be going to the piano. I had had nightmares of my having sacrificed his musical gift for the vanity of a new face. I tried to dismiss the thought, but to no avail. Jermaine climbed up on the piano bench and began to play. However, what he played, I had never heard before in my life. He was playing like an average four-year-old child, not the gifted prodigy that he was. I began to sweat. "Play Beethoven" I whispered. He said he would, but began to play another run of notes that was not anything familiar. I squeezed my eyes shut and tried to calm myself by slowing down my breathing. I prayed. I opened my eyes, put my hands on both of his shoulders, and tried to sound calm. Maybe he could feel my anxiety. I asked him if he could play "Autumn Leaves" he said, "I *am* playing 'Autumn Leaves.'" I began to cry. He no longer had the gift. This went on for another forty-five minutes, until I could take no more. I gently took him off of the piano, caught the elevator up to the eighteenth floor, and went back to our suite to break the news to James and Jamaal.

James was quiet for several minutes and then said that maybe Jermaine was just tired and needed some time, since he had been away from the piano for so long. I knew he was trying to console me, and I didn't believe what he was saying for one moment. I put Jermaine down for a nap, and I, too, went to bed. I prayed for God to give Jermaine his gift back before I drifted into restless sleep. I woke hours later, and it was dark outside. I looked out of the window that Jamaal had earlier claimed as his own and admired the city lights. I immediately thought of Jermaine and went in his room to see if he was stirring. He was in a closet playing with his new toys and his imaginary friends. I spoke to him, and he asked if he could go back and play the piano some more. I told him we could go after dinner.

Later Jermaine and I walked into the quiet ballroom to play the piano. I sat him at the piano and held my breath. He began to play. Still, I did not recognize his music. The nightmare was beginning again. I could not believe this. I asked him to play "Twinkle, twinkle, little star," an easy song. He said he was playing it. I began to cry and was just about to take him off of the piano when a maitre d' walked through the ballroom and said, "Can the little boy have a piece of candy?" I told him that Jermaine could have one. The tall Mexican bent down, positioning himself so that Jermaine could reach the bowl of sourballs. Jermaine chose one, took the wrapper off, and popped the candy into his mouth. "Umm, this is good," Jermaine said. He then spun around on the piano bench and began to play Beethoven's "Moonlight Sonata" in its entirety! God is good! I hugged the maitre d', who looked at me as if I were crazy, and I loudly thanked God (truly a Black thing). Jermaine, in his raspy voice, replied, "Marcy likes this song, 'Moonlight.'" I raced to the wall phone and called our room and told James and Jamaal to come to the ballroom. When they got there, Jermaine was back to his old self and was well into what turned out to be an hour-long concert. He was ready for tomorrow's concert at the hospital. "To God be the glory!"

The atrium of the hospital was beautifully decorated with an art exhibit and the grand piano that Marcy had brought in. The piano had a microphone attached and fresh flowers on it. Cameramen from various television stations were everywhere. The newspapers were there, and the atrium was at "standing room only" capacity. James, Jamaal, Jermaine, and I arrived in time to be interviewed by a couple of newspapers and by two newscasters. Marcy introduced herself, explained how we met, and talked about what Jermaine's surgery meant to the hospital, the International Craniofacial Foundation, and children with facial deformities around the world. Then she introduced me. I quickly thanked everybody in the world for anything they had done to help us and began to tell the audience about my children. I introduced Jamaal and told the audience that he, too, was a pianist and would be performing first. Jamaal performed like the champion that he was, playing flawlessly and charming his audience. I was so proud of him; I was sure that it was not easy being Jermaine's brother. Jamaal played for fifteen minutes, bowed, and began to talk with reporters and well-wishers. Jamaal could hold his own with anyone. I smiled proudly.

Jermaine sat at the piano, and the room instantly became silent. He was dressed in a yellow Hawaiian shirt with matching shorts and navy blue sneakers. His legs swung, freely, from the bench. He was too little for them to reach the floor. His eyes were still swollen from his surgery of a few days ago, and he had staples in his head from ear to ear. He was hard to look at. People looked sympathetic until he struck the first chords on the piano. He played Bach, Beethoven, Chopin, and Liszt as if he had been playing them for years. The audience was mesmerized. I sat beside him on the floor by the piano bench, doing the pedaling for him by hand when the pieces called for it. Someone brought me a pillow to kneel on. Jermaine played for three-quarters of an hour, non-stop, and when he finished, he received five minutes of thunderous applause, complete with standing ovation from hospital staff, visitors, patients, doctors, and newspeople. Jermaine had "kicked butt," and I was honored. "Thank you, God," I whispered. "My baby is back."

The media had a field day with the story of the musical genius from Baltimore. Dallas was abuzz with the talk of Jermaine, his incredible surgery, and his awesome talent. National TV did a story about Jermaine's surgery. I called Baltimore to prepare my family for its airing before they saw Jermaine in person. By this time, while being thankful for all of the generosity that Dallas offered, I was ready to go home. But there was a problem. Jermaine needed additional surgery on his nose because one side was collapsing. This meant that Jamaal and James would be going home while Jermaine and I stayed an additional week. Never had I traveled with Jermaine by plane without my man, and I was scared. I was afraid that with all of the media coverage and notoriety that now surrounded Jermaine, he would be a perfect target for some sick person to abduct. I prayed that God would take away the spirit of fear that encompassed me and let me have faith that Jesus would calm me. He did. I went with a volunteer to the airport to see my family off and then immediately went about the business of thanking God for his mercy as I prepared for the work that Dr. Slayer needed to do on Jermaine's nose.

After about a week, it was time to take Jermaine home. I had been talking to Cookie, so I knew expectations were high. Everyone was anxiously awaiting the arrival of the young maestro with the new face. When the plane finally landed, I scooped the newly nosed Jermaine up into my arms and rushed to the baggage department in search of my family. I panned the sea of people from many cultures in search of the shades of brown in the faces that I loved so much. I felt sweat trickle from my armpits down the sides of my ribcage. I was a wreck. My face was wet with perspiration, and I could feel my hair clinging to my clammy neck. I silently asked God to calm me. James had to work that night, so I knew that his would not be among the faces that I sought, which probably added to my anxiety as I searched frantically for my family. "There they are . . . Jacqui!" I turned to hear the excited voice of my nephew, Tom, who spotted me first. My family began running toward me, and me toward them, like a sappy, corny movie. The reunion was heartwarming; tears of joy streaked all our faces. Cookie and I hugged and cried for at least five minutes. In his low raspy voice Jermaine asked, "How d'ya like my new nose?" We burst into laughter, and Jermaine reached for Cookie to carry him. Terri, my niece, reached for Jermaine so that she could carry him for awhile. Although Jermaine was four, we all carried him everywhere, as if he couldn't walk. People at the airport had gathered around because, by now, Jermaine was being recognized from television. I thanked God for our safe return, my family, and my faith.

Jermaine's surgery was a big deal with the media, and everyone wanted Jermaine to appear on their show. James called it exploitation. I called it positive exposure. After all, it was that "positive exposure" that landed Jermaine the reconstruction surgery that would change his life forever. Soon Jermaine reappeared on national television and at the White House. He became an ambassador for Marcy's Craniofacial Foundation, and I testified on Capitol Hill for Congress to pass a bill supporting assistance for children needing craniofacial reconstruction. It passed. This was a very exciting life, and I soon needed a planner so that I could know where we needed to be and when. I became active in support groups so that I could educate parents about their rights and the rights of their handicapped children. I read everything there was to read about blindness so that I could arm myself and become an advocate for Jermaine—and not a moment too soon.

Jermaine was a student in the Baltimore City Public School System. I learned how to play the game in record time. By the grace of God, his teachers taught me how to get what I needed for him while maintaining some decorum. The school administrators quickly learned that I was a force to be reckoned with; whatever Jermaine needed, I fought to get. My first real battle had been when I wanted Jermaine to be taught Braille when he was three. I was told that he was too young and that was not the protocol. I insisted that if a sighted child could be taught to read at age three, then so could a blind one. After much debate, I won the right for Jermaine to be taught Braille, and he emerged as Maryland's youngest Braille reader. There were other fights with the public schools for which I needed the assistance of the National Federation of the Blind. They became my friends and taught me about the dignity that comes with being a blind person.

Elementary school was, for the most part, good for Jermaine. He had lots of friends and learned a lot. In first grade he met a blind teacher. In addition to being a teacher, she was young, bright, caring, and determined to teach Jermaine what he needed to learn to become a success. She became my inside track and taught me all I needed to know about how and when to let go of Jermaine, and what to ask for at meetings held to determine the educational needs of children with handicapping conditions. She was Jermaine's favorite teacher and even talked me into letting him travel with her clear across the country to enter the Braille Olympics. My family thought that I had lost my mind allowing Jermaine to travel with this ambitious, blind woman. I prayed about it and knew I needed to let him go. Jermaine went to California and won the "surgical" removal of himself from my side. It was a great beginning step toward independence. The teacher and I became fast friends as she taught me to let go, let God, and trust that Jermaine would be fine. She transferred to every school Jermaine attended so that she could make sure he had every opportunity he needed in order to excel and to compete with his sighted peers.

Because I wanted to be up on anything I needed to know that would help Jermaine academically and socially, I took a job as a teacher. I taught Special Education for Baltimore City Public Schools so that I could know the jargon and the loopholes and would be kept abreast of my rights as a parent of a child with special needs. I learned a lot. Yet, in spite of my knowledge of the system, nothing could have prepared me for what Jermaine was about to experience.

After elementary school, Jermaine attended the middle school from hell. The teachers and administration there were neither sensitive nor helpful. In homeroom, Jermaine was seated alone in the middle of the room at a round table. He was ostracized, ignored, and picked on. He was miserable, and so was I. The last straw was when Jermaine began to cry before going to school each morning. Eventually, it came out about a kid who slapped him in the face every day. He never knew when the unprovoked slap would come. The ghetto in me came out immediately. I went to the school to talk with the principal, threatening to beat the aggressor myself or to have my then-17-year-old son Jamaal do it. I even imagined running over the kid with my car when school let out. I was irrational and out of control. My sister Cookie told me to think about what I was saying and convinced me that I would certainly be away from Jermaine for years if I carried out that plan. All I could do was ask God for guidance.

The principal and I talked, along with the school's social worker. They told me how the boy's 15-year-old sister was raising him because his mother was on drugs—yadda, yadda. They went on to say that by victimizing Jermaine, the boy felt he had some power—he really didn't mean any harm, but Jermaine was an easy target. After a quarter hour of this "discount store psychology," I announced that I wasn't concerned about why he did what he did, but that it had better stop or I was calling the police and the media, and heads would roll. I told the principal that I wanted to meet with this child and his mother. She refused, probably wisely, for kicking the mother's butt certainly was my priority. Fortunately, the problem was resolved after the boy, while denying everything, went to sensitivity training classes as dictated by the social worker. After this incident, I got myself elected as president of that school's Parent Teachers Association so that I had an inside edge on what was going on in Jermaine's life. I kept close watch on the middle school and found out later that my impromptu visits put everyone there on alert because of my reputation as a mother who would walk through hell wearing gasoline underwear for her child. The remainder of Jermaine's time at this horrible school was uneventful. When graduation time came, guess who they asked to play the music? Of course. I told Jermaine he didn't have to participate, or even attend. But he was so happy that the kids now thought he was cool that he wanted to do the music and did.

New Beginnings

A good friend of mine has been a nurse for a long time. She convinced me to go to nursing school. I told her all the reasons that I couldn't go back to school, but that I would really love to be a nurse because I'd had a firsthand chance to experience the care that nurses give. She pushed me harder, and it was, truly, one of the best decisions that I could have made. I could see myself as a nurse because I wanted the chance to treat patients as Jermaine had been treated during his stays in hospitals. I had also experienced some encounters from which I wanted to spare others.

The road through nursing school was hard and long. I had two children and a husband. I worked hard and cried long. Nursing school was the hardest thing that I'd done in a while, but I enjoyed the challenge and looked forward to becoming a nurse. While I thought Jermaine's disfigurement and disability were the biggest mistakes ever, I was convinced that everything that I did was a direct or indirect reflection of the lessons that God was teaching me about loving and caring for Jermaine and for others. Jermaine was the center of my life, although God was the center of my joy. My goal was to make sure that Jermaine was blessed with the best life ever. I graduated from nursing school the same year Jermaine entered high school.

Musically, things soared for Jermaine. He performed in Japan that summer and was a real hit. He appeared on local and national talk shows and magazine shows and had numerous articles written about him. Jermaine Gardner became a household word. His dream was now to attend the Baltimore School for the Arts, which is an incredible place for performing artists. This unique institution nurtured Jermaine's already flourishing talent. It was home. Jermaine was respected for the musician that he was. Blindness was not a stumbling block for him. The school simply made the appropriate adjustments. When it was known that Jermaine would be attending, the dean summoned his staff and began to make things happen in preparation for Jermaine's arrival. Doors and offices were "Brailled," additional people were hired, textbooks on tape were ordered, sighted guides were lined up, staff were educated, and students were briefed. Jermaine sailed through as if he had eyes. He was a happy kid, and I was happy because he was cared for and loved by the staff and students at the school. He did great things there and won first place in most of the piano competitions that his teacher entered him in. Jermaine was loving life, and I was praising God for his goodness. Jermaine attended the senior prom with the prettiest girl in the school. She asked him to go to the prom with her. I was shocked, and so was he. It was actually quite funny because Jermaine's friends asked how on earth he landed the most beautiful girl in the school, and he couldn't even see her. His response: "I have skills."

Jermaine graduated from the Baltimore School for the Arts and received numerous scholarships. He applied to the Peabody Conservatory and Oberlin Conservatory of Music in Ohio. He was accepted at both but chose Oberlin because he liked their program and was convinced that they would address his needs there and make his experience memorable. Oberlin made good on that promise. They have treated Jermaine like royalty. Jermaine is now a sophomore. He has two music CDs out. The first one, *The Incredible Journey*, is classical, and the second, *The Night Shift*, is jazz. Jermaine continues to excel musically. I am very proud of his accomplishments and his tenacity. With God's grace, Jermaine will make it, and so will I.

Revelations

What has this experience taught me? Every so often, one is hit with the biggest whammy of one's life in order for lessons to be learned and growth to take place. This score of years has taught me patience, caring, and acceptance of people for who and what they are. This journey has taught me that becoming a nurse has been one of the most rewarding choices that I have made thus far. I am afforded the opportunity to do what I do best—care for people in need and advocate on their behalf. I learned that real beauty is in the eye of the beholder, and most of all, I learned to have a reckless faith in God. Culturally speaking, African Americans as a whole are God-fearing people. After we've thrown a "hissy fit" about some situation, we eventually turn back to God for guidance.

I have learned, regrettably, that many people in the healthcare professions are uncaring—or at least insensitive—when dealing with a parent who has a child with disabilities. Most physicians lacked what was needed to help me endure the shock and the magnitude of the situation that I faced. Caring and compassion seems to be missing from the doctors' "to do" list; they need to become priorities—no matter how busy or uncomfortable doctors are. I feel that more should and could be done in professional schooling and during residencies to convince clinicians that they need to develop some finesse for delivering heartbreaking news to parents and working with them. The social workers were our saving grace. They were responsible for my successfully emerging from all this the way I have. They had oodles of resources, and when they didn't know something, they referred me to someone who did know. The nurses were also generally phenomenal doing what they do, and it gives me great pleasure to be among their ranks.

I never even thought of writing a book before my experience of being the mother of a "fantabulous" child. Now I have a book (Kess-Gardner, 2002) and this chapter. Writing has been extremely therapeutic for me and has, in effect, taught me many things about myself. I realize my work as advocate and supporter of parents with different children is not over yet, and I'm sure that God will let me know where I need to go with this. I have been blessed with God placing so many incredible people in my life. He put them there at different seasons and for different purposes. I am no longer the person I was nineteen years ago, and quite frankly, the person I am now can benefit the world far more than that other person ever could. I thank God every day for this experience, this life, and, most of all, this child. I am most honored to have mothered one of the most talented children in the world. It has been, indeed, an incredible journey. It doesn't get much better than that.

Conclusion

In the harshness of corporeality, babies are either *perfect* or *different*. The word *different* implies an apartness of beings and being from each other—separateness from and unrelatedness to each other (Inwood, 1999). We view and experience differently a common world and see the difference as some other "nature, form, or quality" (*Oxford English Dictionary*, 1999). The difference—the otherness—of other persons extends to communities sharing culture and their daily life and to all humanity (Husserl, 1973). Early in the cultural texture of Jacqui's story, we encounter disharmony when guiding assumptions and metaphors differ and remain implicit (Charmaz, 2000). While Jacqui and James are recoiling from newly birthed Jermaine's disfigurement and are immersed in metaphors of guilt and pollution (Douglas, 1979), physicians assume the metaphor of the objective world of facts, which is extended by the truth that their skill and tools frequently *do* help blind eyes see. It is presumed that patients and their parent surrogates share the same view of the world (Kirmayer, 1988, 1992). To Heidegger (1973), the *Differenz* of being and beings includes a resolution of such chasms of presumption and misapprehension, but they cannot be seen as alike without an a priori understanding of likeness. Biological fact and lived experience of difference lack such connecting. In society, whose very identity depends on a shared "normality," pronounced physical difference is not so much another way of being as it is a sign of negative being.

Issues around stigma appear immediately in Jacqui's story—always in social interaction—from being identified as flawed or spoiled (Goffman, 1963; Jones et al., 1984). Jacqui finds herself renegotiating life with her extended family and community and fending off the angst of not-being-at-home that creeps in with the sinister and unfamiliar (Heidegger, 1962). The gathering of history that is the culture they share has been dealt a heavy blow. Their world is tossed into the unknown, rendered homeless. "It is characteristic of cultural gestures to awaken in all others at least an echo if not consonance" (Merleau-Ponty as quoted in Levin, 1989, p. 271). With the introduction of baby Jermaine's tiny face into a critical corporeal world, dissonance screams liability; yesterday's communicative matrix is threatened with extinction. The family is accosted by callous insinuations that they have caused the aberration. Difference from others, norms, and peers becomes disability and takes on a master status, shaping entire worlds and conferring a devalued personal identity—"blind," "disabled," deviant, ugly rocker of the normal boat, and very, very vulnerable.

In inescapable everydayness, cultural representations of disabled people are reflected most excruciatingly in language (Albrecht & Verbrugge, 2000). Language is not merely spoken but reveals and shows the order of the world, the meaning of being (Heidegger, 1962, 1971). The faintest shadings of words and their tones can soothe or singe the stigmatized, often blaming them for the situation and then again for being stigmatized (Jackson, 1992). One becomes attuned to fear, guilt, and shame as they flood over other statuses and identities in disrupted lives. Language creates a prison into which every aspect of Jermaine and those who share his being and his world are cast and suffer new indignities. Jacqui and her family learn that they cannot escape discovering how others react to them. They question their very worth. They learn how hard it is, when you are feeling vulnerable, to let others know you are in pain. They also learn the power of nonjudgmental support and assertiveness, be they interpersonal, spiritual, or instrumental. Jacqui's story causes one to wonder how it is that people so often express compassion only through apology.

Visible disabilities elicit rude judgments upon their difference. We are social beings, and there is no hiding a craniofacial malformation. With stigma dramatizing difference, loss is magnified. The body as a fragile harmonium (Kleinman, 1995), unified and whole, is fragmented in the tension between difference and sameness, and difference extends to all of it. Music is a sentient metaphor for connecting and separating. Located in aesthetic configurations and therapeutic effectiveness, music ministers both to healing and to finding the self (Bock, 1994; Roseman, 1991). It is no accident that music is ubiquitous in traditional healing rituals (Ember & Ember, 2002; Reichard, 1963). But having found that Jermaine has the gift of music, Jacqui still faces a Faustian choice between her child's endowment and a more socially acceptable face.

Jacqui persists through a maze of explanations and false promises and moves beyond those, for in addition to thrownness and falling, the essentialness of being (in the sense of *Dasein* as Being-in-the-world [Heidegger, 1962]) is existence. And Jacqui determines to make her family's existence harmonious. She distances herself from the exhortation of medical technology by welcoming its tools without letting them determine what happens. Part of this releasement (Heidegger, 1993) comes from learning effective strategies for intervention, and part from learning to let go and let be. To do this, she clasps her faith, for "letting go and letting God" is not an easy choice in a world bound with scientific pragmatism. Jacqui garners strength to nurture knowing and caring and to reject the brashness of objectification. She *wills* the conversations to converge.

Although the disability rights movement has made significant positive changes in recent decades, responsibility for creating and reconstructing identities remains with its proponents (Charmaz, 1995). There are risks in telling the story and drawing attention to the situation. Extroverted Jacqui is more comfortable with this than James, whose solid presence, his being there, is more reticent. Situatedness always includes demographics, such as race and ethnicity, which can further encumber the already burdensome disability experience. Even Jacqui's confidence alludes to awareness of such reality when she is surprised by a woman she considers economically and prestigiously advantaged being content to hold and rock the "Black, blind child" she loves so, for it cannot be forgotten that either attribute can make him potentially less lovable to others. Indeed, part of the beauty of Jacqui's story is in its sheer demolition of old stereotypes. This is a woman who teaches her children classical music from infancy, who thrives in the bosom of kinship, and who still claims to resort to ghetto thinking for survival tactics when the chips are down.

Unconcealment of being happens only when and where "there is hermeneutical opening, a clearing silence, a field of tonality laid out for the disclosure" (Levin, 1989, p. 244). Jacqui's Being resonates in her faith and her family. Her faith involves rebirthing, an existential overcoming and transcending that leads to an understanding of being that need neither be grounded in God nor present-at-hand in mankind to be significant and meaningful. Faith may be seen, as Heidegger saw it, as in between, inasmuch as people need gods or God, and those become as real as anything else projected (Heidegger, 1969, 1973, 1976).

In Jacqui's story, while all but visibly present, James, Jamaal, and Jermaine are themselves little heard from. On the other hand, saying little and having greater tolerance for letting things be do not imply greatly differing worldviews. Likely they are comfortable having Jacqui tell her story her way. "In our personal myths home is the place where we are fully accepted, it is linked with the idea of a woman, mother" (New & David, 1985, p. 54). To Jacqui, giving Jermaine his eye drops and ointment was her job: "That is what mothers do."

Jacqui's gentle allusion to the matrifocality of many African American families (McAdoo, 1988; Stack, 1970; Whitten & Szwed, 1970) as a fact of life and in her relationship with her own mother is also the first and focal point of her turning, the sparking of her spirit to take on immeasurable new challenges.

Jacqui's are not the same issues of oppression as those of other heroines— Pauli Murray comes to mind, with her determination to banish the discrimination she endured as a symbolic "Jane Crow," Black and female (Hartmann, 2002; Murray, 1987; Rosenberg, 2002). But Murray, too, wrote autobiographically (Murray, 1989) and refused to disappear beneath a landslide of rejection and seemingly insurmountable obstacles. In Hegel's philosophy of history, the meaning of ability to exercise human potential in individual action is supplanted by deeper meanings for the whole culture (Rosenberg, 1995), in Jacqui's case the cultures of blindness and disability. If the personal story symbolizes "an existential struggle for honesty and expansion in an uncertain world" (Ellis & Bochner, 2000, p. 749), Jacqui's writing is a powerful symbol of hope. Like music, symbols heal. And much of healing is at the margins, which also serve as points of engagement and unfinished places of social suffering (Kleinman, 1995) in which lived experience is the "breathing of meaning" (Van Manen, 1990, p. 36). Jacqui's story is not over, and it is powerful in its promise.

In "These Are the Children We Hold Dear," the reader experiences a struggle for meaning in the connecting text of family. As a storyteller, Jacqui invites us to live the experience as she lays bare autobiographic layers of the real-life dialectical deviltry of hard realities and raw emotions, faith and doubt, self-consciousness and the pressures of interaction, embodiment and the shaping of tenuous human potential. The story is made so accessible that the truths indeed become inescapable: "we are nowhere but in the present" (Behar, 1996, p. 176), and what matters is what we make of that.

References

Albrecht, G. L., & Verbrugge, L. M. (2000). The global emergence of disability. In G. L. Albrecht, R. Fitzpatrick, & S. C. Scrimshaw (Eds.), *Handbook of social studies in health and medicine* (pp. 293–307). Thousand Oaks, CA: Sage.

Banner, L. W. (1983). *American beauty.* Chicago: University of Chicago Press.

Becker, H. S. (1992). The methodology of a writing observed. In P. T. Clough, *The end(s) of ethnography: From realism to social criticism* (pp. 62–79). Newbury Park, CA: Sage.

Behar, R. (1996). *The vulnerable observer: Anthropology that breaks your heart.* Boston: Beacon Press.

Ben-Ari, A. T. (1995). It's the telling that makes the difference. In R. Josselson & A. Lieblich (Eds.), *Interpreting experience: The narrative study of lives* (pp. 153–172). Thousand Oaks, CA: Sage.

Benhabib, S. (1986). *Critique, norm and utopia: A study of the foundations of critical theory*. New York: Columbia University Press.

Bock, P. K. (Ed.). (1994). *Psychological anthropology*. Westport, CT: Praeger.

Brandes, S. (1982). Ethnographic autobiographies in American anthropology. In E. A. Hoebel, R. Currier, & S. Kaiser (Eds.), *Crisis in anthropology: View from Spring Hill, 1980* (pp. 187–202). New York: Garland.

Brody, H. (1987). *Stories of sickness*. New Haven, CT: Yale University Press.

Cesara, M. (1982). *Reflections of a woman anthropologist: No hiding place*. London: Academic Press.

Charmaz, K. (1995). The body, identity, and self: Adapting to impairment. *Sociological Quarterly, 36*, 657–680.

Charmaz, K. (2000). Experiencing chronic illness. In G. L. Albrecht, R. Fitzpatrick, & S. C. Scrimshaw (Eds.), *Handbook of social studies in health and medicine* (pp. 277–292). Thousands Oaks, CA: Sage.

Chávez, R. C., & O'Donnell, J. (1998). *Speaking the unpleasant: The politics of (non)engagement in the multicultural education terrain*. Albany: State University of New York Press.

Childress, H. (1998). Kinder ethnographic writing. *Qualitative Inquiry, 4*(2), 249–264.

Clampitt, A. (1999). *The collected poems of Amy Clampitt*. New York: Alfred A. Knopf.

Crawford, L. (1996). Personal ethnography. *Communication Monographs, 63*, 158–170.

Denzin, N. (1989). *Interpretive biography*. Newbury Park, CA: Sage.

Denzin, N. (1994). The art and politics of interpretation. In N. K. Denzin and Y. S. Lincoln (Eds.), *Handbook of qualitative research* (1st ed., pp. 500–515). Thousand Oaks, CA: Sage.

Douglas, M. (1979). *Purity and danger: An analysis of concepts of pollution and taboo*. London: Routledge & Kegan Paul.

Ellis, C., & Bochner, A. P. (2000). Autoethnography, personal narrative, reflexivity: Researcher as subject. In N. K. Denzin and Y. S. Lincoln (Eds.), *Handbook of qualitative research* (2nd ed., pp. 733–768). Thousand Oaks, CA: Sage.

Ember, C. R., & Ember, M. (2002). *Cultural anthropology* (10th ed.). Upper Saddle River, NJ: Prentice Hall.

Etter-Lewis, G. (1991). Black women's life stories: Reclaiming life in narrative texts. In S. B. Gluck & D. Patai (Eds.), *Women's words: The feminist practice of oral history*. New York: Routledge.

Fink, E., & Heidegger, M. (1979). *Heraclitus Seminar, 1966–1967*. University, AL: University of Alabama Press.

Frank, G. (2000). *Venus on wheels: Two decades of dialogue on disability, biography, and being female in America*. Berkeley: University of California Press.

Gadamer, H-G. (1996).*The enigma of health: The art of healing in a scientific age* (J. Gaiger & N. Walker, Trans.). Stanford, CA: Stanford University Press.

Goffman, E. (1963). *Stigma*. Englewood Cliffs, NJ: Prentice Hall.

Hankiss, A. (1981). Ontologies on the self: On the mythological rearranging of one's life history. In D. Bertaux (Ed.), *Biography and society: The life history approach in the social sciences* (pp. 203–210). Beverly Hills, CA: Sage.

Harris, L., et al. (1986). *The ICD survey of disabled Americans: Bringing disabled Americans into the mainstream*. Conducted for the International Center for the Disabled and the National Council on the Handicapped. New York: Louis Harris.

Hartmann, S. M. (2002). Pauli Murray and the "Juncture of women's liberation and black liberation." *Journal of Women's History, 14*(2), 74–77.

Heidegger, M. (1962). *Being and time* (J. Macquarrie & E. Robinson, Trans.). Oxford, UK: Blackwell.

Heidegger, M. (1969). *Identity and difference.* (J. Stambaugh, Trans.). New York: Harper & Row.

Heidegger, M. (1971). *On the way to language.* (P. D. Hertz, Trans.). New York: Harper & Row.

Heidegger, M. (1973). *The end of philosophy.* (J. Stambaugh, Trans.). New York: Harper & Row.

Heidegger, M. (1976). *The piety of thinking.* (J. G. Hart & J. C. Maraldo, Trans.). Bloomington: Indiana University Press.

Heidegger, M. (1982). *The basic problems of phenomenology* (A. Hofstadter, Trans.). Bloomington: University of Indiana Press.

Heidegger, M. (1993). *Basic writings: From Being and time (1927) to The task of thinking (1964)* (D. F. Krell, Ed.; 2nd ed.) London: Routledge.

Heidegger, M. (1999). *Contributions to philosophy (from enowning)* (P. Emad & K. Maly, Trans.). Bloomington: Indiana University Press.

Hones, D. F. (1998). Known in part: The transformational power of narrative inquiry. *Qualitative Inquiry, 4*(2), 225–248.

Hurston, Z. N. (1978). *Their eyes were watching God.* Urbana: University of Illinois Press.

Husserl, E. (1973). *Cartesian meditations: An introduction to phenomenology* (D. Cairns, Trans.). The Hague, The Netherlands: Martinus Nijhoff.

Inwood, M. (1999). *A Heidegger dictionary.* Oxford, UK: Blackwell.

Jackson, J. E. (1992). "After a while no one believes you": Real and unreal pain. In M. J. D. Good, P. E. Brodwin, B. J. Good, & A. Kleinman (Eds.), *Pain as a human experience: An anthropological perspective* (pp. 138–168). Berkeley: University of California Press.

Jago, B. (1996). Postcards, ghosts, and fathers: Revising family stories. *Qualitative Inquiry 2*(4), 495–516.

Jones, E. E., Farina, A., Hastrof, A., Markus, H., Miller, D. T., & Scott, R. A. (1984). *Social stigma: The psychology of marked relationships.* New York: W. H. Freeman.

Josselson, R. (1995). Imagining the real: Empathy, narrative, and the dialogic self. In R. Josselson & A. Lieblich (Eds.), *Interpreting experience: The narrative study of lives* (pp. 27–44). Thousand Oaks, CA: Sage.

Jourard, S. M. (1971). *The transparent self.* New York: Van Nostrand Reinhold.

Kess-Gardner, J. (2002). *The incredible journey.* Baltimore: Incredible Journey Productions.

Kirmayer, L. (1988). Mind and body as metaphors. In M. Lock & D. Gordon (Eds.), *Biomedicine examined* (pp. 57–94). Dordrecht, The Netherlands: Kluwer.

Kirmayer, L. (1992). The body's insistence on meaning: Metaphor as presentation and representation in illness experience. *Medical Anthropological Quarterly, 6,* 323–346.

Kleinman, A. (1995). *Writing at the margin: Discourse between anthropology and medicine.* Berkeley: University of California Press.

Kolker, A. (1996). Thrown overboard: The human costs of health care rationing. In C. Ellis & A. P. Bochner (Eds.), *Composing ethnography: Alternative forms of qualitative writing* (pp. 132–159). Walnut Creek, CA: AltaMira.

Krieger, S. (1991). *Social science and the self: Personal essays on an art form.* New Brunswick, NJ: Rutgers University Press.

Laing, R. (1968). *The politics of experience.* New York: Ballantine Books.

Levin, D. M. (1989). *The listening self: Personal growth, social change and the closure of metaphysics.* London: Routledge.

Linde, C. (1993). *Life stories: The creation of coherence.* New York: Oxford University Press.

Macgregor, F. C. (1979). *After plastic surgery: Adaptation and adjustment.* New York: Praeger.

Malinowski, B. (1967). *A diary in the strict sense of the term* (N. Guterman, Trans.). New York: Harcourt, Brace & World.

McAdoo, H. P. (Ed.). (1988). *Black families* (2nd ed.). Newbury Park, CA: Sage.

Merleau-Ponty, M. (1962). *Phenomenology of perception.* London: Routledge & Kegan Paul.

Morrison, T. (1992). Rememory and writing. In P. T. Clough, *The end(s) of ethnography: From realism to social criticism* (pp. 113–130). Newbury Park, CA: Sage.

Murray, P. (1987). *Song in a weary throat: An American pilgrimage.* New York: Harper & Row.

Murray, P. (1989). *Pauli Murray: The autobiography of a black activist, feminist, lawyer, priest, and poet.* Knoxville: University of Tennessee Press.

New, C., & David, M. (1985). *For the children's sake: Making childcare more than women's business.* Harmondsworth, UK: Penguin.

Oxford English Dictionary. (1999). 2nd ed., CD-ROM Version 2.0. Oxford, UK: Oxford University Press.

Polkinghorne, D. (1983). *Methodology for the human sciences: Systems of inquiry.* Albany: State University of New York Press.

Reed-Danahay, D. (1997). *Autoethnography: Rewriting the self and the social.* Oxford, UK: Berg.

Reichard, G. A. (1963). *Navajo religion: A study of symbolism.* Princeton, NJ: Princeton University Press.

Reinharz, S. (1992). *Feminist methods in social research.* New York: Oxford University Press.

Richardson, L. (1994). Writing: A method of inquiry. In N. K. Denzin & Y. S. Lincoln (Eds.), *Handbook of qualitative research* (1st ed., pp. 516–529). Thousand Oaks, CA: Sage.

Ronai, C. R. (1995). Multiple reflections of child sex abuse: An argument for a layered account. *Journal of Contemporary Ethnography, 23,* 395–426.

Roseman, M. (1991). *Healing sounds from the Malaysian rainforest: Temiar music and medicine.* Berkeley: University of California Press.

Rosenberg, A. (1995). *Philosophy of social science* (2nd ed.). Boulder, CO: Westview.

Rosenberg, R. (2002). The conjunction of race and gender. *Journal of Women's History, 14*(2), 68–73.

St. Pierre, E. A. (1997). Circling the text: Nomadic writing practices. *Qualitative Inquiry, 3*(4), 403–417.

Shibayama, Z. (1974). *Zen comments on the Mumonkan.* New York: New American Library.

Stack, C. B. (1970). *All our kin: Strategies for survival in a black community.* New York: Harper & Row.

Stuhlmiller, C. M., & Thorsen, R. (1997). Narrative picturing: A new strategy for qualitative data collection. *Qualitative Health Research, 7*(1), 140–149.

Tedlock, B. (1991). From participant observation to the observation of participation: The emergence of narrative ethnography. *Journal of Anthropological Research, 41*, 69–94.

Tedlock, B. (2000). Ethnography and ethnographic representation. In N. K. Denzin and Y. S. Lincoln (Eds.), *Handbook of qualitative research* (2nd ed., pp. 455–486). Thousand Oaks, CA: Sage.

Tillman-Healy, L. (1996). A secret life in a culture of thinness: Reflections on body, food, and bulimia. In C. Ellis & A. P. Bochner (Eds.), *Composing ethnography: Alternative forms of qualitative writing* (pp. 76–108). Walnut Creek, CA: AltaMira.

Van Maanen, J. (1988). *Tales of the field: On writing ethnography.* Chicago: University of Chicago Press.

Van Manen, M. (1990). *Researching lived experience: Human science for an action sensitive pedagogy.* Albany: State University of New York.

Whitten, N. E., Jr., & Szwed, J. F. (Eds.). (1970). *Afro-American anthropology: Contemporary perspectives.* New York: Free Press.

Yamada, K. (1997). Life's little reminders (Bookmark). Edmonds, WA: Compendium.

3

Personal Dialogue
on Connecting Caring
A Journey

Joanna Basuray

Introduction

This is the story of a life. I am grateful to feminism's bringing autobiography together with reflexive anthropology (Behar, 1996; Richardson, 1997) for the permission it gives me to tell my story as I have lived and am living it. As a personal narrative, my story is autoethnographic and reflexive (Ellis & Bochner, 2000). It illuminates caring and culture as those have shaped and continue to shape me, my learning and my knowing, and my world. Writing both separates me from my lifeworld and what I know, and unites me more closely with that lifeworld and what I know (Van Manen, 1990). While autoethnography implies systematic sociological introspection as I connect the personal to the cultural (Clough, 1997; Ellis, 1991), reflexivity encourages the story of my cultural self to return to deeper examination of interactions between myself and others (Ellis & Bochner, 2000). Caring, in our own cultural contexts, emerges through personal images from our life experiences (Atkinson, 1995).

Folded into this complex interpretation is an ethnographic study of caring and the teaching of caring that serves to link my personal and professional selves. Together these reflect my life experiences within the interwoven caring and cultural context of my understanding of the universe. At the simplest level, this is a study of a human living and communicating among humans (Bateson, 1990). As such, I am always within that which I study, weaving my ideas through language and writing. At more complex levels, each of us is more subtly fashioned and formed by culture and by caring—each a little differently while sharing much of who we are. As do others who practice this self-examination, I ask who I am. I find myself freer to explore issues around caring and culture without the frameworks and dissecting processes that prevail in the traditional academic epistemological and ontological work of health disciplines. It is not that those are unworthy guides, but they lack the fluidity of my life as I live it. I prefer to relate what I trust is an evocative personal narrative (Bochner, Ellis, & Tillmann-Healy, 1997, 1998), one with expressive and dialogic goals. Because autoethnography involves more reflecting by the participant than traditional ethnography's participant observation (Tedlock, 1991), one hopes it might even cause a "stirring in our souls" (Chladenius, 1994, p. 56).

Being autoethnographic, this account of my personal journey is not a text built of evidence marshaled in some additive manner, although I like to think it could be persuasive (Atkinson, 1990). My storytelling refuses to abstract or explain as it prioritizes rhetorical induction (Edmondson, 1984) over any illusions of scientific mastery. Instead of control and goals, I emphasize the journey over the destination and dramatize the motion of relational experiences over time. The story is neither theorized nor settled. Since I am writing for a reader who is also most likely a professional, it is framed within the dimension of those whose business is to support healing.

When approaching research and scholarship, interpretive styles of inquiry assist ably in understanding intangibles of human lives and the expression of human beliefs in cultural landscapes. This is a burdensome endeavor because what gets left out is due either to conscious choice or demonstrates my limits of understanding who I am. But my goal is to share so that the reader will understand my personal life experiences through my lenses—with all their individual tints and cultural facets. A storied life seeks to keep the past alive in the present (Ellis & Bochner, 2000), however incomplete and revisable it might be. I want to use my understandings of the interactions and experiences I've had, but I also want to place historical facts into their appropriate contexts. Autoethnography works for me, displaying as it does multiple layers of consciousness and connecting the personal to the cultural (Hayano, 1979).

Narrative is about living. Layers of writing relay "concrete action, dialogue, emotion, embodiment, spirituality, and self-consciousness"

(Ellis & Bochner, 2000, p. 739) that dialectically reveal the self in relation to history, society, and culture. Ethnography takes that to the textual construction of reality (Atkinson, 1990). This ethnographic enterprise focuses on the dual identity of my reality: I am researcher and subject, public academic and private person, scholar and professional. Although many feminist writers advocate starting inquiry with the self (e.g., Smith, 1979), I realize that my story is neither fully feminist nor traditional, but both. Likewise, it is neither clearly historical nor reflexive, but both. I am a person of the First and Third Worlds. I am all of those, and with our being always more complex than the models would have us, I illuminate caring and culture in all those ways.

As in the image created by a welcoming foyer in a garden or a home, I can say that human caring is easier to find if we open ourselves to understanding others. Openness for me, at times, is analogous to one becoming conscious of one's own breath during spiritual meditation. The universality of caring is ever present when we see the life forces within us, as if we were whole with the universe. The thirteenth-century Sufi philosopher and poet Jelaluddin Rumi believed not only that we are a particle of the whole universe but also that the universe resides in us (Helminski, 1995; Moyne, 1984). I share his sense of humans as caring because we are part of the interdependence of nature and of each other.

I am dust particles in sunlight
I am the round sun

I am morning mist
and the breathing of evening
I am wind in the top of a grove,
and surf on the cliff.

I am a tree with a trained parrot in its branches.
Silence, thought, and voice.

Both candle and the moth
crazy around it.
Rose and the nightingale
lost in the fragrance.
I am all orders of being,
the circling galaxy,

the evolutionary intelligence,
the light and the falling away.
What is and what isn't. You
who know Jelaluddin, you
the One in all, say who I am.
Say I am you. (as cited in Barks & Green, 1997, p.108)

I am a naturalized citizen, a mother of two grown children, and I have had a full professional life as a university professor for the past twenty years. In addition to conventional nursing courses, I teach, present, and write about transcultural healthcare. I also direct my university's Multicultural Institute for faculty development. Thus, caring and culture in health and healthcare and community service have intermingled—personal and professional; past, present, and future; simple and complex—in scripting my life. New meanings of this fusion of caring and culture continually surface. I begin my autoethnography by exploring my cultural background.

I was born to parents in the subcontinent of Pakistan and India. I grew up in postcolonial, partitioned India, in Pakistan, immigrating with my family to the United States during my high school years. My parents represented different geographical and cultural orientations in northern India and Afghanistan. Both from Sayeed Muslim families, they were converted as young adults to Christianity, which implied for my family some integration of Eastern and Western cultures. Thus, already the authenticity of my own voice comes from a dichotomous position. I learned the culture of my family, home, and community, and I learned Western thought through my upper-class education and female socialization, in which the West was idealized in ambivalent naïveté. In my adult education and experience in nursing, and as an immigrant and naturalized citizen, I share my concerns founded in the postcolonial subcontinent with those who encounter entrenched oppression in the nursing profession and elsewhere in society.

In the insidious confusion of traditionalism and colonialism and of Western culture being wedded to Christianity, my family adopted and adapted cultural values and social norms rooted in all those sources. At the core of my reflection I find layers of hegemonic notes of cultural inhibition, suppression, and oppression—"Homo hierarchicus" (Quigley, 1997) with all of that genre's overt and subtle implications. When we identify differences, when we question whether to maintain differences or seek assimilation, when we distinguish the *us*, *them*, and *other*, we cannot help but collide with hegemony. We often do not recognize it, for it becomes accepted as the natural state of things while we debate about minimizing or maximizing disparity. Should we try to erase the lines of difference or celebrate diversity? At what level do we recognize our sameness?

When I teach about multiculturalism, my goal is to recognize differences and make them explicit. I believe those differences exist and are significant and meaningful. Rather than minimize them, I want to know how to deal with them in ways that are not negative. Traits such as ethnicity exist in people and, for all their adaptability and flexibility, are fairly nonnegotiable from the outside. Change may be an ideal, but one has to change from the inside. People do change, for example, in their lifestyles and religious orientations. As an adult in the United States I have observed numerous Christian- or Jewish-born individuals adopt Zen Buddhist lives or Sufism, often with the convert's intense conviction. Some of these converts provide spiritual leadership in the Eastern religions. Change happens. It is wonderful, as can be a stable, unchanging identity. Either can also demand a high toll as we merge with identities born of the varied philosophies around us and evolve into new identities. I might choose to do things very differently while respecting others' choices. It is a giving from the heart that is the basis for culturally sensitive behavior.

Dialectical Roots

Before I was born, the story of my life came together in the form of British and European colonialism and, specifically, oppression and missionary activities. Try to imagine how peoples longing for a sense of equality feel about the promises of Christianity. At the same time missionaries empowered people through literacy, the colonial government suppressed them by maintaining ignorance. The missionaries' activities were in large part separate from those of the government, which merely tolerated them as fellow interlopers in a foreign land (Moorhouse, 1973). Meanwhile, the two ideologies work toward different ends. This type of oppressive phenomenon is best understood through Freire's (1995) description of "cultural invasion" in which "the invaders penetrate the cultural context of another group in disrespect of the latter's potentialities; they impose their own view of the world upon those they invade and inhibit the creativity of the invaded by curbing their expression" (p. 133). That is what happened during British colonization of the Indian subcontinent (Basuray, 1997). But there are always many sides to any story. It is similar to my parents telling their stories to witness for their religion—along with the religious agenda came a rich understanding of lives situated very differently.

The opportunities that missionaries offered appealed to the lower classes of people. The masses were sects that were subsumed under Islam. The lowest castes of Hindus were also desirable targets for conversion (Moorhouse, 1973; Watson, 1982). Missionary promises of Christian brotherhood and heavenly equality were very attractive. Fairness and equality elude peoples within a caste system and can be extremely persuasive, although Muslims were generally more resistant than others to conversion (Basuray, 1997). The missionaries celebrated every Muslim conversion to Christianity.

Having known some of the British and Danish missionaries personally, I am fascinated by their drive and initiative. They seemed to live a dual life away from their countries of origin. They were somehow well prepared for these mission journeys before leaving their homes. Then they ascertained the strength of their beliefs and tested their readiness to survive in a very different environment (Moorhouse, 1992). Once in their mission fields, they were able to adapt and work in ways that involved proselytizing within a complex diplomatic framework. The illiterate natives more likely presumed the missionaries' presence in India was an extension of the British Raj (rule) (Metcalf, 1995; Stokes, 1959)—a helpful but still British version—rather than that of a group from Europe that was undoing the benign neglect that the Raj practiced on the natives' healthcare, economy, and education (Basuray, 1997; Chatterjee, 1993; Hirschmann, 1987; Singha, 1998; Watson, 1985). The missionaries worked in outposts of provinces and cities where the tribal people adhered rigidly to their prescribed principles and moral codes of daily life and work. Traditional roles of family members and community fit the religious beliefs and topography (Mani, 1990; Sen, 2002). People believed in basic survival for themselves, their families, and fellow tribespeople, so offered themselves as honored hosts of invited guests. Overall, intolerance was rife (Miller, 1977).

My mother is a Pathan, born in 1922 in the mountains of Afghanistan. Her mother, my grandmother, died when my mother was very young. As a child, my mother traveled to the valleys of India with her uncle, who traded and took her along on his business trip to an area called Mardan in the northwest frontier province (see Miller, 1977, and Moorhouse, 1992, for more on the area). She lived with her relatives there but fell so severely ill during a smallpox epidemic that her uncle took her to a Danish Lutheran mission hospital in the outpost. The family and local hakims (healers) had tried everything else, and my mother was near death. At the mission, she was fed milk soaked in cotton balls and squeezed into her mouth. It took a long time for her to recover. Her uncle came now and then to check on her, but he was struggling and was often absent from the area, so the missionaries kept her. My mother was happy and content in the missionary living quarters. Assured that she was being lovingly kept, her uncle told the missionaries not to give her to any of the relatives who might come and ask for her. They kept that promise, but eventually he stopped coming. My mother did not know the reason for his disappearance but suspected that he died.

Since she did not have parents, my mother was kept at the missionary compound as an orphan. Others from the extended family knew where she was and that the missionaries were teaching her when she was old enough to go to school. Unlike some, these missionaries only cautiously imposed their religion and their language on those in their care. They schooled my mother in both her indigenous language and in English, preparing her as they did other girls to enter vocational programs such as nursing. All of the missionary-sponsored programs were conducted in English as many of the trained nurses went to work in hospitals that cared for the civil servants of England, for India was a British colony at the time (Basuray, 1997). There were European missionaries all over the subcontinent, most of them from England, Ireland, Denmark, Holland, France, and Portugal. As a Sayeed, my mother did not come from a particularly fundamentalist background, although her tribe was very traditional—in sum, it was rigid without being at all fanatic. Her people were largely illiterate, and the tribe followed Islam with a simple faith (Miller, 1977; Moorehouse, 1992).

While the missionaries rather gently conveyed Christianity in the Danish Lutheran compound, the gardeners, servants, and other workers from the region taught my mother to be Muslim. She learned much of Islam through the local people while participating in the educational and other services provided to local people by the missionary group. But eventually she converted to Christianity and was adopted by the residing Lutheran bishop. It was commendable that, since arranged marriages were the norm in the region and culture, the missionaries tried hard to accommodate their young charges by making nuptial arrangements that were unlike their own. My mother's choice of a husband was influenced by living with Hindu neighbors and by her socialization to Hindus during her nursing education in Delhi.

Meanwhile, many miles away in Agra, India, not far from New Delhi, my father was being converted. He was part of a very large family of land-owning farmers. His father did well and was also a hakim who could cure people. My father was one of the younger children in the family, and after his mother died, a stepmother and an older sister raised him. One of his older brothers left the village and went into town, where he studied for a trade with which he eventually worked for the missionaries on consignment. These were Anglican British missionaries. The missionary principal at the school liked my uncle and encouraged him to send my father for schooling. My father was a creative and rebellious student who, as a teenage Muslim aware of the conflict in which he now lived, became a Christian due to the acceptance and love he experienced at the school. I've always felt that his decision as a young man was very different from that of my mother, who was essentially raised by missionaries and had no close family to go back to. My father had the choice. Many of his older brothers were mullahs (priests) and landowning farmers, and the family was quite traditional. When my father went back home and preached to his family, he was advised by an older brother that, since his action of witnessing his devotion to Christ was blasphemous in the eyes of Islam, my father was now considered a heathen and could be killed. Cast out of his family, my father was taken in by the missionaries, who furthered his education. He became a nurse and, later, a teacher and administrator. In 1965, he was sent to England for training to learn surgical procedures on eyes, as severe eye infections are prevalent in northern India. He began to work as a physician, as a medical intern might do here. He learned both Indian and European classical music. He loved music and played music at home, church, and social gatherings.

My parents got to know individuals who were European government civil servants. These friendships and associations changed my family's lives. In this merging of church and state, my parents became models of Muslim conversion. When I was growing up, this was a novelty, and other converts came to be our guests through the missionaries' networking. We were shown respect, were socialized at parties, and were introduced to European, American, and British guests of the mission hospital and residential compound. We lived in a bungalow alongside those of the missionaries.

My parents were independent; they could say to the missionaries, "I don't need you to feed me; I can do this by myself." Their independence was admired by their closest missionary friends and resented by many others. This was especially true for my mother, who was raised by missionaries from early childhood. In contrast, my parents raised my four siblings and me in a nuclear family separate from both the traditional extended family and the missionaries. They protected us, took care of us, and sent us to private European day schools. They viewed progress for the family as attainable through Western education. It worked out, but they often struggled because of the differences between their indigenous cultures and their new Europeanized Indian social and cultural groups.

In marriage, although my father encouraged my mother to continue to practice nursing, there was also conflict, for he took it upon himself to determine her role as wife, mother, and professional. Although they shared a commitment to education, my parents did not agree on how their marital relationship should work. My mother, strong and individualistic as women tend to be from her tribe, was not about to be second fiddle in the partnership. There was no suppressing her, but she speaks yet of her struggle with the need to leave her children at home for months when professional growth opportunities were offered to her. Yet, she held her own private practice in a clinic in the heart of the city of Peshawar. There she delivered over three thousand babies during her career, managed her practice autonomously, and commuted alone from home. Compared with other women in that time and place, she demanded space and rejected some traits associated with patriarchal North Indian males. Furthermore, she shielded her children from many traditional Eastern ideas and beliefs because they did not fit with what was Christian and Western in her eyes. Note that to my mother, Christianity was Western, not Middle-Eastern. I saw her vacillate sometimes between the two worlds in her choices and adaptation to Western culture.

But most of all, my mother wanted respect as a female. She knew that it was possible. I saw her determination to hold on to her dignity as a respected human being despite her female self. My mother gave us a will and determination to cope that was rooted in her tribal background. The missionaries gave her choices, and she took them. They never tried to give her a European or Christian name, which they routinely did with most of their converts. Leaving her name intact was actually intended to show off her Muslim lineage. Later, after marriage, she took my father's "Muslim" surname.

Meanwhile, in my father I saw a deep appreciation for Western education, which he displayed through his numerous talents and significant intelligence. He was, at the same time, deeply respectful of his Indian heritage, which remained with him always. The missionaries were excited about bringing together these young people of Muslim background. One wonders if they realized how different my parents' cultural origins really were—or perhaps they did, and they knew that Westernization and Christianity were most of what my parents shared.

Connecting Schooling, Culture, and Profession

My professional involvement with diversity was conceived consciously but idealistically. As an undergraduate student in Oklahoma, I began learning, personally and professionally, about cultural congruence in nursing care of clients. In the mid-1970s, there was no formalized focus on the study of multiculturalism in healthcare where I was. I approached multiculturalism with a high level of personal sensitivity, but I was aware of it being limited to my own experience, which was greatly different from the experiences of many around me. Needing to develop more knowledge and my own relationship with multicultural concepts, I engaged in numerous continuing education workshops related to diversity. I leapt forward in my journey toward understanding myself in graduate school. My children were very young at the time, and I sought answers to many questions. Along with intensification of my role as an educator at home and at school came divergent exposures to and inquiries about feminist theories, the nature of oppression, and modes of spiritual journeys. In addition to pediatric nursing, I began teaching transcultural healthcare at the university.

With increasing numbers of immigrants working in the United States since the late 1970s, many of them in the health professions, I empathized with the tremendous challenges experienced by those arriving from postcolonial regions of Asia, Africa, and Central and South America. These barriers were most obvious in educational programs and in gaining license to practice. Five years in Oklahoma and ten in North Dakota taught me about the dynamics of oppression of indigenous peoples, as well as of new immigrants. Early in my journey, I was intrigued by, and found myself wholly sympathizing with, the history and contemporary status of Native Americans. But at that time, I was still *othering* others; it is a phase that I later understood to be essential to my self-knowledge, since I was invisible to my self.

I saw teaching and learning about diversity as a process of unselfconsciously collecting the cultural histories and sociopolitical–religious events of a person's life. Gradually, both my authentic self and my professional posture became rooted in a set of ideologies and then upon a framework for articulating ideas. That led to writing and publishing about colonial oppression and its effect on nursing education in India, and to a dissertation about meanings of caring in the culture of nursing. Most importantly, as paths opened before me, I found myself always selecting, regardless of what other choices might exist, diversity—human diversity both literal and figurative, but always a diversity-related or multicultural topic, approach, or agenda. I developed and have taught a transcultural healthcare course since the mid-1980s. I was amazed as the course became first an anchor point in nursing and then in the general education curriculum throughout the university. This was a fortunate turn of events; many disciplines and universities leave similar courses as electives or special topics courses—with multiculturalism and cultural sensitivity remaining marginalized from the overall curriculum. Teaching and learning in my course allowed me to center myself in deeper self-awareness of who I am and why it is that I am involved in diversity work. I presented papers, led workshops, and gave keynote speeches addressing diversity in healthcare and educational settings and in community organizations. For example, I served as a county human relations commissioner, as a board member of a Catholic church's immigration outreach service. I am entrusted with direction of our campus multicultural institute. I value each of these opportunities to communicate to others the convictions that I hold deeply.

My personal and professional growth contributes significantly to what and how I teach and learn. My first three-credit transcultural nursing course was wrought with anxiety; I felt I was a novice on the subject, despite my experience, my preparation, and the support I received from colleagues. Yet how I teach it today actually increasingly reflects my own persona and growth as a human being. What I have learned—and continuously learn—from both students and colleagues is that diversity is infinitely broad and complex. As individual teachers, we cannot provide a picture that is adequately humanistic and realistic to prepare anyone for diversity-sensitive caring. It is willingness to learn from everyone—the more diverse they are the better—that is crucial to becoming aware of and sensitive to varied perspectives. I discover relevance in those countless perspectives every day, which makes the topic exhilarating for me. I now discuss race, gender, and class with ease in my course. Such controversial topics were originally gently infused via a "back-door" approach, as my activist friends call it. Becoming familiar with a women's studies orientation and studying feminist literature and theory exposed me to more overt, up-front approaches to classism and oppression. This experience was intense and focused, and now I— hardly an in-your-face kind of person—am able to manage the complex nature of the discourse with comfort.

Buber, "Us and Them," Othering, and Gaining Confidence

In my understanding, Buber (1965) made humanism part of the relationship between teachers and students. According to Buber, verbal or nonverbal communication entails mutual dignity and respect for the other in a relationship known as *dialogue*. Individuals in dialogue each possess a personal world, a subjective domain of self. Caring, although not mentioned as such in Buber's writing, is implied in the recognition of the "other" in dialogue as an "I/Thou" relationship in which the element of mutuality and reciprocity is essential. In the "I/Thou" relationship, there is an assumption that "each of the participants really has in mind the other or others in their present and particular being and turns to them with the intention of establishing a living relation" (p. 19). The caring process involves the self as distinguished from the other, and empathy is experienced through shared feelings, knowledge, and aspirations. Giving one's self through one's presence is crucial in the dialogue. Therefore, for Buber, experiencing the relationship, rather than the outcome of the dialogue, is significant. One becomes conscious of this process in teaching and in intercultural health and care.

Buber pointed out that when the relationship is not "I/Thou" but "I/It," the dialogue form becomes Subject-to-Object. A student, for example, may be viewed as the object, to be manipulated or used by the teacher and the educational system. The student is objectified as a number in the class, and individual learning needs or aspirations are ignored. In an interpersonal relationship of "I/It," the "I" is conceived as caring for one's self in relation to one's relationship with others, whereas in the "I/Thou" relationship there is a mutual growth through the dialogue between self and other. Through the reciprocal subjectivity in "I/Thou" one sees openness, characterized by persons connecting with one another in a caring, concerned, and reflective manner. Caring seems inherent in the subjective domain of the relationship and is displayed in the realm between "I" and "Thou." Buber (1965) described this exchange as a between that yields to an openness in which the teacher shows concern for the student and shares a reflective human exchange. Through a dialogical process one reaches a spiritual realm wherein one attains a desirable situation in education. Caring then is grounded in the concrete reality of humanity: "With all deference to the world continuum of space and time I know as a living truth only concrete world reality which is constantly, in every moment, reached out to me" (p. 17). The dialogue is without boundary or limits and includes the past, present, and future, occurring in a concrete world.

Experience is the intersubjective medium in social transactions, situated as it is in local moral worlds (Kleinman, 1995). In using Buber's work in nursing education, I find it important that I encounter students in many different teaching-learning situations, dialogue about their experiences, and let the dialogue become valuable for the personal development and educational progress of the student. Nursing students face innumerable forms of human suffering and joy, which they confront in the company of the teacher as guide. In a reciprocal relationship, the teacher and the student enter a dialogue on caring for others through conferences and discussion about the school assignments. The teacher is able to continue the dialogue by encouraging the students to write and discuss their personal perceptions about caring. Connecting in many ways reduces the line between "I" and "thou," but that line may not be so easily (or safely) expunged between healthcare provider and client. Can one truly prepare for the other?

Rothenberg's (1993) simple declaration that "curriculum is powerful" resonates in transformative curriculum and curriculum design. Over time I see that revisions in my course reflect a movement away from traditional cultural and medical anthropological influences, which were heavy on race and ethnicity. Although anthropology still provides the infrastructure, the course has become increasingly inclusive in the perspectives it represents. I contextualize topics such as power, privilege, domination, subordination, and social roles within sociopolitical, religious–spiritual, and biological dimensions. We deconstruct generalizations in race, gender, and class. I use case studies that look at those issues, and students are asked to bring in moral and ethical perspectives. The learners are also engaged in observation and interview exercises. Written reports and oral presentations foster exploration and discussion of students' thoughts.

It was not always that way. In American culture, discussion of race and racism is virtually taboo. My acculturation to Western ways included that. I found it challenging to frame many topics effectively, but race was the one I feared. I was intimidated by the ages of some students, the social science backgrounds of others. In the early years there was little diversity in my class, with the exception of an occasional individual from Africa who could have taught about race at home and in America as well as I could. I worked very hard to prepare classes. I had students read. I did exercises with them. I learned always to put racism right in the middle of the semester so I was sure not to run out of time. I knew we had to deal with these topics and issues, yet I did not know how. And I did not know how to get the right people in the educational system to support my convictions about diversity. I was rocking the boat. I rocked carefully.

The administrator who finally blessed the course I put together insisted that she did not understand why immigrants didn't try to fully assimilate or completely Americanize. She liked my ideas but never sat in my classroom. I encouraged her support but was not about to try for her conversion to my appreciation of diversity. In the nursing department itself, support was at best mixed. Meanwhile, my experience with the course taught me that my respect for each student's personal worldview allowed the students to deal with each other. Classmates confront a negative or aggressive student in ways that are effective while avoiding the tension generated by the same exchange with someone who is assigning grades. Members of the class learned to make explicit the very constructs that motivated me to create the course.

I began coaching other faculty to teach the transcultural health course. Teachers reach people by teaching in safe and respectful environments. Teaching is interpreting, that is, guiding to understanding (Chladenius, 1994) while acknowledging the limits of expertise (Misgeld & Nicholson, 1992). Students learn and teach each other by "seeing," "writing," and "speaking" in various forms (Good, 1998). The crucial factor is caring. But we care about so many things—our own education and work, teaching and students, raising children, relationships, illnesses, complex mixed marriages—whatever challenges we face. Can we care about more? Sometimes we have to.

Meanings of Caring

My journey, shaped by my culture, led me to begin an ethnographic study of caring, in which new meanings of caring were revealed to me. The following pages describe how my views transformed as I engaged in doctoral studies. Since the 1980s, nursing and healthcare have been besieged by discontented patients, clients, and workers. Given the history of modern nursing and its placement in the social and political economy, the profession had and has much to account for in terms of uncaring institutional frameworks and policies. In my studies, I found that frantic searches for answers had produced a surplus of studies and writing about aspects of caring and noncaring focused on client–patient satisfaction ratings. Innumerable interviews involved students, patients, nurses, and other healthcare providers, including social workers and clinical psychologists. Meanwhile, professional nursing had already established caring as an integral (albeit undefined) component in nursing, indeed as the core, essence, and theoretical basis of nursing (Leininger, 1991; Leininger & McFarland, 2002; Watson, 1985). It seemed that people believed in caring, but it was difficult to observe caring action (let alone assess or measure it) on a wide scale in nursing practice and teaching (Morse, Bottoroff, Neander, & Solberg, 1991; Watson, 2002a, 2002b).

I taught nursing, yet I questioned how caring was being taught to nursing students. I focused on the educational institution and, through ethnography, explored the meaning of caring in a small sample of university-based nurse educators (Basuray, 1993). I wanted to know what it was in nursing education that nurse educators identified as their selective knowledge, and I wanted to know how caring related to that.

As a participant–observer, I spent several semesters with three educators in a nursing baccalaureate program. Caring was explored ethnographically by addressing personal and professional meanings of the phenomenon; observing how caring behaviors were manifested and expressed in the teaching and learning settings of offices, classes, informal interactions, and clinical and laboratory sites; and identifying caring values, beliefs, and attitudes that educators liked to see in their student graduates. Related questions dealt with those values, meanings, and behaviors that educators ascribed to the healthcare institution's role in promoting caring, and the educators' perceptions of their own unique ways of teaching caring in their academic culture. The fieldwork culminated in a complex set of themes for interpretation, which revealed some noteworthy dimensions of the caring concept. These were not limited to professional socialization or workplace ethics but harkened back to personal philosophies on caring, early childhood experiences, and enculturation to caring. The study validated my personal conviction that humans are complex wholes in whom caring is found as culture. The following depicts portraits of three nurse educators' meanings of caring.

Three Nurse Educators' Philosophies of Caring

In the ethnographic study, caring in the personal philosophies and teaching styles of three nurse educators emerged as highly individualized and diverse. This became a critical point, for we speak of nursing as a culture, yet the differences among the three nurse educators were striking. Their philosophies were as different as their cultural orientations. For example, Dorothy, who is African American, was essentially concerned with the ongoing plight of African American clients and her belief that African American nursing students were often maltreated in school. Dorothy's primary approach to teaching caring was through role-modeling and conscientious selection of opportunities to teach students an "open mind" approach to assessing African American clients' health and illness statuses. She focused on making an effort to instill in all her students sensitivity to issues of race.

Mary, who is European American, combined Eastern Taoist philosophy with the Western Christian religious values of the Sisters of Charity. During her young adulthood, she had adopted Taoism and learned to create an inner peace for herself. However, at the same time, she was influenced in her graduate studies by a cognitive behaviorist approach. The result was her espousal of a Taoist–cognitive behaviorism in her teaching and learning philosophy. In practice, for example, Mary adapted Taoism in teaching her students sensitivity and caring behaviors in deliberately planned, noncompetitive learning activities and environments. Her sense of *darshan* (a Hindu religious term for making contact with or communicating with God) was through her untiring devotion to caring for the students. Her methods of teaching were conscientiously planned with decisive explanations of her rationale for actions.

Veronica, also European American, based her philosophy of caring overtly in Western Christian religion. She was an evangelical Christian who had committed her daily activities as an educator to the Christian love doctrine. Caring, in Veronica's eyes, was her religious obligation. She believed that action is critical in living a Christian life and expressed this belief in interactions with her students. Student behaviors provided cues for her to join selected students as a "sojourner" in their spiritual journeys. However, she could not describe the "calling behaviors or cues" but merely cited them as something she "just knew." Even in a public university, Veronica used the term "Christian student" to refer to students who interacted with her regarding their spiritual development.

Veronica enjoyed teaching an elective course on "spiritual care" in nursing. She focused on developing students through a religious/spiritual orientation and wanted other educators to be generally more nurturing and loving—characteristics she believed are lacking in the school environment. Veronica's religious beliefs were contextualized in a Christian way of life but exemplified in nursing actions. Unlike Dorothy and Mary, caring was exclusionary for Veronica, because caring was limited to Christian belief-in-action. Students, who often saw caring from a different belief system, were sometimes seen as not sharing the behaviors that exemplified caring. Veronica believed that by taking action that is guided by Jesus Christ, she met the goal of promoting "His presence." Her participation in Christian Nurses Fellowship retreats and publication of essays based on her convictions served as demonstrations of Christian enactment of her philosophy on caring.

Themes of Inquiry: Early Socialization and Caring

For the three nurse educators who participated in the ethnographic inquiry, practicing caring through their teaching activities was critical to their beliefs about caring. The "caring" terminology, if used, was more implicit than deliberate; the nurse educators assumed that caring was inherent in nursing and that it emerged through actions. When these educators described caring, each emphasized different meanings and approaches. There has been little exploration of individualized experiences with and meanings of caring in the healthcare literature. In several studies, caring expressions and meanings expressed by faculty were strongly patterned (Appleton, 1990; Miller, Haber, & Byrne, 1990). Those studies addressed the pedagogical context of caring, presenting humanistic expressions of caring in nurse educators as related by graduate students (Appleton, 1990) and through faculty and undergraduate students combined (Miller, Haber, & Byrne, 1990). In my study, the most striking finding was the diversity in how caring is valued, operationalized, and taught by nurse educators.

The meaning of caring and the expressed caring beliefs of nurse educators are a function of numerous influences, including personality, cultural background, religion, organizational cultures, and bureaucratic support. Early life experiences contribute directly to the formation of caring ideology, for caring is "essentially a culturally learned and expressed behavior" (Leininger & Mcfarland, 2002, p. 57). For Dorothy, a sense of security in her church community and the nurturing and loving teachers of a historically black liberal arts college were positive encounters in the African American culture she knows well. Situations in nursing during military service and a master's degree program provided a sense of caring through a large network of friends and associates that extended beyond African American culture. Noncaring lurked in the treatment she observed other African Americans receiving from white clinicians.

Mary's rigid and somewhat unhappy childhood led her to eventually forge her own ideology of caring from two separate philosophies. Her cultural roots in traditional Catholicism led her to accept what she interpreted as a "tough love" bureaucracy in the school at which she taught. This facet of bureaucratic management was acknowledged as oppressive, yet Mary accepted it and used Taoist practices to endure the stress it generated. She also sought clinical teaching sites in which she could maintain control of her teaching and learning environment.

Veronica traced her idea of caring to early childhood. For her, caring developed as both natural (innate) and nurtured by her family and relatives. Compassion and expression of caring were valued in her youth and remained important to her, as was observed in her practice of recovering Christian students from "insensitive" nurse educators. Veronica, like Dorothy, openly criticized the "businesslike" environment of the nursing school culture, which both saw as nonsupportive of their personal beliefs about caring. Veronica used spiritual beliefs rooted in evangelical Christianity to guide the Christian students. In teaching the elective course on spirituality, she defined spirituality and caring as one concept.

Rewards in Teaching Caring and Juxtaposed Dichotomies

Patterns of similarity among the nurse educators lie in the deep sense of reward and gratification they find in their teaching. They see their contribution as bringing about "growth" in students, as well as "change to a more caring self." This satisfaction was injected with an element of self-sacrifice in each nurse educator's approach, yet it was rewarding to be designated "best teacher of the year" or asked to pin the students at graduation; each viewed such accolades as confirmation of the effect of their caring. Dorothy cherished the gratitude demonstrated by a group of students through a special gift. Although Veronica took pride in her caring activities, she denied personal credit and viewed herself as an instrument of Jesus Christ. Thus the impact of the reward was external for Veronica, while for Dorothy and Mary, credit was internalized. All three held growth in the student to be the desired outcome, whether it was manifest as cultural sensitivity, spiritual growth, or competence in practice.

The organizational culture of the particular school played a significant role in the merging of the themes. Each nurse educator saw herself as a caring faculty member. Each emphasized a need for nursing administration to be caring toward faculty and students. Each woman independently developed a mechanism to convey her agenda for caring, although all three felt the hegemonic constraints imposed by micromanagement and administrative emphasis on structure and function. None considered the culture of the school conducive to caring. They recognized the challenge of socializing students to a professional ideology in the context of conflict between the educators' need to express caring and the reality of the academic culture. Students being taught to be caring nurses must somehow learn to face and cope efficaciously with the reality of uncaring bureaucracy in their academic and workplace environments, but their experience with enduring hegemony in the context of school and hospitals does little to instill trust in nurses' power to instigate positive change.

Valuing Caring in the Culture of Clinical Practice

The ethnographic study of three nurse educators demonstrated partiality and incompleteness related to the value they placed on clinical nursing practice. Experienced clinicians themselves—wearing the lenses of nurse educators—each put forth a self-proclaimed and biased view of clinical practice, as well as evidence of the complex relationship between clinicians and clinical practice (Benner, 1984; Gaut, 1983; Sarason, 1985; Street, 1992). Benner and Wrubel (1989), expressing concern for caring in nursing practice, stated that nurse scholars (who frequently are also nurse educators) too often ignore the nursing knowledge they derive from the practice component of nursing.

In my interactions with the three nurse educators, there was a presumption of power obtainable through knowledge both theoretical and didactic. Scholarly achievements were revered, and students served to demonstrate excellence in nursing. Yet, in this study, it was the activity associated with caring that took precedence for the nurse educators. In clinical practice, role-modeling was highly valued. For instance, Mary's commitment to coaching each of her students was planned, organized, and implemented for optimal clinical practice.

There is a need for more meticulous examination and understanding of the meanings, values, and expressions of caring in the culture of nursing. Although caring is proclaimed to be the core of the nursing culture, little is known of how nurse educators, as groups or individuals, develop or share their meanings of caring in the nursing profession. Greater consideration of the phenomenon is necessary if we are to understand philosophies and theories of caring. How do personal ideologies of caring converge with or detract from a common meaning of caring? Is there need for a universal meaning of caring? There seem to be multiple understandings and interpretations of the phenomenon, depending on who uses what type of lens.

It is important to note that the nurse educators in the study reflected on and discovered their meanings of caring. In the inquiry, the tacit nature of caring emerged through interviews and informal ongoing conversations in which each nurse educator articulated her own definition and meanings of caring. Self-disclosure was critical to that revealing. Is such sharing a personal academic exercise for each educator in practice-based professions? Can it be comfortably modeled with students? The inquiry became part of my search for caring in my life. The study became a pivotal point in my understanding of caring through scholarship and self-reflection. From that point, my life and profession began to transform for me. I became more confident in articulating the subject and increasingly sensitized to universalistic concerns about caring.

Culture, Needs, and Oppression

As nurse educators, we talk often about ethics in class, trying to bring together health-related content and cross-cultural aspects of healthcare. We speculate about those circumstances with which we really disagree as healthcare professionals, posing possible interventions and resolutions—and often leaving without solid answers. It is the dialogue that is important. *We have to face, and teach our students to face, the reality of differences.* We need to communicate well, learn to negotiate, and resolve differences and conflict. Today's students are often comfortable with making demands; many are not as inclined to suffer silently as their predecessors seemed to be. Sometimes a student will tell the faculty about not having enough food or a place to stay. An environment is needed in which needs can be recognized, assertiveness supported, and perhaps the manner of request shaped for effectiveness in other contexts.

In my time at the campus Multicultural Institute, there seems to be no end to unanticipated problems. For example, international students may come to the United States with serious health needs and hope for a good healthcare system—while many of our American students have no health coverage. Students can misinterpret our efforts, as we might theirs. One of the deans allowed an international student, when he first arrived, to use his phone to make a call to his home country. The student was then confused when he was held responsible for later calls made from university office phones. For a long time, faculty had more trouble dealing with the students who were members of American minority groups than they did international students, who were often viewed as rather quaint.

Culture is as complex as caring is. Frequently, differences within groups are as significant as those between them. Perhaps few Americans

would notice this, but I am accustomed to being in places where someone will stop and point out that I am not Bengali, although my married
name was Bengali. I would find myself in a group of westernized people
who are not thinking about the different places from which we have
come and the different routes we have taken, but only that he or she
is Bengali and I am not. Each of us is insular in our identity; we identify
the differences, however slight, between us and some other person or
aggregate—until something or someone we view as *more* different
comes along.

Here is a simple example of how easily race and class become confused, and how change and progress get confounded with oppression.
Neem bark and leaves are materials readily available in the Indian subcontinent. People have used them for centuries, probably millennia, to
clean their teeth. Worldwide, Indians are known to have beautiful, clean
white teeth. Rich and poor used neem, which also has antiseptic properties and is a traditional Ayurvedic medicine for the stomach and skin
irritation in communicable diseases. Along comes a Western toothpaste
company. A van goes from village to village to show a propaganda video
to market the toothpaste. The company uses Indian agents and hands
out candy to the children. Samples of the toothpaste are given to villag-
ers, who are encouraged to spend part of their small incomes every
month on a substitute for what is available economically from their own
backyards. Is it better to cut oneself off from such changes and stick
with the traditional ways? Or to give in to change that carries with it
costs, both seen and unseen? These are questions about change and
tradition, about caring and culture, about responsibility for self and
others.

Times change. Positions of understanding change. Yet "the other"
remains—perhaps suffering deep disharmonies among outward displays
of sociocultural solidarity, but still somehow (if only vaguely) identifiable
as "other" (King, 1995; Vidich & Lyman, 2000). Differences are no
longer thought to be innate. Critical racial theory, unapologetically challenging scholarship that would depersonalize and dehumanize, raises
important questions that challenge mainstream orthodoxy about the
control and production of knowledge (Delgado, 1995; Ladson-Billings,
2000). Yet somehow the liminal status of people of color still more often
than not remains beyond the normative boundaries of self and other,
knower and known (Bell, 1992; King, 1995).

I am committed to teaching and practicing multiculturalism. I am energized by it. With ethnography's methodologies emancipated, I am committed to writing my story. Initially, I found myself looking at the other" because I could not tell the students how I lived and felt every day, although I had come to realize that they wanted stories—disclosures. At the same time, I feared their categorization of my experience, their assessment of it in their terms, and their stereotyping. Could I portray myself fairly? What parts could I share without opening myself up to being stereotyped? I began slowly, at first giving the students "good stories." Then I started giving them case studies; they were really my own case studies, but I gave them other nationalities. A scenario might focus on how difficult it is to find a mate when you look and think differently from everyone around you, or perhaps you are merely *assumed* to think differently *because* you look different. Or perhaps you assume you look different because you think differently.

The Ways of Social and Cultural Oppression

I belong to no specific religious community. My own frameworks both shape my needs and conflict with them. I try to keep distance in my involvement, not to suffocate. I love the sense of familiarity and peace that comes with tradition, but I don't want it to be deterministic. I no longer need a building to meditate, or a social club to feel like I belong. I want to impart stories to my children, not dogma.

I grew up immersed in Christian catechism. My husband grew up with Hindu religion and related mythology—great, wonderful stories of classical Hindu tradition. He married me, a non-Hindu and a Pakistani. Yet he needed me to understand his own Hinduism. He knew I did not want him to try to make me into a Hindu, and he did not want me to try to make him something he is not. When the children came, we used our common sense and gave them stories. I would actively participate in Hindu religious ceremonies. But then Easter would come, and I would feel somber, or on Christmas Eve, I would feel a strong loss even though I had the house decorated, as if something was missing. I would ask my Hindu husband to accompany me to carols and church services. There was always that potential for conflict. I felt that if I did "the church thing" with the children, it would distance them from their father. I sampled many churches, rejecting them because they would indoctrinate my children to think in a particular way and direction. Eventually

I found a Unitarian Universalist program and a teacher who thought it was wonderful when my seven-year-old son drew a dragon for their Noah's Ark. I knew it was the place for our children as long as it was a place that was not constraining. Years later, when they were in their late teens, the day came when my son and daughter both completed their religious education programs.

As a teenager in the United States, I quickly acculturated. My siblings and I soon made our ways to college. We were prepared by knowing English, which helped a great deal. And my parents were educated, and we all valued education. But for my parents, there was much to give up and much to take in to accommodate to this new place, even welcomed as we were in Oklahoma. Although we were not Baptist, a Baptist hospital greatly facilitated our resettlement. Upon arrival, we lived in an old, unused wing of the hospital. We had some beautiful donated furniture along with a few donated hospital pieces in our home for years. We were invited to join the Baptist church, but my father was an Episcopalian lay deacon, and feeling he had to hang on to what he could from his past, he wanted to find an Episcopal church and involve himself in it through the music as well as the service.

Over time, my father became an independent entrepreneur with a small business in our family's new adopted hometown, but it was still hard for my parents to adapt. My younger sister suffered by observing my parents' struggle. We grew up as the model, integrated, successful, patronized, and *different* (which underlined the image of success because it was deemed exceptional) family. I learned to see myself and our family through those Western eyes.

I was socialized in a traditional society where the oppressor and the oppressed both understood and deferred to "class" in the sense of prestige—family names or group affiliation, education and occupation—rather than owning extensive property or having money. I came to the United States having read 18th-century British novels and attended operas with the elite of many backgrounds. In this country, I wanted to embrace the new culture quickly, and I did not realize how much I was a reserved Pakistani woman with a neo-Victorian upbringing. For instance, I was raised never to look a man in the eye if he is older than I am. It remains an unconscious reflex, although I work on it. I alter my behavior according to whom I am with: I dress conservatively in the company of older Indian men.

Despite my youth, I carried these values with me to this country;

they remain with me and always will. People have different expectations. When I worked with an emergency room team, my colleagues initially would not take me with them to the Irish bars where they hung out because I was too proper and didn't use the four-letter words they did at work. Finally, as I loosened up, I began to join them for "let your hair down" sessions. I had to learn not to depend so much on my husband to guide my living. At the same time, I had to negotiate that too.

Integration

Integrating self, cultures, meanings, and understandings of caring— it is an intriguing concept. When our family came to the United States, stereotypes took positive forms; we were expected by our hosts to be educated and civilized. The local newspaper's Sunday special edition heralded our arrival with photographs and a lengthy story by a freelance writer. Five years later, the community again celebrated our family as we took the oath of citizenship. New foreign-born arrivals from Asia and the Middle East were often introduced to us. We were generally viewed as somewhat arrogant perhaps, but as professional, despite having dark skin. Our home environment quickly became international, due to our model family status and the presence of an airfield and colleges that enrolled foreign students not very far away.

I saw my father as gracious and giving, as helping the poor and supporting charitable causes. The rules were changed for him here in this country, though. It was a culture shock for him. Suddenly a nurse who was a woman (and most were women) could be his boss. That was something he never quite got used to. Both of my parents went back to school here. They were well into their 50s, and they were mistreated for their differences. My mother lost her confidence. Feeling incompetent in English literacy, she took an entire series of adult learning classes at the public library. A Chinese American nurse and a caring faculty person in Tulsa helped her get through her nursing program of studies.

In many parts of this country, people are accustomed to seeing others as black or white. Falling outside those handy categories, Asians are usually expected to look Chinese. People don't know what to make of me. My facial features are reminiscent of various ethno-racial and cultural heritages; I have been spoken to in Hebrew, Arabic, and Mexican Spanish, as well as a mélange of Asian languages.

What type of lenses do I wear now as I consider caring in my life? I still go back to Buber, but since the use of "I" and "thou" leads to the opaque and dangerous ground of "us" and "them" (Westerners and Orientals, perhaps, or Easterners and Occidentals?), I am attracted to Jung's confluence of East and West (Jung, 1933, 1946; Jung & Kerényi, 1949). I try to be sensitive to all suffering, but I know I cannot change, let alone fix, everything that begs for intervention. I try to be integrated in the sense of being authentic, of having integrity. I can think multiculturally without liking or disliking particular individuals. I learn a lot from different people, including some who are remarkably difficult to get along with. I firmly believe that we must deal with issues around morality in education today—issues around universalizability, impartiality, and impersonality (Vetlesen, 1997). This brings me back to caring. I try always to acknowledge individuals. People have stories to share, knowledge gained from their experience. We do not have to agree. The hardest part is to practice what I preach and to avoid stereotyping.

Adapting Gender and Culture

I am still writing and sorting out the meanings and significance of my life experiences. In seeking ways to articulate some of those, I found myself identifying with the term *improvisation* as Bateson (1990) described it in the lives of four women she studied. My story at times seems improvised in its interpretation and presentation.

What meanings do I give to my improvisations? Is this a universal phenomenon for women regardless of variations in culture? Other than the juxtaposition of my ethno-racial background with that of my middle-class professional life and living in the West, I might say that I've easily identified with the descriptions of improvisation by females as written by Western authors. I ascribe much of the familiarity with what I read and hear in large part to the near universality of patriarchy. Cultures display their inherent characteristics in their cultural values and social norms. My socialization to society's prescribed female role and eventually to marriage included all manner of improvisations. Some of those were eagerly initiated by myself—especially in my young adult life in my role as my future husband's girlfriend, as his wife and the mother of his children, and as a daughter-in-law, a sister-in-law, and a member of both kinship and ethnic-based personal social networks.

Because I'm very much my father's daughter, my world evolved into an adjustment to patriarchy. I've learned to get along with older men and to work with older men without conflict. And yet, my need to be myself led me to question the oppressive side of patriarchy. I discussed many of those phenomena with selected older male friends for their perspectives and, at times somewhat accusingly, with my husband. He came to symbolize the male personification of traditionalism and patriarchy, not only in our marital relationship but in my improvised life. I attribute this to our divergent socializations, his great attachment to his family and their community, and his adherence to traditionalism. Outside of marriage, in contrast, he empowered females who sought his help in the bureaucratic world.

Paralleling all this was my expectation to be professional as my parents were, to be independent and earn my own pay, and, most important of all, to be recognized as a well-performing, successful, respected person. As soon as I married, my priorities began shifting to meet my husband's social needs. Late-night work shifts (common to clinical roles) were not desirable. My friends at the emergency room where I worked were not his type. I needed to be ready to travel to attend gatherings in Indian communities. Presentation of self, educational status, family name, types of jobs, and chastity were altogether an expectation of both the Indian subcontinent and the Midwest. The married state for me involved appearing Bengali and becoming as Bengali as possible in dress, food, language, and behavior. My cherished and well-preserved Pakistani clothes were not an option. Neither was meeting someone from Pakistan. On top of that, cocktail discussions about politics and culture were entrenched with conservatism and expressions of prejudiced views, which were occasionally insensitively anti-Pakistani.

Over time, I found a sadness in the many improvisations and compromises that I so wholeheartedly and eagerly worked hard at making. They were, more often than not, concessions immersed in learning about Hindu ways. Learning Hinduism for its own sake was enjoyable. For years I attended the reformed Hindu Rama Krishna society worship services and seminars. My active interest in Hindu ways was praised, yet, as a Pakistani national, I was never totally accepted by my husband, his family, or his peers. I was hidden away. My struggle was always apparent, yet I chose not to pay attention to friends' and relatives' questions and comments—their poignant queries. "Why don't you sing a Pushto song for us?" "Why don't you make a Pakistani/Peshawari dish for us next time?" "I'd like to see you in your national/provincial dress— do you have any?" "Have you traveled back home?"

In my parents' home, I had been seen as open, caring, compassionate, moody, and energetic. I painted during early education and even in high school. Later, in the early days of my marriage, my siblings encouraged me to paint again and to make my own friends. I tried the friends but never cultivated friendships. I always let go when I did not get my husband's interest or approval; his social and professional endeavors came first. The tug and pull came from both sides. If I did well in Bengali or Indian cultural displays—cooking, dressing, behaving, and speaking— then the praises increased, and more of me was demanded. I felt useful and needed, and my social status increased. I felt as if I was engaged in a sport: the higher I raised the bar, the more I challenged myself to achieve good results and win acceptance from my husband and the community. Compromise. Improvise. Achieve. After a quarter century of this, my husband's family's acceptance of his bride never came.

When a teaching job was offered to me early in our marriage, I was encouraged to take it for the better working conditions and increased prestige it promised. My in-laws especially appreciated this change, as they held a low opinion of nursing in India (Basuray, 2002). When the dean of the nursing college encouraged me to go for a master's degree, I consulted with my husband, who optimistically supported me. Part of my success in my studies was due to the emotional encouragement that he gave me—although that was also about showing his parents how he was developing me as a professional with status. They in turn acknowledged him for his self-sacrifice and benevolence in letting me leave town and family to pursue education.

During the first semester, I found myself with my young son in another state, and my husband in North Dakota with two aged parents. It was traumatic for them, for my son, for me, for all of us. But I continued living in my husband's world. I gave away my firstborn, at the age of 15 months, to my sister-in-law on the East Coast to keep for us. She had publicly announced in the Bengali community her desire for a son and was willing to keep my child. She had always been antagonistic toward me since our marriage and remained an unaccepting family member. Later, when I embarked on doctoral studies, my husband encouraged me emotionally and intellectually, along with displaying some resentment at my success.

Unlike many women around me who accepted their improvisations quietly or at least gracefully, I sought the counsel of friends—most of them female, but a few males who arrived late in the picture. My awakening began when I found my rebellious voice; it spoke one day, and I began to change at a more rapid pace. I credit this change in part to my doctoral studies; I now knew that it was permissible to rebel. I began discussing my issues with my husband; he responded—ever intellectual and empathetic—with gifts of novels and articles written on women's issues by women (especially from the subcontinent). Today, I continue that journey, though more boldly. At the start, my steps were small and taken cautiously, with some fear of falling into the crevices of extremism. Now I readily assure myself that I am gravitating toward a balanced view. I understand better the deep roots culturally embedded in one's worldview and how each individual interprets cultural tradition in the context of his or her own personal life experiences. Still, despite the understandings—or perhaps because of them—I am eager to move on, reclaiming along the way some aspects of the early days that delighted or soothed me. "The other" has become myself, and I am being-for, caring for and caring about this new persona.

Friendship has become an important focus of my life. I feel open to others and am perceived as such by persons of both sexes who wish to cultivate friendships. Becoming is a beautiful experience. I previously paid little attention to the support and interest that professional women invest in friendship. These women, many of whom are successful by anyone's criteria, seem to enjoy sharing my journey toward self-growth. They are leaders, friends, and mentors offering friendship and unconditional caring, despite their own battles in the world of female professions shadowed by traditional hierarchy and patriarchy. Other friends are nonprofessionals who care to help me develop myself by quietly supporting my efforts, praising or advising me.

I shyly brought men, colleagues, and others in higher positions into my world. Some are from the Indian Bengali community or my church work organizations. As I mellowed in the eyes of my siblings and parents, they too opened their arms to help. I slowly open myself to receive the help of others, finding warmth and affection in the care people have for others. My growth has allowed me to build bridges and friendships for the work of the Multicultural Institute, which can be very challenging to promote openly in an academic institution.

The Spiritual Journey of Care: I and Thou, the Personal and the Professional

Western monotheism is sometimes held accountable for a determinative shaping of biomedicine, even as it is practiced in non-Western societies (Kleinman, 1995; Unschuld, 1989). The notion of a single god legitimates that of a singular, underlying, universalizable truthful (however elusive) unitary paradigm, just as genderized religion (that is, God as male) has shaped female stature in Western culture (Fessenden, 2002). The cultural ramifications are obvious. In some ways, Eastern cultures are more flexible, the sacred and the profane less distinguishable. Indeed, the entire cosmos (replete with gods and goddesses) is more likely viewed as sacralized (Eliade, 1959). My spiritual journey is the most private of all subjects for disclosure at this point in my life, but I feel I can articulate it with some understanding and can deal with the criticism often proffered in the West when one does not tread a single, focused path.

In my youth, I had a particularly strong interest in Judaism, in part due to intense curiosity about Pakistan's ban on publications about the holocaust. After arriving in the United States, my older sister gave me a copy of the novel *Exodus* (Uris, 1958). After that, reading and watching documentaries on the holocaust became an obsession. I traveled to Israel with my family. There, through social and political lenses, I became more sensitive to the state of Israel and its policies toward Arabs who reside with or beside them. I respect those who keep the history of destruction (from the atom bomb to the Native American and Nazi holocausts) in our memories so that crimes against humanity are not repeated. At the same time, I am reminded of Paulo Freire's (1995) warning that the vicious cycle of oppression can easily be maintained when newly emancipated leaders oppress their own people. This I observe all around us.

In Eastern spirituality, the opening to the higher plane does not so much represent passage from the human to suprahuman as it honors the freedom of transcendence (Eliade, 1959). There are mythical images of "shattering the roof" (perhaps a cultural variation of "rocking the boat"), for figuratively destroying the personal cosmos one inhabits opens new possibilities for living and understanding the universal, and for integrity in this life. Friends and sojourners have introduced me to yet more approaches in understanding spirituality and humanism. Recently, through one who is quite eclectic in his approach, including Gnostic Christianity, Buddhism, and Hinduism, I became aware of the Sufis in a more serious and beautiful way. Here I am, thirty years in the United States of America, and only now do I get close to a topic I grew up knowing about, albeit distantly and vaguely. I hear Sufis spoken of in respectful tones by my family, our friends, and our community and described as purists, seclusive, scholarly, passive, god-loving, and mystical—as transcendent.

Presently, as I become more at ease with my work in the Multicultural Institute, I am taking on new issues and concerns about diversity and the university community's involvement in such concerns as the plight of refugees and asylum seekers in the United States. I now work on their healthcare issues, which leads me to seek ongoing education in health law and its cultural variations. Healthcare in the United States leads the world in powerful technology and scientific research. In this open society, there is space for combining Eastern and Western thought through alternative and complementary healthcare practices, such as Ayurvedic medicine, yoga, and Chinese medicine (Cant & Sharma, 2000; Unschuld, 1987). While new healthcare options are a novelty to many, traditional viewpoints regarding care and caring are also making inroads (Baer, 2001; Aspen Reference Group, 2002). In discourse on "sensitive" and "congruent" multicultural education and practice, I observe new ways of addressing caring and culture and of resolving conflicts through strategies conceptualized in humanism.

Conclusion

There is always tension in ethnography with its characteristic shifting of voices and contrasting exemplars and expositions (Atkinson, 1990). The persuasive force in autoethnography is in its multileveled interplay of experiences and responses, examples and discourse—but lack of explicit theorizing. Every experience enriches reflection on the meaning of life, but experiences are diachronic, and even repetition does not ensure equivalence in significance or meaning. In the final interpretation, the self is indistinguishable from the story it constructs out of inheritances, experiences, and desires (Freeman, 1993, 1998; Kerby, 1991). In a sense, in autoethnography the writer and individualism's "invisible hand"

(Rosenberg, 1995) co-participate in dialogue that sensitizes the inquirer to the reality that her understanding and knowing is anything but passive. Learning, for me, is the praxis born of interacting, caring, and culture: my stressful life with a mother-in-law and sisters-in-law taught me about our cultural differences; my in-laws reflect other traditions.

Differentiating work relationships framed in classism and the social–philosophical dichotomies observed in nurses from middle-class America prompted me to explore discourses on patriarchy and ideological disunity. Unitarian teachings taught me to broaden my Christian religion and spiritual views. Academia and ongoing inquiry into countless interpretations of caring and culture allow me to actively participate in society. I accept the Taoist teachings that interpret dualistic thinking as an illness. In Taoist thought, caring exists when we see ourselves as inseparable from the universe. I long for the ability to be able to articulate my life experiences within a non-dualistic thought pattern. However, even as I move toward understanding the oneness of being, I am bound by Western society's dualistic pattern for framing and expressing my thoughts. My life is the field, the story is both academic and personal—and as yet only partially understood and surely incomplete. But I am living and learning. Three nurse educators showed me that there is no single way of caring. Their exemplars of caring are signs that my caring is my way—complex, always incomplete, and rife with new possibilities.

References

Appleton, C. (1990). The meaning of human care and the experience of caring in a university school of nursing. In M. Leininger & J. Watson (Eds.), *The caring imperative in education* (pp. 77–94). New York: National League for Nursing.

Aspen Reference Group. (2002). *Holistic health promotion and complementary therapies: A resource for integrated practice.* Gaithersburg, MD: Aspen.

Atkinson, P. (1990). *The ethnographic imagination: Textual constructions of reality.* New York: Routledge.

Atkinson, R. (1995). *The gift of stories.* Westport, CT: Bergin & Garvey.

Baer, H. A. (2001). *Biomedicine and alternative healing systems in America: Issues of class, race, ethnicity, and gender.* Madison: University of Wisconsin Press.

Barks, C., & Green, M. (1997). *The illuminated Rumi.* New York: Doubleday Dell.

Basuray, J. (1993). *Meaning of caring in nurse educators: An ethnography.* Unpublished doctoral dissertation, School of Education, University of Maryland, College Park.

Basuray, J. (1997). Nurse Miss Sahib: Colonial culture-bound education in India and transcultural nursing. *Journal of Transcultural Nursing, 9*(1), 14–19.

Basuray, J. (2002). India: Transcultural nursing and health care. In M. M. Leininger &

M. R. McFarland (Eds.), *Transcultural nursing: Concepts, theories, research and practice* (3rd ed., pp. 477–491). New York: McGraw-Hill.

Bateson, M. C. (1990). *Composing a life.* New York: Plume.

Behar, R. (1996). *The vulnerable observer: Anthropology that breaks your heart.* Boston: Beacon Press.

Bell, D. (1992). *Faces at the bottom of the well.* New York: Basic Books.

Benner, P. (1984). *From novice to expert: Excellence and power in clinical nursing practice.* Menlo Park, CA: Addison-Wesley.

Benner, P., & Wrubel, J. (1989). *The primacy of caring: Stress and coping in health and illness.* Menlo Park, CA: Addison-Wesley.

Bochner, A. P., Ellis, C., & Tillmann-Healy, L. (1997). Relationships as stories. In S. Duck (Ed.), *Handbook of personal relationships: Theory, research and interventions* (2nd ed., pp. 307–324). New York: John Wiley.

Bochner, A. P., Ellis, C., & Tillmann-Healy, L. (1998). Mucking around looking for truth. In B. M. Montgomery & L. A. Baxter (Eds.), *Dialectical approaches to studying personal relationships* (pp. 41–62). Mahwah, NJ: Lawrence Erlbaum.

Buber, M. (1965). *I and thou.* New York: Macmillan.

Cant, S., & Sharma, U. (2000). Alternative health practices and systems. In G. L. Albrecht, R. Fitzpatrick, & S. C. Scrimshaw (Eds.), *The handbook of social studies in health and medicine* (pp. 426–439). Thousand Oaks, CA: Sage.

Chatterjee, P. (1993). *The nation and its fragments.* Princeton, NJ: Princeton University Press.

Chladenius, J. M. (1994). Reason and understanding: Rational hermeneutics. In K. Mueller-Vollmer (Ed.), *The hermeneutics reader.* New York: Continuum.

Clough, P. (1997). Autotelecommunication and autoethnography: A reading of Carolyn Ellis's "Final negotiations." *Sociological Quarterly, 38,* 95–100.

Delgado, R. (Ed.). (1995). *Critical race theory: The cutting edge.* Philadelphia: Temple University Press.

Edmondson, R. (1984). *Rhetoric in sociology.* London: Macmillan.

Eliade, M. (1959). *The sacred and the profane: The nature of religion (The significance of religious myth, symbolism, and ritual within life and culture).* New York: Harcourt, Brace & World.

Ellis, C. (1991). Sociological introspection and emotional experience. *Symbolic Interaction, 14,* 23–50.

Ellis, C., & Bochner, A. P. (2000). Autoethnography, personal narrative, reflexivity: Researcher as subject. In N. K. Denzin & Y. S. Lincoln (Eds.), *Handbook of qualitative research* (2nd ed., pp. 733–768). Thousand Oaks, CA: Sage.

Fessenden, T. (2002). Gendering religion. *Journal of Women's History, 14*(1), 163–169.

Freeman, M. (1993). *Rewriting the self: History, memory, narrative.* London: Routledge.

Freeman, M. (1998). Mythical time, historical time, and the narrative fabric of self. *Narrative Inquiry 8,* 27–50.

Freire, P. (1995). *Pedagogy of the oppressed* (Rev. ed., M. B. Ramos, Trans.). New York: Continuum.

Gaut, D. (1983). Development of a theoretically adequate description of caring. *Western Journal of Nursing Research, 5*(4), 313–324.

Good, M. J. D. (1998). *American medicine: The quest for competence.* Berkeley: University of California Press.

Hayano, D. (1979). Auto-ethnography: Paradigms, problems, and prospects. *Human Organization, 38,* 113–120.

Helminski, C. (1995). *Rumi: Daylight*. Watsonville, CA: Threshold Books.

Hirschmann, E. (1987). The necessary delusion: Racism as a pillar of empire. *Towson State University Lecture Series, 5*, 1–9.

Jung, C. G. (1933). *Modern man in search of a soul*. New York: Harvest Book/Harcourt Brace Jovanovich.

Jung, C. G. (1946). *Psychological types*. London: Kegan Paul, Trench, Truber.

Jung, C. G., & Kere'nyi, C. (1949). *Essays on a science of mythology* (R. F. C. Hull, Trans.). New York: Littleton Scott.

Kerby, A. (1991). *Narrative and the self*. Bloomington: Indiana University Press.

King, J. E. (1995). Culture centered knowledge: Black studies, curriculum transformation, and social action. In J. A. Banks & C. M. Banks (Eds.), *Handbook of research on multicultural education* (pp. 265–290). New York: Macmillan.

Kleinman, A. (1995). *Writing at the margin: Discourse between anthropology and medicine*. Berkeley: University of California Press.

Ladson-Billings, G. (2000). Racialized discourses and ethnic epistemologies. In N. K. Denzin & Y. S. Lincoln (Eds.), *Handbook of qualitative research* (2nd ed., pp. 257–313). Thousand Oaks, CA: Sage.

Leininger, M. (1991). *Culture care diversity and universality: A theory of nursing*. New York: National League for Nursing Press.

Leininger, M., & McFarland, M. R. (2002). *Transcultural nursing: Concepts, theories, research and practice* (3rd ed.). New York: McGraw-Hill.

Mani, L. (1990). Contentious traditions: The debate of the sati in colonial India. In K. Sangari & S. Vaid (Eds.), *Recasting women: Essays in colonial history* (pp. 88–126). New Brunswick, NJ: Rutgers University Press.

Metcalf, T. (1995). *Ideologies of the raj*. Delhi, India: Cambridge University Press.

Miller, B. K., Haber, J., & Byrne, M. W. (1990). The experiences of caring in the teaching–learning process of nursing education: Student and teacher perspectives. In M. Leininger & J. Watson (Eds.), *The caring imperative in education* (pp. 125–135). New York: National League for Nursing.

Miller, C. (1977). *Khyber, British India's North West Frontier: The story of an imperial migraine*. New York: Macmillan.

Misgeld, D., & Nicholson, G. (1992). *Hans-Georg Gadamer on education, poetry, and history* (L. Schmidt & M. Reuss, Trans.). Albany: State University of New York Press.

Moorhouse, G. (1973). *The missionaries*. London: Eyre Methuen.

Moorhouse, G. (1992). *To the frontier: A journey to Khyber Pass*. New York: Henry Holt.

Morse, J. M., Bottoroff, J., Neander, W., & Solberg, S. (1991). Comparative analysis of conceptualizations and theories of caring. *Image: Journal of Nursing Scholarship, 23*(2), 119–126.

Moyne, J. (1984). *Open secret: Versions of Rumi*. Watsonville, CA: Threshold Books.

Quigley, D. (1997). Deconstructing colonial fictions? Some conjuring tricks in the recent sociology of India. In A. James, J. Hockey, & A. Dawson (Eds.), *After writing culture: Epistemology and praxis in contemporary anthropology* (pp. 103–121). London: Routledge.

Richardson, L. (1997). *Fields of play: Constructing an academic life*. New Brunswick, NJ: Rutgers University Press.

Rosenberg, A. (1995). *Philosophy of social science* (2nd ed.). Boulder, CO: Westview.

Rothenberg, P. (1993, Spring). The inclusive curriculum and its critics. *Transformations, 4*(1), 4–7.

Sarason, S. B. (1985). *Caring and compassion in clinical practice.* San Francisco: Jossey-Bass.

Sen, S. (2002). The savage family: Colonialism and female infanticide in nineteenth-century India. *Journal of Women's History, 14*(3), 53–79.

Singha, R. (1998). *A despotism of law: Crime and justice in early colonial India.* Delhi, India: Oxford University Press.

Smith, D. (1979). A sociology for women. In J. Sherman & E. Beck (Eds.), *The prism of sex: Essays in the sociology of knowledge* (pp. 203–267). Madison: University of Wisconsin Press.

Stokes, E. (1959). *The English utilitarians and India.* Delhi, India: Oxford University Press.

Street, A. F. (1992). *Inside nursing: A critical ethnography of clinical nursing practice.* Albany: State of New York University Press.

Tedlock, B. (1991). From participant observation to the observation of participation: The emergence of narrative ethnography. *Journal of Anthropological Research, 41,* 69–94.

Unschuld, P. (1987). Traditional Chinese medicine: Some historical and epistemological reflections. *Social Science and Medicine, 24*(12), 1023–1029.

Unschuld, P. (1989). *Approaches in traditional Chinese medical literature.* Boston: Kluwer.

Uris, L. (1958). *Exodus.* New York: Random House.

Van Manen, M. (1990). *Researching lived experience: Human science for an action sensitive pedagogy.* Albany: State University of New York Press.

Vetlesen, A. J. (1997). Introducing an ethics of proximity. In H. Jodalan & A. J. Vetlesen (Eds.), *Closeness: An ethics* (pp. 1–19). Oslo, Norway: Scandinavian University Press.

Vidich, A. J., & Lyman, S. M. (2000). Qualitative methods: Their history in sociology and anthropology. In N. K. Denzin & Y. S. Lincoln (Eds.), *Handbook of qualitative research* (2nd ed., pp. 37–84). Thousand Oaks, CA: Sage.

Watson, J. (1985). *Nursing: Human science and human care: A theory of nursing.* Norwalk, CT: Appleton-Century-Crofts.

Watson, J. (2002a). *Assessing and measuring caring in nursing and health science.* New York: Springer.

Watson, J. (2002b). Metaphysics of virtual caring communities. *International Journal for Human Caring, 6*(1), 41–45.

Watson, K. (1982) *Education in the Third World.* London: Croom Helm.

4

Prejudice, Paradox, and Possibility

The Experience of Nursing People from Cultures Other Than One's Own

Deb Spence

Introduction and Background

Nursing a person or people from a culture other than one's own is a dynamic and complex phenomenon. William Saroyan (as cited in Moore, 1994) suggests that "the very little difference between one person and another . . . is what makes the difference so precious" (p. 199) and, certainly in Western cultures, individual difference is highly valued. Internationally, too, the nurse providing care is expected to promote environments in which the values, customs, and spiritual beliefs of the individual are respected (Fry, 1994). Also essential to human coexistence is the sense that alongside such differences there is common understanding among cultures with respect to human care. Madeleine Leininger's theory of Culture Care (Leininger, 1991, 1995) argues forcefully that both diversities and universalities need to be accommodated by culturally congruent nursing: "The roots of culture care are deep and widespread. It requires that health personnel discover the similarities and differences in a sensitive and competent way in order to provide meaningful health care service" (Leininger, 1995, p. 115).

The International Council of Nurses (ICN) *Code of Nursing Ethics*, adopted in 1973 and reaffirmed in 1989, states further that the need for nursing service is universal and that professional nursing service is

140

not restricted by nationality, race, creed, color, age, sex, politics, or social status. Nurses are primarily responsible for those who require nursing care, and people in need of care have a right to receive such care regardless of religious and other considerations (ICN, 1989).

In the context of New Zealand nursing, however, Ramsden (1997) challenges these codes of ethics for seeming to deny difference. Arguing that nursing practice must be "culturally safe," as defined by the client, she suggests that people should be nursed *"regardful* of all that makes them unique, rather than *regardless* of color or creed" (p. 116). The challenge is indeed a valid one. But are these philosophies necessarily antithetical? The following couplet by Pat Parker (1978) seems to exemplify the paradoxical nature of respect for difference:

The first thing you must do is forget that I'm black,
The second, you must never forget that I'm black. (p.68)

Perhaps, as Lacan (1978) suggests, the most paradoxical facts are the most instructive. Perhaps the truth reveals itself most fully, not in dogma but in the paradox, irony, and contradictions that distinguish compelling narratives (Lopez, 1989).

Inspired by Schon's (1983) work on the reflective practitioner and confronted as a nurse–teacher by disparities between the real and the ideal of nursing practice, I believed that exploring the meaning of cross-cultural nursing experiences would contribute to the discipline's knowledge. I wanted to explore the phenomenon of nursing people from cultures other than one's own, and I chose an interpretive approach informed by the tradition of philosophical hermeneutics because of its congruence with the dynamic, situated, and intersubjective nature of nursing practice (Spence, 1999).

Hermeneutics: Philosophy, Methodology, and Method

Research informed by philosophical hermeneutics recognizes the situated nature of human existence. Being human means being in the world with others past and present, oriented toward a future. Knowledge therefore arises through the dialectics of history, culture, and language. Understanding evolves in an ongoing cyclical manner, metaphorically described as the hermeneutic circle (Dilthey, 1961; Gadamer, 1975; Heidegger, 1927/1962; Taylor, 1985b; Wachterhauser, 1986).

Interpretations of experience are shaped reciprocally through the interaction of past and present traditions in an ongoing manner. Thus, in
relation to the experience of nursing someone from another culture, the
meaning of each new encounter is interpreted in light of the whole of
one's previous experiences. This *part–whole* dialectic impacts simultaneously at personal, interpersonal, professional, and societal levels.
Nurses' practice experiences are always *part* in terms of their experience
of life as a whole. The nurse as an individual is a part in the sense of
relating within the wider community in which he or she lives and is also
a part within the *whole* of the nursing profession. In each of these part–
whole relationships, provisional understandings develop and grow in a
potentially infinite process of fusion. Multiple layers of meaning coexist
and interpenetrate, and for those who are open to new and different
interpretations, striving for understanding is an ongoing project.

Philosophical hermeneutics, as articulated by Gadamer (1975, 1976,
1996), Taylor (1985a, 1985b) and Hekman (1986), facilitates the exploration of meanings in context. Research using such an approach comprises the following interrelated features: making sense of experiential
phenomena through speech and language, articulating the cultural and
historical horizons of the participants, explicating pre-understandings or
prejudices in relation to the interpretive project, and describing
the essential qualities of a phenomenon in ways that extend previous
understandings.

Making Sense of Experiential Phenomena Through Speech and Language

Both Gadamer (1975) and Taylor (1985a) argue that language facilitates understanding. When trying to make sense of their situation, human
beings pose questions and fumble for answers. Through language, they
reflect on the adequacy or otherwise of their interpretations, and in accepting, rejecting, and refining their articulations, they are able to move
from inchoate experiences to ones that more clearly define and facilitate
ongoing understanding and expression. Language embodies tradition by
transmitting meanings pre-reflectively. It also enables reflection on past
experiences and is the medium through which past and present understandings fuse to enable the development of understanding.

Taylor (1985b) describes hermeneutic interpretation as an "attempt
to make sense of an object of study" and suggests further that "the object

must, therefore, be a text or text analog, which is confused, incomplete, cloudy, seemingly contradictory—in some way or another unclear. The interpretation aims to bring light to an underlying coherence or sense" (p. 15). According to Gadamerian philosophy, the goal of interpretation is not simply to retell events as they happened. The researcher–interpreter enters a dialogue with the data, not only asking certain questions but also listening critically for questions that arise from interpreting the texts. A willingness to work between "the familiarity and strangeness" of texts is required in this form of inquiry because "the true locus of hermeneutics is this in-between" (Gadamer, 1996, p. 295). At the same time meaning is given, meaning also remains hidden. Thus analysis requires reflexive engagement within the hermeneutic circle of understanding (Koch & Harrington, 1998).

The texts in my study primarily consisted of New Zealand nurses' accounts of their practice experiences. In order to comprehend these experiential accounts, other texts in the form of nursing's professional literature, media reportage, sociological writing, and New Zealand history, art, and literature contributed to the interpretation by way of contextualizing the experience.

Articulating the Cultural and Historical Horizons of the Participants

Nurses are cultural and historical beings. Their practice reflects the values, interests, and expectations of those with whom they live and interact. New Zealand nurses share understandings with their international counterparts, yet they have also been influenced by understandings that relate specifically to events in New Zealand. The traditional humanitarian philosophies of caring and providing a service that is not restricted by nationality, race, color, age, sex, politics, or social status (ICN, 1989), for example, persist alongside new insights and emphases. New Zealand nurses have responded to a strong bicultural movement toward eliminating social inequalities that are racial in origin. In 1992, the introduction of Kawa Whakaruruhau, or cultural safety,[1] in nursing and midwifery education (Ramsden, 1990; Nursing Council of New Zealand, 1992, 1996, 2002) heightened awareness of the potential for nursing's contribution to more equitable health outcomes. It also created uncertainty and tension within the nursing profession and between nurses and their wider community. Certain experiences, both as a clinician and teacher, in relation to the implementation of Kawa Wha-karuruhau prompted my interest in the phenomenon of nursing people from cultures other than one's own (Spence, 1999, 2001a).

Explicating Pre-Understandings or Prejudices in Relation to the Interpretive Project

Researchers and participants bring their own prejudices or back-grounds of understanding to any research question. What matters to the researcher in relation to the research topic influences the questions asked and not asked of the research participants during data collection. Meanings are disclosed, checked, and co-created through the processes of question and answer. The construction of meaning continues through researcher interaction with the data as further levels of interpretation are developed during analysis. Then readers of the research contribute their interpretations to the research findings.

Hermeneutic researchers need therefore to be mindful of that which has previously been held to be true. If connections between meanings and actions are to be clarified, then assumptions about differing mean-ings and their significance must be carefully questioned. Heidegger (1927/1962) uses the term *pre-understandings* to describe the temporal nature of human understanding, and Gadamer (1975) similarly uses the term *prejudice* when referring to one's background horizons or frames of reference. It is important to note that prejudice, in this context, does not imply something negative or needing elimination. Prejudices are the conditions whereby something is experienced as having meaning. They are not necessarily erroneous or unjustified but rather "constitute the initial directedness of our whole ability to experience" (Gadamer, 1976, p. 9). Prejudices enable and constrain interpretation. In hermeneutic research it is therefore important to clarify, as much as possible, the direction and limitations of the researcher's guiding interests.

Bringing Pre-Understandings to the Surface

A researcher's being interviewed prior to commencing data collec-tion assists identification and documentation of assumptions and expec-tations held in relation to a research topic. The aim is not to *bracket* or set these aside but rather to bring them to the surface through dialogue so that they are more amenable to scrutiny.

As a teacher and nurse, I have been actively involved in the implementation of cultural safety in nursing education. I enjoy the humanness (Travelbee, 1971) and diversity of people and have strong views about justice and equality. Firsthand experience of the complex, controversial, and unpredictable nature of cross-cultural nursing prompted me to explore this topic. In 1993, I undertook a pilot study that focused on how cultural safety was being interpreted and implemented in practice. The study confirmed that the introduction of cultural safety was a contentious issue, and it reinforced my belief that nursing must continue the work of addressing racism in its practice. On the basis that little was known about the values, attitudes, and actions of New Zealand nurses toward people from other cultures, I concluded that an exploratory descriptive study using a hermeneutic approach would be useful and appropriate. I wanted to know what it was like to nurse people from increasingly diverse cultural backgrounds at a time when the attention being given to cultural issues was challenging expectations both within nursing and within New Zealand society. I also suspected that valuable knowledge and expertise lay embedded within the practice of nursing (Benner, 1983, 1984), and I wanted to bring those understandings to the surface.

Ongoing Exploration of Prejudices

By talking with people outside one's circle of familiarity, one can increase one's understanding of personally held prejudices. I consciously sought nonfemale, nonnurse, nonteacher, and non-Pakeha sources of dialogue.[2] Of particular value were my business-oriented husband, a Maori woman with whom I shared an office, and one of my research supervisors, a male sociologist (Spence, 1999).

Proponents of rigorous hermeneutic research (Denzin, 1996; Koch & Harrington, 1998) also recommend that researchers keep a reflexive journal that documents ongoing self-appraisal in relation to the research process. Throughout the study, I documented my experiences as a researcher in a large journal, filling four such journals during the five-year journey. I recorded the decisions I made regarding method and my rationale for doing so. I described my reactions to the participants' stories, the literature I read, and media events pertaining to cultural issues. Using Peshkin's (1988) notion of "warm and cool spots" (p. 18), I wrote about situations and ideas that encouraged me, as well as those about which I preferred not to hear. There were times, for example, when I noted my disappointment at the seeming inability of participants to see the patient's perspective. In relation to one transcript, I jotted:

Nurse X mentions client vulnerability but does not seem to recognize the need for nurses to take more responsibility or make efforts towards compromise and flexibility. It's hard trying to avoid being judgmental about nurses' attitudes and their capacity to be culturally sensitive. (Spence, 1999, p. 84)

Although knowing the difficult circumstances in which this nurse worked, I found myself expecting that the nurse should overcome these barriers in order to meet patients' individual needs. This was a "cool spot" that, along with others, later facilitated articulation of the *things that matter* when nursing a person from another culture.

At a midpoint in the analysis phase, a colleague interviewed me again, this time to surface and record the nature of my changing understandings in relation to the topic. Regular conversations with fellow interpretive researchers also served to clarify both methodological and substantive interpretations (Smythe, Spence, & Gasquoine, 1995). Other important challenges came from clinical colleagues. For example, a comment that not all nurses can, or do, attempt to meet patients' cultural needs prompted me to explore the data for instances when nurses did not seem to make such an effort. I wondered what *not striving* looked like when nursing a person from another culture, and this wondering helped me to illuminate the possibility of different directions and intensities within the theme *striving (toward right)*. It also prompted me to reconsider the contradictions inherent in the phenomenon as a whole, thus facilitating comprehension of the essential place of paradox in cross-cultural nursing.

Describing the Essential Qualities of a Phenomenon in Ways That Extend Previous Understandings

The purpose of research informed by philosophical hermeneutics is to illuminate the manner in which a phenomenon has meaning in context. The process of textual interpretation is one of constant elaboration and synthesis through questioning, exploring words and their contextual meanings, and confronting contradictions. Reading, thinking, writing, and rewriting are essential parts of this process. Patiently employing these practices, the researcher situates, clarifies, challenges, and refines the ideas generated through interaction with the data. Rather than being the final act in the research process, writing is an essential way of giving appearance and body to thinking (van Manen, 1990), because it facilitates the reflective activity that hermeneutic interpretation requires.

Also important is the manner in which ideas are communicated in writing. Words need to be selected carefully and often need explanation. For example, the term *stranger* is common in literature pertaining to cross-cultural interaction. Gudykunst and Kim (1992), Ogletree (1985), Schutz (1971), and Simmel (1950) each refer to "other" as a "stranger." Yet a stranger is a person who is "foreign," "alien," or "peculiar" in some way, and the term *stranger danger* engenders fear for personal safety; thus there is a tendency to avoid strangers.

Nurses have a professional responsibility and social mandate to assist all patients requiring their services. Background philosophies of humanism, holism, and caring motivate nurses in the Western world to come to know their patients individually (Tanner, Benner, Chesla, & Gordon, 1993). Thus priority is placed on reducing distance, and the phenomenon of strangeness is short-lived. I therefore selected the word *difference* rather than *stranger* because the associations with danger and distance were fewer. Moreover, the multifactorial nature of difference meant that the issue was one of degree and that strangeness might, on occasions, be part of difference.

In an effort to stay close to the phenomenon, I also sought to *show* more than *tell* when presenting the findings. Narrative descriptions, interview excerpts, literature, poetry, and researcher journal entries were used to produce a text that vividly portrayed the experience of nursing people from cultures other than one's own. I found that using questions helped to convey the tensions inherent in the experience and, consistent with hermeneutic openness to other possibilities, the terms *yet, although, but,* and *at the same time* helped to illuminate the paradoxical nature of the phenomenon as interpreted.

The Issue of Rigor in Hermeneutic Research

The value of any research depends on the readers' certainty that the processes, findings, and implications stated are trustworthy or rigorous (Gasquoine, 1996; Koch, 1994). If knowledge is the result of a dialogical process between the self-understanding person and that which is encountered, be it text or the expressions of another person, then decisions regarding the rigor of a work are expressions of agreement or commendation, rather than depictions of the interpretation as "correct" or "right" (Smith, 1990). Van Manen (1990) suggests therefore that rigor has less to do with adhering to rules and procedures than it has to do with remaining faithful to the spirit of qualitative inquiry. Particular criteria can be stated, but they can be applied only loosely because they are ultimately tied to the social practices of dialogue and negotiation (Sandelowski, 1993; Smith, 1990).

The strategies recommended for enhancing rigor through writing include treating facts as social constructions, emphasizing showing rather than telling, using multiple viewpoints, varying one's narrative strategies, and explicating one's moral position vis-à-vis radical societal change (Denzin, 1996; Koch & Harrington, 1998). Of utmost importance, however, is the notion that incorporating reflective accounts into the research product enables the reader to decide whether or not the research is plausible.

Data Collection and Analysis

Following approval by Massey University's Ethical Review Committee, 17 participants were selected using intermediary colleagues through professional networks. Their anonymity was maintained through the use of pseudonyms. Twelve participants described themselves as "Pakeha" or as "New Zealanders of European descent." Two said they were "New Zealanders of Maori/Pakeha descent," one stated she had Irish ancestry, and the other mentioned Nga Puhi heritage.[3] One person was Samoan. Another was, in her words, "Eurasian from Singapore," and the final participant was born and schooled in England but had received her nursing education in New Zealand as a mature student. Their employment settings included acute medical and surgical wards, district and public health nursing, pediatrics, mental health, midwifery, and private sector nursing.

Loosely structured interviews using broad, open-ended questions were tape-recorded. The initial question focused on a recent situation in which the participant had nursed someone from another culture, and subsequent questions probed the feelings experienced and sought clarification of the meanings interpreted. The nurses were also invited to reflect on aspects of personal and educational background that they believed influenced the ways in which they practiced. Most participants were interviewed twice. Two focus group interviews were conducted to cross-check and clarify experiential meanings, and several participants also contributed written stories.

Recognizing the need to explore the cultural and historical horizons of the interpreters of the experience (Hekman, 1986), I reviewed the literature to identify the philosophical bases of nursing and placed particular emphasis on the evolving interpretation of the term *culture*. Reviewing curricula documentation, media discussion of cultural safety, and race relations together with New Zealand's sociological and historical literature further enhanced understanding of the phenomenon of interest.

After transcribing the interviews and rereading each participant's interviews together, I wrote descriptions of overall impressions to gain a sense of the whole for each participant. Then, returning to the transcripts, I highlighted significant passages, writing interpretations and questions in the margin. The transcriptions, overall impressions, and interpreted statements were then returned to their owners for validation and further comment. Subsequent telephone conversations served to clarify these interpreted meanings. Bringing the experiential texts and literature together generated further questions. It was by reading, questioning, and experimenting with meanings progressively that the themes and their interrelationships were crystallized through the processes of writing and rewriting.

Nursing People From Cultures Other Than One's Own

In order to illuminate the experience of nursing people from cultures other than one's own, I drew heavily on the experiential narratives of nurses working with people from diverse cultural backgrounds. Registered nurses from the Auckland region were asked to describe their thoughts, feelings, and actions in relation to the phenomenon of interest. The other major source of data comprised the literature contextualizing the nurses' experiences. The ideas presented in relation to the phenomenon are therefore constituted culturally and historically by meanings deriving from being a nurse in New Zealand (Spence, 2001b).

The Evolving Meaning of Culture in New Zealand Nursing

Prior to the mid-1900s, culture was interpreted primarily as *racial other*. Indigenous and settler cultures were perceived to differ in terms of their physical characteristics and levels of civilization. Despite their altruistic intentions, New Zealand nurses were, for the most part, certain of the superiority of their values, beliefs, and practices. Then, inspired by nursing's quest for professional status, nurses in the middle twentieth century began to extend their education in the areas of social science and the humanities.

An appreciation of the relevance of anthropology to nursing began in the 1960s in the United States. Papers by Jewell (1952) and Zborowski (1969), for example, challenged the belief that people should be treated the same, regardless of nationality and cultural background. The establishment of the Council of Nursing and Anthropology in the United States in 1969 demonstrated nursing's interest in cultural issues (Morse, 1988), and in the 1970s, research published by Madeleine Leininger (1970, 1978) introduced the notion of transcultural nursing. However, the theory of culture care that Leininger advocated did not impact significantly in New Zealand. During the 1970s, culture was only minimally recognized under the umbrellas of holism, humanism, and the World Health Organization's definition of health. Nicola North's (1979) monograph exemplifies early development of cultural awareness in New Zealand nursing. The focus of change in this work, though, was the nurse rather than social structures, and its impact was adversely affected by an insufficient groundswell of support.

In the 1980s, prompted by a visible resurgence of Maori interest in the Treaty of Waitangi[4] and legislative encouragement of bicultural developments in education and health, changes began to appear in the cultural emphases of New Zealand nursing publications (Abbott, 1987a, 1987b, 1987c; Hoult, 1984; Sherrard, 1984). Then, in 1988 at a nursing *hui*[5] sponsored by the Department of Education, a Maori student is reported to have asked: "Why can't we go a step further than cultural sensitivity and have cultural safety?" (Wood & Schwass, 1993).

Although cultural sensitivity was acknowledged as essential in nursing, its tendency toward neutrality could not guarantee an end to discriminatory practices. Appropriating the term *safety* highlighted the need for nurses to demonstrate in practice that they were not only academically and clinically competent, and ethically and legally safe, but also that they were culturally safe (Dyck & Kearns, 1995). This notion was supported and extended at subsequent *hui*, prompting the development of a model of education based on negotiated and equal partnership

(Ramsden, 1990). Strategies were also identified to assist the recruitment and retention of Maori nurses. Thus Maori visions of partnership and participation, deriving from the Treaty of Waitangi, melded with nursing philosophies of holism and humanism. In addition to the acknowledged importance of physical, emotional, and legal–ethical safety, cultural safety became a further criterion for the delivery of safe nursing care in New Zealand.

The model for Negotiated and Equal partnership outlined by Ramsden (1990) is founded on a sociopolitical definition of culture. Cultural safety programs focus on attitude change through a process of education that analyzes history and power relationships and seeks change in which the consequences for health are negative. Although access to appropriate services is sought for all culturally different New Zealanders, redressing the long-term consequences of colonialism and monoculturalism for Maori as indigenous people is a priority.

Controversy in New Zealand's media between 1993 and 1996 contributed to the confusion and uncertainty among nurses about the meaning and the implementation of cultural safety (Murchie & Spoonley, 1995; Ramsden, 2000), yet the nursing profession has continued to critically evaluate its practices, and new guidelines have been published by the Nursing Council of New Zealand (1996, 2002). *Culture* in the 1996 document is defined as "the sharing of meaning and understanding" (Nursing Council of New Zealand, 1996, p. 40), and the evaluation of cultural safe practice emphasizes the recipients' experience of care: "Cultural safety is an outcome of nursing and midwifery education that enables safe service to be defined by those who receive the service" (Nursing Council of New Zealand, 1996, p. 10).

The principles of cultural safety are argued to apply in all situations in which there are potential power and status imbalances between the nurse and the patient. Thus culture has meaning in terms of the ways in which patients' cultural understandings may differ from the cultures of nursing and midwifery. Cultural safety programs assist the development of attitudes and behaviors that accommodate and show appreciation of the ways that ethnicity, age, gender, disability, and socioeconomic position impact upon a patient's ability to relate to the healthcare offered. In addition to achieving a shared understanding, culturally safe practice therefore seeks to empower the recipients of health and disability services (Nursing Council of New Zealand, 1996).

In summary, the nature of New Zealand nurses' understanding of culture has moved from being well intentioned but assimilationist to being anthropologically focused on acquiring knowledge about health beliefs and patterns of behavior, toward a more explicitly political interpretation that recognizes and seeks to eliminate health inequalities that are racial in origin (Spence, 2001b). Assisted by the Treaty of Waitangi, nurses in Aotearoa/New Zealand are extending their understanding of culture,[6] and it is against these background horizons that the phenomenon of nursing a person or people from cultures other than one's own has been interpreted.

Clarification of Key Terms

The term *culture* was purposefully not defined prior to commencing the study reported here. Rather, its meaning emerged in the course of the research, unfolding in a way that is amply described by Ritchie (1992), who stated: "The real stuff of culture in any of its meanings is messy, confusing, paradoxical . . . unclear . . . allowing alternatives and interpretations on some occasions and not on others" (p. 99). The words *other* and *another* are used in the sense of meaning difference. They are not meant to marginalize or put down difference with connotations of cultural supremacy. In this study, *other* refers to a person's (usually the patient's) difference from the nurse.

Research Findings

Representation of the nurses' experiences is described in the themes *Encountering difference, Experiencing tension(s),* and *Striving (toward right).* Common to and pervasive throughout each of these themes are the notions of *prejudice, paradox,* and *possibility.* An overarching theme of *Working with Prejudice, Paradox, and Possibility* thus illuminates the coalescent and contradictory nature of the phenomenon as a whole (Spence, 2001a).

Encountering Difference

Nursing a person or people from cultures other than one's own begins by encountering difference. Encountering difference describes what announces a person as being from another culture and illuminates the significance attached to this descriptor. Nurses understand people from other cultures in relation to themselves, that is, "as different from me," in both a personal sense and in terms of group membership. Such understanding also has a temporal relationship. Difference may be anticipated. Difference is experienced in the moment of happening and can also be understood more deeply on reflection. A name can announce a person as different in the form of a written referral read before the meeting takes place. Differences are also recognized immediately upon meeting in their physical sense. Language, skin color, dress, and gestures are not passed over as they might be in encounters with people from one's own culture. In addition, differences continue to be experienced from a distance as nurses mentally revisit cross-cultural events seeking to more fully understand their meanings and implications.

Encountering difference is also relational. It means experiencing oneself as a nurse in relation to a person who is culturally other. Difference in this study was revealed most often as meaning ethnicity with priority given to Maori because of the Treaty of Waitangi and the poorer health statistics of Maori people (Pomare & de Boer, 1988). Amanda explains: "When I stop and analyze myself transculturally, it's usually in terms of me nursing a Maori patient. For some reason that seems to have higher priority for me, so that is probably most of what I will talk about."

In the Northern Region of New Zealand, Maori constitute 14% of the population, in comparison with 62.3% Pakeha/European. A further 9.8% identify as being from the Pacific Islands, 8% are "Asian," and 6% are "other" (Walker, 1998). Thus, the 23% of the population who are neither Maori nor Pakeha/European are more numerous than are Maori. Yet the nurses' greater emphasis on Maori suggests that being Maori is a difference that matters.

In addition to ethnicity, difference has meaning in relation to gender, social class, education, occupation, and place of domicile. Jo notices that Indian males are less receptive than other men to female nurses:

In my experience they get on much better if they have a male nurse. If you're female they're not going to tell you anything. It's just: "Get down there, woman, I want my lunch." . . . That's not to say they're all like that. It's just that I've found it works better with a male nurse. They'll talk on a deeper level.

These are practice observations from a psychiatric setting, and Jo's generalization suggests that similar situations have been experienced previously. Although the patient's responses differ from that to which she may feel entitled, Jo is neither offended nor expecting all Indian men to be the same. In addition to considering ethnic difference, Jo is taking the man's illness into account. Of utmost importance is this person's need to relate therapeutically to someone. Jo knows that challenging or rejecting the man's behavior might compromise his progress toward health. She therefore accepts that it is in his interest to be nursed by a male. Thus, although inclusive of gender, nationality, and illness, the difference that matters is that of the person's vulnerability.

Cultural variations relating to rural and urban socialization experiences are also recognized:

I notice quite a difference in people who are brought up in the city. This is really generalizing, but city people seem to be more forward about asking for things or telling you something is not right . . . whereas I've found people who are from the little towns, in the middle of nowhere, sort of just sit there quietly.

The concern again is that the care of those who are less assertive may be compromised. Even within the same city, differences are acknowledged to exist. Comparing district nursing in the poorer areas with experiences in affluent areas, Beverley explains that people in more affluent areas "expect you to be there at 9 AM and if you're not there by five past, they're on the phone finding out where you are. They have quite rigid expectations of you."

Socioeconomic difference is also recognized in other ways. Jane remembers attending a community meeting in which discussion centered on ways of breaking the poverty cycle occurring among Maori people:

Ultimately it came back, not to a specifically ethnic culture, but to the culture of where you live. It might be that in the area you live, everyone is unemployed, that they are on benefits and that there is that dependency cycle. . . . Often that's a stronger culture than someone's ancestral roots.

Of greatest significance, however, was the potential for such differences to prevent effective communication and thus to jeopardize standards of care. Beverley, for example, finds it difficult to "know how much they're taking in." Lara worries "that they lie there frightened and not understanding," and Amanda explains that when there is a language barrier she has to simplify things more, and the information is compromised: "I think, 'Gosh, Is this really giving them all the information in a really informed way?' That's the difference that seems greater."

Questions also arose as to the meanings of identity and difference. It was the difference between the nurses' culture and the patients' culture that was pivotal. Culture was difficult to define because of its multifaceted and evolving nature. Thus, it was difference, rather than culture, that mattered. Nurses experience greater uncertainty when nursing people from other cultures. Difference brings about difficulty because the nurse cannot assume that the patient will share, or be able to understand, the background horizons that inform nursing practice. For instance, Theresa knows that misunderstanding is possible even when the same words are used. The word *sick*, for example, is likely to mean being spiritually unwell to someone from Samoa, rather than feeling nauseated as it may to the nurse. Health priorities also sometimes differ.

For a small section of the community I work with (predominantly Maori and Pacific Islanders), there's apathy towards health care. I've looked at it from the view that it's not a priority for them. School sores [impetigo], for example: Often the family have lived with those for a long time and can't see the importance of treating them. . . . They know they will heal eventually and they don't worry about the scarring.

Difference presents as difficulty because the task of finding solutions that meet diverging expectations is far from straightforward. Jane talks of "treading the fine line," of always having to consider others affected by a decision and what the outcomes might be. Furthermore, this meaning has implications for the patient because difference is anticipated to constrain establishment of the nurse–patient relationship regarded by nurses to be so fundamentally important in the delivery of nursing care. People from other cultures are therefore perceived to be more vulnerable; paradoxically, nurses find a greater need to communicate and establish trust alongside their increased difficulty of doing so.

Experiencing Tension(s)

Tension is an ever-present part of the experience of nursing someone from another culture, and congruent with hermeneutic philosophy, *experiencing* in this theme means being in a world of multiple meanings and shaping and being shaped by differing understandings that are always evolving. Born of a moral imperative to engage willingly with others and to assist those in need (Bishop & Scudder, 1990; Henderson, 1966), nurses experience tension intrapersonally, interpersonally, and in their relationships with the wider community. They come into closer contact with individual differences than do people from many other occupational groups. The fact that nursing care is often intimate and intrusive in nature (Lawler, 1991) further increases the tension for both parties in the encounter. Placing the *body* centrally in nursing, Lawler suggests that nurses must know about the taken-for-granted rules that govern the body in society. But when nursing a person from another culture, questions arise as to which rules and whose culture. Consciously and unconsciously, nurses must live with and work through these and other differences.

Experiencing has meaning in terms of reflecting on past encounters, as well as relating in the moment to others perceived to be different. The notions *tension* and *tensions* describe the subjective and intersubjective nature of the experience. Experiencing tension therefore means being played by one's emotions and ethical responsibilities, both personally and professionally. It means having to make decisions about to whom, when, and how best to respond. Tugged in one direction and then in another, nurses may be certain of their purpose yet uncertain of the most appropriate way of achieving that purpose (Spence, 2001a).

Such tension is experienced on multiple levels simultaneously. Intrapersonal conflicts are derived from competing social discourses and priorities. Aware of the increased vulnerability of many persons from other cultures, nurses often feel concern on behalf of these patients. They worry about them and want the best for them. Yet, when the client's values differ from those of the mainstream, the nurse often feels torn or caught between the social views predominating and those of the patient. Tension is experienced in the form of the ongoing dilemma of how best to accommodate everyone's expectations.

I think the biggest stresses that I find are situations like the man down the far end of the ward with troops and troops and troops of visitors before visiting hours. Kids everywhere—all about two feet high with lovely hard shoes on and it gets to the stage where, as much as you want to be culturally sensitive, you are being insensitive to everybody's else's needs, and that's the sort of situation that drives me nuts.

The families get angry and agitated. They say, "Oh, but I've come from up north and my Dad's sick," and I think, "But everybody else in the ward is sick too and your children are running up and down the corridors" and I do feel like tearing my hair out because no matter how sensitive I try to be, sometimes it feels like a kick in the face.

I think, "Here we are helping your Dad. We've let you come in before visiting . . ." and I feel abused and taken for granted.

This story does not describe an isolated experience. Theresa is generalizing as she recounts "situations like the man down the far end of the ward" and openly acknowledges the stresses they induce. The extra people, their noise, the length of the ward, and the demands being made seem overwhelming, and in trying to meet the cultural needs of some clients, Theresa risks undermining the needs of others who require rest in a well-managed environment. There is a sense that Theresa feels she is losing control and that there is little chance for improvement. The design of the ward does not fully support its users' needs. It has long corridors and no carpets, and there are rules that must continually be explained and either enforced or relaxed. Anxious and frustrated, Theresa hopes, but does not communicate her expectation, that the visitors will understand and appreciate both her situation and that of the other patients; thus, achieving reciprocal understanding is unlikely.

Theresa is in an acute hospital setting. In her second year post registration, she is the nurse in charge on this shift. The responsibilities she feels create tension, the intensity of which is exemplified in her language. The word *troops* is used repetitively to describe the visitors, and kids everywhere, "two feet high," add vividly to a picture of disorder. Her ironic use of "lovely, hard shoes" reveals feelings of frustration, and the violent metaphors, "driving me nuts," "tearing my hair out," and "a kick in the face," suggest significant levels of emotional stress and negative tension. Yet they may also constitute carefully expressed negative prejudice.

Shaped culturally and historically, both as a member of the nursing profession and as a nurse employed in an acute care context, Theresa has embodied the need to prioritize the physical safety of her patients. However, she also wants to meet their health needs more holistically and to do so in a way that is equitable. Theresa accepts responsibility for the patients' well-being. She is in charge of the ward, and her role is that of ensuring the smooth delivery of nursing care to everyone. But tension is inevitable where values and priorities differ (Gudykunst & Kim, 1992), and it is exacerbated when decisions are required as to whose values and which priorities take precedence. While it is possible to provide a broad range of nursing interventions more in accordance with notions of holism in a well-staffed and philosophically supportive working environment, this is problematic in the present climate of cost containment and medically dominated healthcare. New Zealand's re-structured health delivery system is "dominated by corporate interests and sustained by the power of a select group of providers, notably physi-cians" (Tilah, 1996, p. 20). Englehardt (1985) suggests that the position between doctors, patients, and employing institutions creates difficulties for the nurse. Perhaps Theresa's feelings of tension relate to being *caught in-between* in this way?

Associated with similar interpretations of practice is the notion that nurses have their own legitimate area of authority and expertise. The clinically focused research of Benner (1984) and Benner and Wrubel (1989) describes, very specifically, how nurses can make a critical differ-ence for patients and their families. Bishop and Scudder (1991) argue, therefore, that in addition to being *in-between* in the negative sense described by Englehardt, it is also possible for nurses to use their situa-tion to advantage. Bishop and Scudder conclude that "practising nurses experience nursing primarily as a moral and personal human endeavor" and that "the in-between stance" can also be construed as a position of "privilege" from which nurses can "foster the team decisions required in health care ethics" (Englehardt, 1985, p. 68). How easy is it for nurses to advocate for patients from other cultures in the manner suggested by Bishop and Scudder? Is it possible that, when living through dilem-mas in the moment, feelings of frustration and anxiety may be related to the tension between feeling caught and being unable to negotiate an outcome that satisfies the needs of all parties? Do nurses simultaneously experience both forms of *in-between*? Is this the meaning of tension in cross-cultural nursing practice?

Referring to immigrants from other cultures, the following state-ment by Anne illuminates a tension between society and nursing:

Yes, part of me thinks "why are we bringing all those refugees into the country?" Yet when I visit a Somali family that doesn't come into it. I'm glad they're here and safe. That one-to-one relationship is where nursing is at.

In nurse–patient interaction, the lack of knowledge by both parties about each other's expectations contributes feelings of dissonance; stress is increased further by inflexible and unaccommodating environments and people. In an ante-natal clinic with predominantly Maori and Pacific Island clientele, Pamela experiences tension relating to the clinic's failure to accommodate difference: It's obvious . . . because when they walk in at 9:15 for a 9 a.m. appointment the first thing they get is a lecture. The clinic might have one or two posters on the wall but it's European."

Alongside the tensions, however, are experiences that are cherished. Anne talks about "something lovely" when working with Samoans that she finds difficult to express: "I can't put it into words—a richness and gentleness that they have. When I go and sit with a Samoan woman, talking about her child, it can be a magical thing." Tara feels great when an Indian man tells her that she is "a good nurse" and that he likes coming back, and Jo feels valued when she walks in the door, and "immediately someone is hanging off your arm."

Although many experiences are affirming and serve to encourage the nurse, these positive feelings are encountered paradoxically with less positive feelings. Feelings of anxiety, ignorance, embarrassment, concern, doubt, anger, guilt, fear of rejection, frustration, and powerlessness are interspersed with feelings of privilege, admiration, satisfaction, and joy. When Anne summarizes the experience of nursing people from other cultures by saying, "there is a whole gamut of experiences, rich and frustrating," she is describing the demanding, challenging, frustrating, and rewarding nature of this work.

Striving (Toward Right)

Nursing, in the face of difference and its related uncertainties, requires greater effort than does nursing people from one's own culture. The participants in this study repeatedly used the word *trying* when describing their efforts to provide appropriate care. They spoke, for example, of "trying to be as unthreatening as possible," "trying to learn Maori protocol," and "trying to be there" for patients and families. Jane talked about "doing my utmost for the family [explaining that] there are times when I go further than the job involves." Jo said: "There are a lot more things that I don't take for granted. There is a lot more learning . . . watching body language, what they do, trying to pick up on how they are feeling." Anne, referring to cross-cultural communication difficulties, explained that: "It takes more energy and time." Although *trying* was the word most frequently used by the participants, I believed that its cumulative meaning demanded a stronger descriptor. The term *striving* was selected because it more adequately captured the diverse and ongoing nature of the nurses' efforts.

In this theme, the meaning of nursing a person from another culture as striving (toward right) is revealed through the interrelated notions of "striving as a hermeneutic response," "striving as conscious and deliberate action," "the being and doing of striving," *and* "struggling against hindrances."

Striving as a Hermeneutic Response

Puzzled by the diverse and ongoing efforts made by the participants, I wondered why they continued to try. It seemed as if those who stayed rather than left the nursing profession were compelled to continue their efforts. Levinas (1984) suggests that the face of the other makes an appeal, or ethical demand, and van Manen (1999) speaks of "caring-as-worrying" when exploring the meaning of caring in nursing. Referring also to Levinas's notion of "other," van Manen suggests that in being face to face with other, one is "taken hostage" in a way that is initially beyond one's control. In a similar way, the person from another culture, by being present, asks something of the nurse. The person not only asks for care but also that his or her heritage and condition be respected (Shabatay, 1991). Striving as a hermeneutic response therefore describes a pre-reflective call of caring responsibility to other (Berman, 1994).

Striving as Conscious and Deliberate Action

Nurses also strive because there are personal and professional standards of practice to be maintained. Striving as conscious and deliberate action derives from the values brought by the nurse to cross-cultural encounters. Anne speaks of patient well-being as her major goal: "I would put well-being above everything." Teresa believes "practicing holistically is the essence of nursing," and Lara says, "the way I behave has to do with basic respect for people and that they are different. I would leave nursing if I had to clump them all together." Without exception, moreover, each of the participants also found the nurse–patient relationship to be central in the practice of nursing.

The nurses in this study strive because they believe that establishing interpersonal relationships is crucial to the purpose of nursing and that being accepted personally by patients assists the development of a good working relationship. They strive to actively uphold their beliefs about the rights of all patients to receive care that is equally respectful. Their stories also provide evidence of hope for a better future for New Zealand and its people.

Amanda speaks, for example, of

trying to make an effort. . . . Yes. I really want to be part of this country so I believe I have put in an effort. . . . I feel accountable because if we have a Treaty . . . then I feel I have to uphold my end of it.

Born in New Zealand, Amanda describes herself as a Pakeha New Zealander. Underpinning her efforts is an awareness of bicultural issues and hopes for the positive accommodation of cross-cultural differences. Thus, Amanda strives consciously and deliberately toward this end.

The Being and Doing of Striving

Striving also encompasses the nurses' *trying to be* and *ways of doing* when nursing a person from another culture. The being is not separate from the doing, and both are oriented toward *getting it right*. Nurses strive toward a standard of care that meets the patient's and their own expectations as well as those of the providing institution. The *being* of striving underpins the *doing* aspects of striving. It comprises the essential, often taken-for-granted attitudes such as willingness, respect, compassion, self-awareness, and openness toward others.

It's an approach. It's a way of being a nurse. A lot of it is the way I go about things. The way I am as a person. You might not be able to put into words exactly what it is, but it's about the way you talk or act.

Striving can show itself through creative use of the imagination. There are times when the nurse uses strategies of visualization to assist the understanding of the patient's situation. Beverley imagines that the patient is someone of special importance:

The way I nurse people is to look at them as if they are a relative of mine and to think, "How would I like my mother to be treated?" . . . I try to keep that attitude, so that I have compassion and feeling for what I am doing.

Lara uses herself as the yardstick: "I have sometimes thought, 'Imagine myself in that situation. Whatever that person is feeling is real for them.' And if I were lying there, I wouldn't want to be told this, that, and the other thing." Tara draws specifically on a past experience:

I felt sorry for her not being able to understand English. . . . I have been in that situation. I can understand how difficult it is to learn. So, even though I was frustrated, I thought "What if it were me? It would be the same."

In each of these situations, the nurses seem to be searching for an aspect of familiarity among the differences. They are striving within their imagination, both retrospectively and prospectively, for something within their personal experience that will help begin their relationship with the person from another culture.

Changing things in oneself is another aspect of striving toward right. Changing involves adapting and compromising in an effort to meet multiple needs and expectations. Sometimes it means becoming more like the patient. Anne feels herself "change" when she visits Maori homes. "I think I sort of try to become a bit more Maori when I go to a Maori home. It's like part of me takes on, not consciously, but being a bit more like them, I suppose." She then reflects that this happens similarly in her own culture. "When I go to an employer meeting, I'm different again."

It would seem that, even though nurses value uniqueness and difference, there are times when they make themselves more like others in an effort to foster the building of relationships. A recent exploration of nurse–patient interaction by Aranda and Street (1999) refers to nurses' references to the term *chameleon*. Used by Australian nurses to describe the way in which they alter their approaches to people and practice "in order to become the sort of nurse the person required" (p. 75), the notions of *empathy* and *being a chameleon* support the behaviors described above. Also congruent with this study's substantive findings is the inherent tension between the nurses' desire to be genuine and their need to be congruent with patients' wishes without subjugating their professional responsibilities.

The doing of striving is exemplified by *little* or *basic things* that are cumulatively important: "being around a bit more," "listening," "thinking about how to use space." It means "identifying what is important for the person rather than following guidelines written by someone else," "seeking permission," "using a person's name correctly," and "not calling the shots." These are thoughtful, seemingly simple yet critically important nursing behaviors.

However, striving coexists with "non-striving," or "deficient and neglectful modes" of concern (Heidegger (1927/1962). Discussing the role of the cultural liaison service, Amanda knows that this service is misused.

We just abuse them. . . . On the admission form . . . you tick and date that you have contacted them. We're quite good at passing the buck. . . . We assume that once we've introduced them and we've got the whanau[7] room for them to stay in, then everything will be all right.

Amanda is referring to the occasions when nurses minimize their involvement in meeting patients' cultural needs by referring them to a specialist service. She is describing the everyday world in which other matters claim nursing attention.

Struggling Against Hindrances

There are numerous hindrances to striving in the cross-cultural context. Nurses struggle with their own negative prejudices, the multiple demands of their job, and the constant need to prioritize. Constraints of time and cost relate to accessing the interpreter service. The attitudes and priorities of other members in the health team require consideration, and the conflicting and contradictory nature of wider society is also always present.

Working with Prejudice, Paradox, and Possibility

Exploration of the phenomenon of nursing a person or people from cultures other than one's own is further revealed in the coexistence and interplay of prejudices, paradox, and possibilities at intrapersonal and interpersonal levels as well as in relation to professional and other social discourses. Gadamer (1996) articulates the notion of prejudice in terms of the unconscious judgments and prior understandings that influence interpretation. Our prejudices originate from past experiences and influence our ongoing interpretations. They enable us to make sense of the situations in which we find ourselves, yet they also constrain understanding and limit the capacity to come to new or different ways of understanding. It is this contradiction that makes prejudice paradoxical (Spence, 1999, 2001a).

Paradox describes situations that initially seem to be incongruent but on closer examination are proved to have connection. In the context of this study, paradox describes the dynamic interplay of numerous tensions. Nurses may, for example, feel bound to nurse all patients regardless of differences in ethnicity, class, and gender, as nursing codes of ethics have specified (ICN, 1989). They must also accept and actively uphold differences between individuals and groups of individuals (Lipson & Meleis, 1985; Meleis, 1996; Ramsden, 1995).

The ethical command to respond to all persons equally is a powerful, enabling prejudice. Nurses also find necessary an understanding of the ways in which people's specific nursing needs vary and a concomitant capacity to provide care differently in accordance with these needs. Paradox acknowledges the existence and interpenetration of opposites, not as dichotomies, but as variances, checks, and juxtapositions that recognize the contribution and relevance of more than one understanding.

Allen (1995) reminds us that being a nurse means participating in services that do not meet the key health needs of large sections of the community. He argues that nursing needs to engage in analysis and critique of the political and social conditions of practice. Yet the traditions embodied existentially (Gadamer, 1996), in this case by women as nurses (Rodgers, 1994), do not make the involvement in politics easy. If equitable outcomes are to be achieved in healthcare, egalitarian ideals need to be understood in relation to the numerous factors that reduce this possibility.

In this study, possibility acknowledges the infinite nature of understanding. The potential for new and different understandings derives from the human capacity to interpret and communicate. Gadamer (1996) refers to "true prejudice" as that which prompts questioning and thus keeps open the possibility of new understanding. Yet such questioning is paradoxical for in posing a question, both openness and limitation coexist because the openness to a question is limited by its horizon. Even questioning that is inclusive of what can be seen and not seen remains partial and is infinitely ongoing. Possibility therefore describes potentialities, which are diverse, and truth, which is infinite. It predicates a condition of openness that always operates within a limited horizon. In relation to nursing a person from another culture, possibility can therefore mean getting it right, getting it wrong, and simultaneously getting it both right and wrong.

Stories From Practice That Help Explicate

The nurses in the following stories live and work with prejudice, paradox, and possibility. Although the specific form and relative emphasis of these three notions varies, each is always present, and together they describe a wholeness that extends and enriches the previously articulated thematic descriptions.

Alice: Not Helping / Wanting to Be Better Prepared

I particularly remember looking after a Lebanese gentleman and his family. He had come in with an acute illness and a potentially fatal prognosis and neither he nor his wife spoke a lot of English, although they understood a limited amount. Their sons spoke and understood English well.

I noticed that any staff involved in looking after this man seemed to get pulled into a very intense caring relationship with the family—more intense than I've seen with other cultures and I didn't think it was just them as individuals. It seemed to me that people from that part of Europe or the Middle East were more passionate. Their facial expressions, they wanted so much. They were what I call "emotional people," wearing their hearts on their sleeves, and I wondered if looking after Italian people might be similar.

What really struck me was that there were no resources. I didn't know who or where to turn to for information on how to care for these people in a cultural sense. They seemed easily offended. If you didn't accept food when they offered it to you, no matter how fast you were speeding down the ward, or how many drips or things you had in your hands, they got very offended. It was almost as if they wanted you to really like them because if you didn't, they thought they wouldn't get good care. And maybe where they come from, that is what happens.

Then, for a time, I couldn't look after this man. He had developed some nasty infections that placed my other patients at risk. But trying to explain this to the family—that it wasn't that I did not want to look after him. They were very hurt and wouldn't talk to me. I'm sure there was a major cultural component. It was more than a family in grief. I knew they didn't understand and I tried to support them. But time, in work hours didn't allow searching for things and it wasn't the interpreter service that I needed. I felt I needed to be better prepared.

In this story the interplay of the previously described themes is highly visible. Encountering difference has meaning for Alice in terms of the perceived greater demands being made on the nursing staff by this family. Alice experiences tension in the form of feelings of confusion, frustration, and guilt. Aware that she does not understand the meaning of the family's expressions, she wants to be better prepared and tries to find resources to assist her. Like the family, she too strives to be understood and liked; yet she is unable to help and feels harshly judged because the family cannot understand her position.

The prejudices that constrain cross-cultural understanding in this scenario outweigh those that enable. Alice seems to assume that because the sons are fluent in English, the family should be able to understand and accept the priorities and practices of the healthcare system with which they are engaging. Although there is evidence that Alice questions her interpretation of the family's more passionate expressions, she attributes to cultural difference greater significance than the possibly universal emotional pain of a potentially fatal prognosis. In interpreting their behavior in terms of difference, she paradoxically sees, but does not see, the family's pain. Furthermore, in seeking resources to improve her knowledge of cultural difference, Alice seems to have overlooked the potential for her own relationship with the family to provide this information. Her busyness with "drips and things" and fears of "infection risk" appear to have unwittingly precluded the development of trust with this family. Styles (1991) suggests that nurses, more than any other group of professionals, experience the paradoxes, dilemmas, and challenges at the jagged interface between science and service. Perhaps, in prioritizing medical science and technology, Alice is underplaying the importance of human care processes in nursing (Watson, 1988).

Yet the issues are not as simple as they might seem. Overlapping hermeneutic circles of understanding and misunderstanding coexist. There is, on the part of the nurse and the family, *reaching out*, while at the same time there is *calling or pulling back*. The family wants support and needs care. The nurse similarly wants to support and needs to give care. But there is lack of understanding by both parties. Confusion exists on the part of the family in relation to the nurse's behaviors. The nurse is also struggling to understand the responses of the family.

Forrest (1989) notes that when situations become difficult, nurses often distance themselves from the patient by providing limited or routine physical care. In "being busy" one can avoid the deeper and more challenging levels of involvement. However, it is only when we strive to understand others' perspectives that we can begin to discover concerns that are critically important to us as well (Taylor, 1994). Lampert (1997) suggests that mutual understanding becomes possible through the dialectical relationship between identity and difference. A hermeneutics of conflict is therefore important because it alerts us to the presence of different interpretations. In the next story, sharing conflicting horizons is evident. Distance is recognized through contact, and the interpretation exemplifies the coexistence of both conflict and agreement.

Lara: Knowing, Not Knowing, and Coming to Know

As a nurse in a women's health clinic, Lara is uncertain about whether or not a Chinese woman will be included on the afternoon operating list. The woman is seeing her counselor again. Perhaps the decision to terminate the pregnancy is a difficult one? Then, when her place on the operating list is confirmed, Lara learns that the problem is not one of ambivalence on the woman's part. The husband, who strongly opposes the termination, had been berating his wife since their arrival four hours earlier. In her late 40s, this woman has had two terminations and a child in China. Two more children have been born in New Zealand but of the three, only one is a boy. Through an interpreter, the woman has explained that her husband, irrespective of her age and feelings, wants this pregnancy to continue because having a larger family is acceptable in New Zealand, and the baby might be another boy.

The story, from Lara's perspective, is as follows:

The woman looked exhausted and worn when she came through to meet me pre-operatively. She was thin, and her skin was wrinkled and dry, accentuating her tiredness. As I spent time with the very helpful interpreter, discussing the expectations for self-care post operatively, the woman sat patiently but very sadly. Her frequent eye contact was unusual and now and then she spoke directly to me as if expressing from the heart what was happening to her. Through the interpreter, I learned that she thought the decision to terminate would probably destroy her marriage.

But there was another problem. Unfortunately I had to tell the woman that she had a chlamydia infection. Giving such information is always difficult and it's worse when the person is in a stable relationship. There are huge implications for those who are certain of their own fidelity. The woman took it all in and then sadly turned to me saying [that] she didn't expect her husband would listen or take the prescribed antibiotics.

This patient was in crisis. Feelings of injustice flooded through me. I found myself judging the husband for being selfish, nonsupportive and abusive. Regardless of their cultural beliefs this woman was being punished unfairly. And all this in a different world.

Then, again through the interpreter, I learned of her feelings of guilt at having taken up so much of our time and of her shame that something so private had come to involve so many people (the charge nurse had previously been with the interpreter). I felt deeply for her. At this hugely distressing time, one that would have implications for the rest of her life, she was explaining that she had not received this sort of attention during the terminations in China. Although she seemed greatly to appreciate our support, she was embarrassed that the care had been so concentrated and lengthy.

The woman left immediately [after] she recovered post operatively. I understood her need to go quickly. I respected that she had had enough and I admired her courage. Of the many people I have nursed, this woman and this experience have remained unique.

The prejudices that enable Lara's actions are again both personal and professional in origin. The intensity of Lara's emotional response to the woman's situation reveals the importance of personally held values pertaining to justice and equality. Matters such as the child's gender, the age at which pregnancy may no longer be safe for women, and whether husbands have the right to be unfaithful yet authoritarian in relation to their wives create tension in Lara. There is evidence of heightened awareness and concern on her part, and she is alert to information that will help her to decide how best to respond in this situation.

Lara's nursing background provides skills in observation. She listens and watches, relying heavily on the contribution of nonverbal cues to assist her developing understanding. Lara notices characteristics in the woman that prompt her continued engagement. Eye contact and the direct appeal by the woman to her, rather than to the interpreter, communicate an intensity and passion that are interpreted by Lara to mean crisis for the woman. Recognition of the woman's social and emotional needs means that attention is given to aspects of care beyond the physical nursing requirements associated with a termination of pregnancy.

In this scenario, the combination of personal and professional skill and concern is enabling. Yet the prejudices involved can just as easily obtrude and limit the capacity to respond appropriately. Inherent in the development of professional expertise is the possibility that the more technically expert the nurse becomes, the harder it is to "switch off" this embodied expertness in order to be authentically present (Lashley, Neal, Slunt, Berman, & Hultgren, 1994) with the patient. The constant struggle to combine the being and doing aspects of nursing is evident in the subthemes *experiencing tension* and *striving*. From a personal perspective, difference has meaning for Lara in terms of conflicting values, especially in relation to women's rights. She struggles to accept that these are her values: that they may not be shared, and in striving to remain open and present for the woman, she learns that there are times when people may be helped most by a carefully made decision not to intervene further.

The experience is tension filled and paradoxical. The interplay between knowing and not knowing is constant. Lara knows she will have a role in the woman's care and has beliefs, based on her professional education and experience, about what is "best" in relation to this, but she is uncertain about the woman's specific needs and thus does not know what the woman expects and requires of her. Lara knows, therefore, that she needs to know more, and in the process of coming to know, she develops new understandings.

Also present is the tension inherent in the call to meet patients' social and emotional needs for well-being. It could be argued in this situation that responsibility for the social and emotional needs of this woman lies with the counselor rather than the nurse, and indeed having to retell her story clearly added to the woman's distress. Yet it is Lara's personal and professional prejudices that enable her continued engagement with this woman. Perhaps not recognized is the impossibility of ever fulfilling such expectations, but without contact with this woman's difference, Lara would not have learned the inappropriateness of the support she offered. Paradoxically then, the coexistence of *knowing, not knowing,* and *being unknowing* makes possible a new and different knowing.

Munhall (1993) suggests that "the art of unknowing" is an essential pattern of "knowing" in nursing (p. 125). Unknowing is described as a condition of openness that minimizes the risk of premature closure to other possibilities. The nurse needs to be unknowing in order to hear the other person's perspective. An "air of mystery" and an "attitude" that is "open to alternative interpretations" is adopted (Munhall, 1993, p. 127), and in coming to "know" the patient's world, the nurse's knowing is temporarily suspended. Yet the idea that one's assumptions and beliefs can be held in abeyance is limited by the impossibility of standing outside one's own horizon or frame of reference. Do we therefore become prisoners of ethnocentrism (Taylor, 1995)? Can understandings change and develop as argued by the proponents of Gadamerian philosophy?

Taylor (1995) suggests that the possibility of coming to know another's perspective lies in being able to articulate and question our implicit understandings. Identifying and contrasting these "home understand-ings" (p. 150) with those of another person reveals them to be one possibil-ity among others. The hope that ethnocentrism can be overcome therefore derives from the potential for these contrasts to challenge and go beyond previous understandings.

Speaking of the possibility that in challenging others' understandings we may also challenge our own, Taylor contends further that under-standing is inseparable from criticism, which in turn is inseparable from self-criticism. It is possible that Lara, in reexamining her own values, comes to see with renewed understanding the tension between women's rights to justice collectively and one woman's rights as an individual to choose her course of action. When Lara hears of the woman's shame and embarrassment at the lengthy and concentrated care being offered, it is also possible that Lara reevaluates nursing notions of holism for their appropriateness. Lara seems to recognize that in showing concern for the woman's social and emotional needs she, like the husband, is contributing to the woman's suffering, albeit in a different way.

Lara's compassion and her capacity to listen and hear and to see personal and professional values in a new light, together with the respect and admiration developed for the woman in this story, are crucial in enabling Lara to let go, yet remain hopeful, in this situation. Moreover, it is through engaging with and reflecting upon coexisting differences and tensions that the paradoxes become evident. Lara's horizon of un-derstanding grows beyond what it was. A sufficiently common under-standing develops that allows both horizons to be, and this experience, although not fully satisfying for Lara in terms of getting it right, is epi-phanic for the learning it provides.[8]

This story amply illustrates that foreign cultures are potentially an important source of learning and, furthermore, that pre-understandings do not necessarily "lock us into ethnocentric prisons" (Taylor, 1995, p. 149). Inherent in encountering others as different is the possibility of exposure to new understandings. If we respond to our feelings of uncer-tainty and dissonance by reexamining our implicit beliefs, changes in understanding become possible. If we work consciously to identify and articulate the contrast between these prejudices and those of the other person, "distortive understandings" can be reevaluated. Broader and new possible understandings therefore arise through comparisons and contrasts that "let the other be" (Taylor, 1995, p. 149). Moreover, as is seen in the next story, the memorable nature of the event suggests that self-understanding is also enhanced through contact with others who are different.

Jane: A Precious Moment

The following experience, which triggers the vivid recollection by Jane of "a precious moment," took place four years prior to its telling. For Jane, the moment was special because, although she and her patient's mother, Sulu, came from different worlds, they were united by a common goal in which ethnic boundaries lost their significance. They were *"just human beings together."*

Sulu, Samu's mother, was born and educated in a Samoan village. She is married and has little money but is strongly supported by her religion and the Samoan community. For her, New Zealand, the hospital, and the intensive care unit are new and difficult. Jane is older than Sulu. She is Pakeha, is single, and has a career that enables her to feel confident within an intensive care environment.

I knew Samu from one month old until he died at 18 months, caring for him on almost every shift. I was there at every milestone. I watched him gain head control, learn to sit, say his first word, and I was as proud as his parents of the achievements he made. My love for him was like love for my brother.

As the trust between his mother, Sulu, and I deepened, she was able to confide in me some of the stressful times in her marriage. We grew, learning from one another. I grew as a person and she developed confidence in the technical aspects of Samu's care, becoming able to accept and understand machines bleeping, tubes and central lines in different places, ileostomy bags, etc.

I was at home the night he died suddenly. A nurse rang to tell me the news and that Sulu wanted me to come in. I went completely numb. Then I felt hot all over. I couldn't hear my partner's question, only stammering "I need to get to the hospital." We drove in silence.

I went to the whanau room where Samu's family and church members were gathering. Other nurses who were on duty were there. I remember slipping off my shoes. There were lots of shoes and the people, lining the four walls, were looking at me.

I saw Sulu holding Samu. He had his best Sunday wear on—a little tuxedo and tiny black patent shoes. Sulu beckoned and I haltingly took steps to get there. Everything around me dulled. As I knelt before her, all I could see was the two of them together. Then Sulu leaned forward asking if I wanted to hold Samu and, stunned by this gesture, I cried. I couldn't see a thing but felt his warmth as she placed him in my arms. All the machines and tubes were gone. Samu was free at last. I didn't speak and can't remember how long I held him.

Life is so precious and he had enriched my life. His mother was giving me the opportunity to grieve and say goodbye. I have never forgotten that closeness and acceptance of death. It was a precious moment.

Stories like this offer a glimpse of the meaning of a shared humanity that encompasses difference. Levinas (1987) speaks of something passing from one to another as human beings are seen as being in need. Beverley Taylor (1994) suggests that nurses and patients relate to one another as different people with unique backgrounds, yet they are often able to find commonality in their humanness. In describing this commonality as "ordinariness in nursing" (p. 33), a paradox emerges in that the ordinary can also be seen to be extraordinary. Travelbee (1971) argues that the emotions of "love, tenderness and compassion are readily comprehended by individuals from all cultures and backgrounds" (p. 19), and Paterson and Zderad (1988) describe the human capacity of "becoming more" (p. 15). Drawing on Buber's (1958) notion of "I and Thou," Paterson and Zderad (1988) state that "man becomes more through his relations with others" (p. 44).

Within this story these authors' ideas each have meaning in terms of possibility, yet the experience may be regarded as atypical for several reasons. Jane's use of the term *caring for* rather than *nursing*, the analogy "like love for my brother," and the request that she come from home immediately after Samu's death suggest that this is not an everyday nursing encounter. Numerous factors have combined to contribute to the epiphanic nature of the experience. Samu's illness, the availability of a whanau room, and the prolonged period of contact between the family and staff supported the development of trust and reciprocal learning. Jane's knowledge of child development, her technical expertise, and her willingness to teach are enabling prejudices that derive from her nursing background. The notion of "brotherly love" implies a genuinely rewarding relationship, and as is evident in nursing literature, *caring* has been reclaimed as centrally significant to the profession of nursing (Benner & Wrubel, 1989; Leininger, 1978; Watson, 1985). These philosophies coalesce with Jane's personal capacity for compassion and concern. But in addition to this, Jane feels enriched. Her understanding of the meaning of life and death deepens at Sulu's feet.

In Peshkin's (1988) language, this was a "warm" story. It was one that I responded to positively and was a sort that I would like to see more often because of its positive outcomes. The experience of exploring its meanings was therefore enjoyable, and yet it also engendered feelings of regret: in my experience, the opportunity for sustained engagement with patients was rare in acute care settings.

Jane's and Sulu's backgrounds were very different, and had it not been for Samu's illness, their paths would have been unlikely to cross. Jane values the experience for what she learned from it. She also believes, and is pleased, that the learning has been reciprocal. Yet pleasure and sadness are intertwined. Perhaps she and Sulu had lived through similar tensions. Each had experienced shock, hope, friendship, and loss, although they had done so from different vantage points.

Slunt (1994), with reference to Paterson and Zderad (1988), contends that "beautiful moments give meaning to nursing" (p. 57). Gadamer (1986) speaks, too, of "the relevance of the beautiful" and the potential for unexpected encounters with beauty to illuminate truth. Plato, in *Phaedrus*, describes the beautiful as "that which shines forth most clearly and draws us to itself, as the very visibility of the ideal. In the beautiful, presented in nature and art, we experience this convincing illumination of truth and harmony, which compels the admission: 'This is true'" (as cited in Gadamer, 1996, p. 15):

The work of art transforms our fleeting experience into a stable and lasting form of an independent and internally coherent creation. It does so in such a way that we go beyond ourselves by penetrating deeper into the work. (p. 53)

Jane's "precious moment" simply and powerfully expresses something profoundly universal. It offers an assurance that truth and beauty can be encountered in the pain and disorder of reality. It also reminds that, as human beings, we are continually faced with the challenge of learning from each other. The words in this story seem both to *express us* and speak to us. The story illuminates a unity that values difference, that stimulates and nourishes thought and human community. Gadamer (1996) suggests that encounters with art do not leave us feeling the same about life as previously. "The ontological function of the beautiful is to bridge the chasm between the ideal and the real" (Gadamer, 1986, p. 15). In this story, there is genuineness and shared understanding that makes the world seem brighter and less burdensome. Later in our conversation, Jane talks about nursing transcending cultural difference.

"For me, nursing transcends all different cultures because we go in caring and I think that's the one thing all people look for." Is this the "possibility" toward which nurses strive? Are these the beautiful moments that encourage and inspire both learning and the continued commitment toward others in nursing?

Conclusion

These stories have highlighted some of the intrapersonal conflicts experienced as nurses try to integrate personal and professional aspects of their being when nursing people from other cultures. The stories also exemplify attempts to reconcile interpersonal aspects of nursing within a highly political, sociocultural context and illuminate some of the prejudices influencing nursing practice. Prejudice, paradox, and possibility coexist and interpenetrate the themes of encountering difference, experiencing tension, and striving (toward right).

In each of the stories, there is a conscious awareness of difference. There is also evidence of nurses' efforts to develop effective relationships with patients from other cultures. Difference is encountered as difference from the nurse in terms of cultural values and expectations. Difference creates anxiety and tensions that remain a barrier to a greater or lesser extent, depending on the success or otherwise of the establishment of interpersonal trust. The prejudices that facilitate getting it right when nursing a person from another culture include attitudes of respect, concern, openness, and commitment, but equally important are the nurse's self-esteem and clinical competence. Confidence in one's identity is enabling: nurses who possess a strong sense of self-worth and commitment to others experience less tension and are more able to continue striving. A lack of knowledge about culture-specific health beliefs and practices can be a limiting prejudice. Yet, in most cases, the tension associated with this deficiency prompts or enables action that reduces the limitation. Using highly developed skills of observation and interpersonal communication, effort is expended toward coming to know each person's particular needs for nursing.

Concerned for the vulnerability of their patients, the nurses work to reduce that vulnerability. Questions are asked of themselves and of others. Efforts are made to communicate both with the patient and with other people significant in the situation. But in each situation the constraints and opportunities differ. Time availability, attitudes, and the capacity for communication vary. Although nurses may feel confident in terms of their technical skills, they tend to be less confident about their ability to adequately meet the needs of people whose values and beliefs differ from those of the mainstream. Nurses feel uncertain about whether and how they will be accepted by the patient. Their embodied ways of being may not be appropriate, and their environment may not easily facilitate practice that accords with other cultural values.

Despite the sometimes overwhelming feelings of uncertainty experienced in cross-cultural situations, nurses continue to strive both to achieve personal satisfaction and the satisfaction of their patients as individuals. When Jane describes trying to be "so flexible you're not even a shape," she is referring to the need to be open and ready to listen and respond. Gadamer (1996) suggests that the person who listens is fundamentally open. Such readiness opens the possibility for entering the *play*, a questioning and inquiring mode of being that is directed toward escaping the thrall of one's prejudices. Possibility, in this thesis, recognizes that there will undoubtedly be tensions, misunderstandings, and distortions, but this does not mean that pursuing different understandings is impossible; nor does the infinite nature of this process mean that such engagement is without value, because movement between opposites is an inevitable part of the human condition (Rowan & Reason, 1981).

Getting it right involves accepting the invitation to reflect, to reconsider one's responses to another, and, through reflecting on experiences with others, to obtain new insights about self that in turn enable seeing others with fresh understanding (Taylor, 1995). When nursing a person from another culture, therefore, possibility means being alive to the way understanding shapes, disrupts, and facilitates effective practice. It means being willing to wonder, being open to positive and negative judgments, and moving with ever-changing horizons (Gadamer, 1996). It also means being open to the possibility of seeing good in another person's ways, even when these conflict with one's own. The recognition of "two goods" becomes possible where previously "we could only see one and its negation" (Taylor, 1995, p. 163). The possibility of coming to understand others and of continuing one's self-development arises through engaging with people who are culturally other.

The findings of this study recognize that assumptions and values are intrinsic to practice. A nurse's prejudgments or prejudices exist along-side—interpenetrating and at times opposing—other interpretations in-herent in cross-cultural encounters. Statements such as "I don't think I'll ever be comfortable saying: 'Yes, I know how this culture works'" and "I'm convinced you've never got it 'sussed'"[9] (Spence, 1999, p. 177) encapsulate the paradoxical nature of nursing someone from another culture. Being oneself in a way that enables others also to be themselves, under circumstances that are intrinsically never fully knowable, is never likely to be free of tension. Nurses seem, perhaps more so than others, to be faced with learning to live within the play of uncertainty and paradox.

This chapter has explored the anxieties, uncertainty, and satisfaction inherent in cross-cultural nursing, illuminating the often contradictory and ambiguous nature of such work. It offers the notions of prejudice, paradox, and possibility as descriptive of the experience of nursing peo-ple from cultures other than one's own. The findings constitute a contri-bution to the dialectic between science, humanity, reflective practice, professional dialogue, and practical wisdom (Lumby, 1996). They are offered with the expectation that they will provoke further contempla-tion and other possible meanings, for in hermeneutic inquiry all under-standings are open to growth and change. As Gadamer (1996) stated, "It would be a poor hermeneuticist who thought he could have, or had to have, the last word" (p. 579).

Acknowledgments: Sincere thanks go to my colleagues Liz Smythe and Judith McAra-Couper for their encouragement and support during the development of this paper.

Notes

1. *Cultural safety* is defined as "the effective nursing of a person/family from another culture by a nurse who has undertaken a process of reflection on his/her own cultural identity and recognises the impact of the nurse's culture on his/her own nursing practice" (Nursing Council of New Zealand, 1996, p. 9).

2. *Pakeha* is the Maori term given to New Zealanders of European or non-Maori descent. *Maori* is a collective term given to the tribes indigenous to Aotearoa/New Zealand.

3. The Nga Puhi is a northern tribe of Maori descended from Rahiri and based traditionally in the Hokianga region.

4. The Treaty of Waitangi, signed by some Maori and the British Crown in 1840, is the constitutional and legislative structure of New Zealand is founded on this document.

5. *Hui* is the Maori term for a meeting or gathering of people for a purpose.

6. *Aotearoa* means the land of the long white cloud—the name given by Maori to New Zealand.

7. *Whanau* is the Maori term for family. In this context it refers to a room with facilities made available, by the institution, to family supporting ill relatives.

8. *Sussed* is a colloquial term meaning "fully understood."

References

Abbott, M. (1987a). Taha Maori in comprehensive nursing education. *New Zealand Nursing Journal, 81*(8), 25–26.

Abbott, M. (1987b). Taha Maori in comprehensive nursing education. *New Zealand Nursing Journal, 81*(9), 28–31.

Abbott, M. (1987c). Taha Maori in comprehensive nursing education. *New Zealand Nursing Journal, 81*(10), 27–29.

Allen, D. G. (1995). Hermeneutics: Philosophical traditions and nursing practice research. *Nursing Science Quarterly, 4*(4), 174–182.

Aranda, S., & Street, F. (1999). Being authentic and being a chameleon: Nurse–patient interaction revisited. *Nursing Inquiry, 6,* 75–82.

Benner, P. (1983). Uncovering the knowledge embedded in clinical practice. *Image: Journal of Nursing Scholarship, 15*(2), 36–41.

Benner, P. (1984). *From novice to expert: Excellence and power in clinical nursing practice.* Menlo Park, CA: Addison-Wesley.

Benner, P., & Wrubel, J. (1989). *The primacy of caring: Stress and coping in health and illness.* Menlo Park, CA: Addison-Wesley.

Berman, L. (1994). What does it mean to be called to care? In M. Lashley, M. Neal, E. Slunt, L. Berman, & F. Hultgren (Eds.), *Being called to care* (pp. 5–16). Albany: State University of New York.

Bishop, A. H., & Scudder, J. R. (1990). *The practical, moral and personal sense of nursing: A phenomenological philosophy of practice.* Albany: State University of New York Press.

Bishop, A. H., & Scudder, J. R. (1991). *Nursing: The practice of caring.* New York: National League for Nursing.

Buber, M. (1958). *I and thou* (2nd ed.; R. G. Smith, Trans.). New York: Scribner.

Denzin, N. (1989). *Interpretive interactionism.* Newbury Park, CA: Sage.

Denzin, N. (1996). The facts and fictions of qualitative research. *Qualitative Inquiry, 2*(2), 230–241.

Dilthey, W. (1961). *Meaning in history: W. Dilthey's thoughts on history and society* (H. P. Rickman, Trans.). London: George Allen & Unwin.

Dyck, I., & Kearns, R. (1995). Transforming the relations of research: Towards culturally safe geographies of health and healing. *Health and Place, 1*(3), 137–147.

Englehardt, J. H. T. (1985). Physicians, patients, health care institutions and the people in between: Nurses. In A. H. Bishop & J. R. J. Scudder (Eds.), *Caring, curing, coping* (pp. 62–79). University, AL: University of Alabama Press.

Forrest, D. (1989). The experience of caring. *Journal of Advanced Nursing, 14,* 815–823.

Fry, S. T. (1994). *Ethics in nursing practice. A guide to ethical decision making.* Geneva, Switzerland: International Council of Nurses.

Gadamer, H. G. (1975). *Truth and method.* New York: Seabury Press.

Gadamer, H. G. (1976). *Philosophical hermeneutics* (D. E. Linge, Trans.). Berkeley: University of California Press.

Gadamer, H. G. (1986). *The relevance of the beautiful and other essays* (N. Walker, Trans.). Cambridge, UK: Cambridge University Press.

Gadamer, H. G. (1996). *Truth and method* (2nd ed.; J. Weinsheimer & D. G. Marshall, Trans.). New York: Continuum.

Gasquoine, S. (1996). *Constant vigilance: The lived experience of mothering a hospitalised child.* Unpublished master's thesis, Massey University, Palmerston North, NZ.

Gudykunst, W. B., & Kim, Y. Y. (1992). *Communicating with strangers* (2nd ed.). New York: McGraw-Hill.

Heidegger, M. (1962). *Being and time* (J. Macquarrie & E. Robinson, Trans.). Oxford, UK: Basil Blackwell. (Original work published 1927)

Hekman, S. J. (1986). *Hermeneutics and the sociology of knowledge.* Notre Dame, IN: University of Notre Dame Press.

Henderson, V. (1966). *The nature of nursing.* New York: Macmillan.

Hoult, S. (1984). Teaching for cultural awareness in a vocational education course. *Tutor, 29,* 14–17.

International Council of Nurses (ICN), Council of National Representatives. (1989). *International code for nurses.* Geneva, Switzerland: Author.

Jewell, D. (1952). A case of a "psychotic" Navajo Indian male. *Human Organization, 11,* 32–36.

Koch, T. (1994). Establishing rigor in qualitative research: The decision trail. *Journal of Advanced Nursing, 19,* 976–986.

Koch, T., & Harrington, A. (1998). Reconceptualising rigor: The case for reflexivity. *Journal of Advanced Nursing, 28*(4), 882–890.

Lacan, J. (1978). *Le seminaire 11.* Paris: Seuil.

Lampert, J. (1997). Gadamer and cross-cultural hermeneutics. *Philosophical Forum, 29*(1), 351–368.

Lashley, M. E., Neal, M. T., Slunt, E. T., Berman, L. M., & Hultgren, F. H. (1994). *Being called to care.* Albany: State University of New York Press.

Lawler, J. (1991). *Behind the screens: Nursing, somology, and the problem of the body.* Melbourne, Australia: Churchill Livingstone.

Leininger, M. (1970). *Nursing and anthropology: Two worlds to blend.* New York: John Wiley.

Leininger, M. (1978). *Caring: An essential human need.* Thorofare, NJ: C. B. Slack.

Leininger, M. (1983). Cultural care: An essential goal for nursing and health care. *AANNT Journal, 10*(5), 11–17.

Leininger, M. (Ed.). (1991). *Culture care diversity and universality: A theory of nursing.* New York: National League for Nursing Press.

Leininger, M. (1995). *Transcultural nursing: Concepts, theories, research and practices* (2nd ed.). New York: McGraw-Hill.

Levinas, E. (1984). Emmanuel Levinas. In R. Kearney (Ed.), *Dialogues with contemporary continental thinkers: The phenomenological heritage* (pp. 47–70). Dover, NH: Manchester University Press.

Levinas, E. (1987) *Collected philosophical papers* (A. Lingis, Trans.). Boston: Martinus Nijhoff.

Lipson, J., & Meleis, A. (1985). Culturally appropriate care: The case of immigrants. *Topics in Clinical Nursing, 7*(3), 48–56.

Lopez, B. (1989). *Crossing open ground.* New York: Vintage Books.

Lumby, J. (1996, August 28–30). *Evidence and nursing practice.* Paper presented at the Evidence and Health Practice Conference, Christchurch, New Zealand.

Meleis, A. I. (1996). Culturally competent scholarship. *Advances in Nursing Science, 19*(2), 1–16.

Moore, T. (1994). *Echoes of the early tides.* Pymble, N.S.W, Australia: HarperCollins.

Morse, J. M. (1988). *Recent advances in nursing: Crosscultural nursing,* no. 20. Edinburgh, Scotland: Churchill Livingstone.

Munhall, P. L. (1993). "Unknowing": Toward another pattern of knowing in nursing. *Nursing Outlook, 41*(3), 125–128.

Murchie, E. R., & Spoonley, P. (1995). *Report to the Nursing Council of New Zealand on cultural safety and nursing education in New Zealand: Cultural Safety Review Committee.* Wellington, NZ.

North, N. (1979). *The nurse, the patient, and culture.* Unpublished monograph, New Economy Research Fund (NERF) Studies in nursing, number 7.

Nursing Council of New Zealand. (1992). *Kawa Whakaruruhau: Guidelines for nursing and midwifery education.* Wellington, NZ: Author.

Nursing Council of New Zealand. (1996). *Guidelines for cultural safety in nursing and midwifery education.* Wellington, NZ: Author.

Nursing Council of New Zealand. (2002). *Guidelines for cultural safety, the Treaty of Waitangi and Maori health in nursing and midwifery education and practice.* Wellington, NZ: Author.

Ogletree, T. W. (1985). *Hospitality to the stranger.* Philadelphia: Fortune Press.

Parker, P. (1978). For the white person who wants to be my friend. *Movements in black: The collected poetry of Pat Parker.* Ithica, NY: Firebrand Books.

Paterson, J., & Zderad, L. (1988) *Humanistic nursing.* New York: National League for Nursing Press.

Peshkin, A. (1988, October). In search of subjectivity—One's own. *Educational Researcher,* 17–21.

Pomare, E. W., & de Boer, G. M. (1988). *Hauora Maori standards of health.* Wellington, NZ: Department of Health and Medical Research Council.

Ramsden, I. (1990). *Kawa Whakaruruhau: Cultural safety in nursing education in Aotearoa.* Wellington, NZ: Ministry of Education.

Ramsden, I. (1995). Own the past and create the future. In K. Irwin & I. Ramsden (Eds.), *Toi Wahine: The worlds of Maori women* (pp. 109–115). Auckland, NZ: Penguin Books.

Ramsden, I. (1997). Cultural safety: Implementing the concept. The social force of nursing and midwifery. In P. Te Whaiti, M. McCarthy, & A. Durie (Eds.), *Maii Rangiatea* (pp. 113–125). Auckland, NZ: Auckland University Press, Bridget Williams Books.

Ramsden, I. (2000). Cultural Safety / Kawa Whakaruruhau Ten Years on: a personal overview. Nursing Praxis in New Zealand. 15(1), 4–12.

Reason, P., & Rowan, J. (eds). (1981). *Human inquiry: A sourcebook of new paradigm research.* New York: John Wiley.

Ritchie, J. (1992). *Becoming bicultural.* Wellington, NZ: Huia.

Rodgers, J. (1994). *A paradox of power and marginality: New Zealand nurses professional campaign during war: 1900–1920.* Unpublished doctoral dissertation, Massey University, Palmerston North, NZ.

Sandelowski, M. (1993). Rigor or rigor mortis: The problem of rigor in qualitative research revisited. *Advances in Nursing Science, 16*(2), 1–8.

Schon, D. A. (1983). *The reflective practitioner: How professionals think in action.* New York: Basic Books.

Schutz, A. (1971). *The stranger.* The Hague, The Netherlands: Martinus Nijhoff.

Shabatay, V. (1991). *The stranger's story*. New York: Teachers College Press.

Sherrard, I. (1984, November). Cross-cultural studies. *New Zealand Nursing Journal*, 22–23.

Simmel, G. (1950). The stranger. In K. Wolff (Ed.), *The sociology of Georg Simmel*. New York: Free Press.

Slunt, E. T. (1994). Living the call authentically. In M. E. Lashley, M. T. Neal, E. T. Slunt, L. M. Berman, & F. H. Hultgren, *Being called to care* (pp. 53–64). Albany: State University of New York.

Smith, J. K. (1990). Alternative research paradigms and the problem of criteria. In E. G. Guba (Ed.), *The paradigm dialogue* (pp. 167–187). Newbury Park, CA: Sage.

Smythe, E., Spence, D., & Gasquoine, S. (1995, December 9–10). *Doing phenomenology: The story of our journey*. Paper presented at the Asia-Pacific Human Science Research Conference, Monash University, Melbourne, Australia.

Spence, D. (1999). *Prejudice, paradox and possibility: Nursing people from cultures other than one's own*. Unpublished PhD thesis, Massey University, Albany Campus, Auckland, NZ.

Spence, D. (2001a). Prejudice, paradox and possibility: Nursing people from cultures other than one's own. *Journal of Transcultural Nursing, 12*(2), 100–106.

Spence, D. (2001b). The evolving meaning of "culture" in New Zealand nursing. *Nursing Praxis in New Zealand, 17*(3), 51–61.

Styles, M. (1991). *Keynote address: Controlling nursing's destiny*. Paper presented at the Royal College of Nursing's Annual Conference, Brisbane, Australia.

Tanner, C. A., Benner, P., Chesla, C., & Gordon, D. (1993). The phenomenology of knowing the patient. *Image: Journal of Nursing Scholarship, 25*(4), 273–280.

Taylor, B. (1994). *Being human: Ordinariness in nursing*. Melbourne, Australia: Churchill Livingstone.

Taylor, C. (1985a). *Human agency and language*. Philosophical papers, vol. 1. Cambridge, UK: Cambridge University Press.

Taylor, C. (1985b). *Philosophy and the human sciences*. Philosophical papers, vol. 2. Cambridge, UK: Cambridge University Press.

Taylor, C. (1995). *Philosophical arguments*. Cambridge, MA: Harvard University Press.

Tilah, M. (1996). The medical model to the management model: Power issues for nursing. *Nursing Praxis in New Zealand, 11*(2), 16–22.

Travelbee, J. (1971). *Interpersonal aspects of nursing*. Philadelphia: F. A. Davis.

van Manen, M. (1990). *Researching lived experience*. New York: State University of New York Press.

van Manen, M. (1999, April 7-10). *Don't worry, be happy!—Reflections on caring*. Paper presented at the 5th International Qualitative Health Research, University of Newcastle, Australia.

Wachterhauser, B. R. (1986). *Hermeneutics and modern philosophy*. Albany: State University of New York Press.

Walker, D. R. (1998) *People in the Northern Region: A demographic profile from the 1996 census* (pp. 1–61). Auckland, NZ: Health Funding Authority, Northern Office.

Watson, J. (1985). *Nursing: The philosophy and science of caring*. Boulder: Colorado Associated University Press.

Watson, J. (1988). *Nursing: Human science and human care: A theory of nursing*. New York: National League for Nursing.

Wood, P. J., & Schwass, M. (1993). Cultural safety: A framework for changing attitudes. *Nursing Praxis in New Zealand, 8*(1), 4–15.

Zborowski, M. (1969). *People in pain*. San Francisco: Jossey-Bass.

5

Cultivating Stories of Care

Billie M. Severtsen

Introduction

Caring is usually taught to student nurses by means of a conceptual package. Students learn the definition of caring, identify nursing practices meeting the criteria of caring, and apply those practices to specific patient situations. Caring, when taught and learned this way, purports to ensure an objective standard of caring nursing. In other words, educators believe that what is caring in nursing practice can be standardized and judged as meeting the criteria of caring in most patient situations. They believe that transhistorical and transcultural aspects of caring can be identified for all patients through this process.

My contention, based on ongoing research and long experience as a nurse educator, is that the context-free objectivity sought in the conceptual model of caring is elusive at best. Caring does not conform to a one-size-fits-all paradigm. For caring practices to be effective, they must be recognized as caring by patients, viewed through the specific lens of the patient's culture, his or her concerns, and whatever else gives meaning in the patient's world. What is perceived by one patient as caring may be viewed as oppressive, patronizing, or irrelevant by another. In contrast to caring viewed as a generic concept, caring taught as a reflective process allows nurses, students, teachers, and patients to think deeply about specific shared lived experiences of caring. Through such reflection, nurses begin to identify the caring embedded in nursing and other healthcare situations, imbued as these situations are with background meaning, culture, and language.

Culture, or the sum total of ways of living built up by a group of humans and transmitted from one generation to another, is generally thought of as applicable to an ethnic group. This definition is also applicable to other groups such as caregivers and persons who are ill (Leininger, 1981). A particular culture carries with it its own values and language, which can be identified as specific to the world or culture of illness and of care giving. Higgins (1981) notes three other elements that must be considered in making a contextual study of culture. These are labor, which refers to the nature of people's ranges of productive activity (what do they do?); time, which addresses when the observed behavior is taking place (when illness happens and care giving is needed); and space, which refers to where and under what circumstances the behavior takes place (the environment where caregivers and patients interact).

In part 1 of this chapter, the concept of caring and its historical development in nursing is explored. Traditional or conventional approaches to teaching and learning about caring are contrasted with the reflective approach advocated by Benner and others. In part 2, a specific reflective methodology is explicated that has proven useful in teaching and learning about caring in nursing. This method or pedagogy, called the Recollective Pathway, is examined in detail. Narratives of students who learned about caring in this way are examined to illustrate and interpret the attributes of the pedagogy. In part 3 of the chapter, the culture of ill persons and the culture of caregivers are explored within the context of learning in the Recollective Pathway pedagogy. Leonard (1994) has stated that "persons, in the phenomenological view, have not only a world in which things have significance and value but qualitatively different concerns based on their culture, language and individual situations" (p. 50). Therefore, it can be argued that culture, language, and one's individual situation together become a powerful lens that one can use to identify what is significant or what holds meaning for specific patients, nurses, and teachers. Hence, culture is of paramount importance in deciding what is or is not a caring practice.

Part I. Historical Development of Caring

To examine caring, it is useful to examine the historical development of this idea as it appears in nursing literature. Although caring has always been associated with nursing, specific definitions, characteristics, and applications in practice were lacking until the middle of the past century.

Caring: Traditional or Conventional Approaches

Caring has been associated with nursing ever since nursing was identified as a vocation. Religious nursing orders have cared holistically for the sick since their inception. Caring, traditionally thought of as a female attribute, has been compared and contrasted with the "masculine" attribute of curing, traditionally associated with the practice of medicine. As early as 1966, Joyce Travelbee wrote extensively about what it means for a nurse to care. She linked the concept of caring to "interpersonal aspects of patient care" and defined caring in the following way: "to care is to experience some degree of attachment toward the object of one's caring and concern" (p. 72).

Travelbee's notions about interpersonal aspects of nursing and caring were predicated on the idea that a nursing curriculum should provide students with knowledge incorporating concepts about interpersonal caring: "It is believed essential that students in nursing develop an understanding of the knowledge underlying the skills; i.e., the major emphasis must be on the why rather than on the how" (Travelbee, 1966, p. vi). Note how Travelbee supports the idea of learning a theoretical construct before practicing it in a clinical situation. She advocates having students demonstrate a thorough theoretical knowledge of caring, drawn from theory, as a prerequisite to working with that concept as they practice nursing with their patients.

Madeleine Leininger, a nurse anthropologist who refers to caring as "an essential human need," provided crucial leadership and collaboration in early discussions about integrating caring concepts into nursing education. Leininger (1981) noted that, traditionally, caring as a concept was not taught but merely enfolded into the overall practice of nursing as something that students were supposed to inherently know. Caring was assumed to be part of what students already did with their patients. Leininger challenged that assumption; she considered caring as important a concept for nurses to know about as "curing medical diseases" or "understanding medical diagnostic techniques" (foreword). She advocated examining caring rationally and academically, the way diseases or diagnostic techniques are studied. This is, of course, the traditional scientific view or method.

Bevis and Watson (1989) wrote a guide for a caring curriculum in nursing and proposed an "ethic of care." Peter Morley, an anthropologist, posited that caring is linked with "human reciprocal altruism" (Morley, 1981, p. 149). These scholars held that caring should be taught as a concept in schools of nursing based on its being at least as important as other aspects of nursing care that were discussed conceptually. "Caring is the central and unifying domain for the body of knowledge and practices in nursing" (Leininger, 1981, p. 3). Both Watson, with her ten "carative factors" (1981, p. 9), and Leininger, with her numerous "caring constructs" (1981, p. 13), implied that caring could be operationalized in some way as a set of behaviors that could be observed and measured. Were that the case, a science of caring free from contextual variables might be identifiable.

It is clear that, historically, nursing leaders and theorists thought of caring as a concept that could be defined with specified characteristics. They conceived of caring as a generic kind of action that nurses would use with patients. By examining the concept of caring, they sought to understand the parameters of the concept and demonstrate its utility in the practice of nursing.

Today outcome-based assessment is generally hailed as the optimal way to measure whether specific nursing topics have been effectively learned. For example, in a chapter in a current nursing fundamentals text, the author sets out various specific conceptualizations of caring and cites studies that review caring from the perspective of nursing practice. Changes in the healthcare system that constrain caring nursing behaviors are then explicated, and the chapter closes with caring outcome guidelines that nurses can use in interacting with patients (Lindeman & McAthie, 1999). Elsewhere, the concept of caring in nursing is explored as it is revealed in research and literature (Paterson & Crawford, 1994). Definitions, objectives, attributes, and constraints of caring are critically analyzed. The authors are interested in finding out what is known and what needs to be known about caring in an effort to fully develop the generic concept of caring as it applies to most nursing situations.

Caring: Reflective Approaches

Patricia Benner and Judith Wrubel, drawing heavily on the work of Hubert Dreyfus, Martin Heidegger, Richard Lazarus, and Maurice Merleau-Ponty, identified caring as embedded in the hidden significant work of nursing as a caring practice. . . . Caring is a basic way of being in the world—caring sets up what counts as stressful and what coping options are available. . . . Nursing is viewed as a caring practice whose science is guided by the moral art and ethics of care and responsibility. It is argued that caring as a moral art is primary for any health care provider. (Benner & Wrubel, 1989, p. xi)

Benner and Wrubel's approach to caring differs from those of earlier authors in that they view practice as theory instead of perceiving theory as the essential precursor to the practice. Instead of teaching caring conceptually as separate from practice, the authors talk about caring as embedded within the practice of nursing. This means that the practice itself must be examined or reflected upon to discover or uncover the caring within it. Other authors joined Benner and Wrubel in asserting that caring is embedded within the practice of nursing rather than existing as a generic concept that can be applied to every patient or every situation. Critical of any attempt to describe caring as a set of context free variables, Dunlop (1994) viewed caring as always tied to each individual patient situation—not free of the context of patient and family circumstance. Increasingly, caring is viewed as showing itself in specific crisis situations, in the stories of patients, families, and healthcare workers, and in philosophical reflections on caring practice (Phillips & Benner, 1994).

Caring as practice and the phenomenological interpretation of nursing was further explored by Bishop and Scudder (1991, 1996). Those authors, like Benner, look at caring as embedded within nursing practice. Like Watson, they affirm an ethic of caring, but unlike Watson's early writings they view caring as phenomenological, as seen within specific situations or incidents in a context of shared cultural practices and language.

Additionally, following the pioneering example set by Leininger in 1981, many nursing conferences have been devoted to the topic of reflective caring. These meetings have explored caring as healing (Gaut & Boykin, 1994), caring as explicated in the feminist perspective (Neil & Watts, 1991), caring as seen in chronicity (Watson & Ray, 1988), and caring as revealed in public policy (Boykin, 1995).

Caring as Generic Concept or Reflective Process

Reflective process is contrasted in this section with the generic concept idea of caring. Reflective process refers to the actions of contemplating the caring embedded in nursing practice, and reflective pedagogy refers to the process of teaching and learning reflective process. Whereas a generic idea of caring purports to apply to most nursing situations, reflection or contemplation of caring embedded in practice makes caring a specific, situation-based enterprise.

Consider the following example to illustrate the difference between caring viewed as a concept and caring seen as embedded in the situation: A student attending a nursing class told other students of his experience nursing a patient who was one-day postoperative for a nonmalignant bowel obstruction. The patient had a nasogastric tube connected to suction for bowel decompression. The student nurse noticed that the patient was having "really more pain than I thought she should be having." The patient told him, tearfully, that the day was her wedding anniversary and that she was sad because she couldn't appropriately celebrate the occasion with her husband. The student, after reflecting on the situation and consulting with the patient's husband, purchased a cupcake from the hospital cafeteria, placed a candle in it, and presented it to the patient and her husband. The student remarked as he told his story,

I'm not exactly sure why I thought that a faked anniversary cake would make a difference. But I wanted to do something so that she wouldn't feel so sad about missing her anniversary celebration. When I checked with her husband, he thought it was a great idea. So I went ahead and bought the cupcake.

The patient was surprised and pleased with the student's cupcake gift. She and her husband shared the cupcake, the patient by blowing out the candle on it and the husband by eating it. The student indicated his surprise to his group of classmates upon finding that, within an hour of blowing out the cupcake candle, the patient's pain had decreased from a reported 8 on a 10-point pain scale to 4 without administration of any traditional pain alleviation measures. "I thought the anniversary 'cake' would cheer her up, but I didn't realize that it would really decrease her pain," he told his classmates.

In this example, the student offers his experience with the patient and her family to other students in the class. It can be argued, of course, that the story is just another example of caring through attending to the psychosocial needs of the patient. But the argument can also be made that the situation serves as a paradigm story for reflection and the impetus for a conversation between teacher and students about possibilities of caring within this lived experience.

Reflecting upon this example to uncover the caring embedded within it means that many of the basic assumptions that students, teachers, and patients have about each other are to be reexamined to ascertain if the assumptions really reflect the way things are. One such assumption made by conventional pedagogy (coming as it does from natural science) is that people are basically the same. The "generic" patient is treated as an object upon which the nursing interventions will be implemented (Benner & Wrubel, 1989, p. 35). If this view is subscribed to, caring constructs or attributes can be identified that will apply to all people, since all people are the same. Reflective pedagogy, by contrast, views persons as different from each other, primarily because of culture, language, and lived experiences. The culture through which persons acquire their basic values and enter into the culture of *patient* or *nurse* fundamentally influences whether they perceive certain actions or interventions as caring or uncaring. Heidegger's (1962) phenomenological view of persons points to this difference. He states that humans find all of their possibilities and potentialities from shared background practices and familiarity. These are acquired from being-in-the-world of one's culture and society. Therefore, it is possible for people to have both shared and individual interpretations of their world. Heidegger (1962) states that this shared understanding comes to be in "the clearing"; and furthermore, "to say that (human being) is 'illuminated' means that as being-in-the-world it is cleared in itself . . . in such a way it is itself the clearing" (p. 171).

It is important to understand that encounters within a clearing are possible only because of our shared background understanding. To summarize Heidegger's thought concerning phenomenology, Dreyfus (1984) cites three theses:

1. Human being is a self-interpreting activity. This is the hermeneutic circle.
2. This activity involves an understanding of what being means, and it is this understanding that opens a clearing (for human beings' encounters). All members of society share a preontological understanding of this interpretation.
3. Everyday practices and everyday awareness take place inside this clearing that governs what everyday human activity takes for granted. These practices embody specific cultural ways . . . all of what counts as real for us. (p. 73)

In the student's story, he, the patient, and her husband are engaged in self-interpreting activity concerning this situation. They each have an individual interpretation of what is going on and a shared interpretation of their world at this point in time. Their understanding of the postoperative recovery period and the anniversary date opens a clearing, allowing them to engage in the usual practices associated with postoperative recovery and to contemplate possibilities for remembering the anniversary in some way. The clearing allows the three participants to move from perceiving the anniversary as an ordinary or taken-for-granted day to an understanding of the possibilities and potentialities for celebrating the date in this unusual situation.

Embodied intelligence, background meaning, concern, and the situation itself are four attributes that contribute to the ability of persons to be self-interpreting. Benner and Wrubel (1989) define embodied intelligence as intelligence of the body (p. 43); embodied intelligence makes possible skilled activity of the body such as recognizing a familiar face or object. It involves the recollection of previous bodily experiences so that present activity is possible without conscious attending. Benner and Wrubel (1989) remind us:

Embodied intelligence is an integral part of the highly complex skills of the jazz pianist or of the expert nurse. All of these are part and parcel of the kind of beings we are. That is, we are the kind of beings who have an ontological capacity to respond to meaningful situations. (p. 43)

Embodied intelligence makes it possible for people to inhabit a world of meaning. It gives them the capacity to feel at home in their world. It also makes possible the ability to form a culturally skilled habitual body. As our bodies become acclimated to a particular activity, we acquire a kind of automatic pilot so that, for instance, we do not have to consciously think the specific thought of how close to stand to another.

In the student's story the patient feels at home with the knowledge that a certain day is her anniversary and that the significance of the anniversary event should be celebrated. In her current status, as a member of the culture of patient in a hospital, unable to eat or drink, she experiences disruption of her comfort or *at home-ness* with her anniversary date. She is unable to celebrate the date as she had done previously, and she is not enough of an expert with hospitals to devise another solution. The student is a member of the culture of nurse. He is moved by the patient's tears and by her story of the missed anniversary. He wonders if her distress is related in any way to her physiological pain. Part of nurse caring is to assess the patient's comfort level and to intervene, if possible, when a patient is in pain. The student does not have to think about whether or not he should try to help this patient with her pain. His motivation to try to assist the patient with her pain is taken for granted by all three participants.

For the student nurse the desire to relieve the patient's pain and the idea that the pain may be related to the anniversary date predominate over the idea of maintaining a professional distance from an event such as the anniversary date. Just as the patient does not consciously think "Maybe this nurse can help me" but rather assumes that he will be of assistance, the student doesn't think "Perhaps I should see if I should address the issue of pain for this patient." The student intuitively knows because of shared culture, language, and life experiences and is at home with the idea that it is his responsibility to help the patient deal with the pain and that all possibilities for identifying and addressing this problem need to be explored.

The second attribute enabling persons to be self-interpreting is background meaning. Background meaning has to do with the perception of reality given us by a particular culture with its attendant values. The family, the subculture, and the culture to which the person belongs provide background meaning to the individual. Benner and Wrubel (1989) state:

Background meaning, according to Heidegger, is neither subjective, nor propositional. Rather, background meaning is what a culture gives a person from birth; it is that which predetermines what counts as real for that person. It is a shared public understanding of what is. Background meaning is not itself a thing; it is, rather, a way of understanding the world. Although it does not exist as a thing itself, it is what allows for the perception of the factual world. Merleau-Ponty has offered the analogy of background meaning to a light. You do not see the light, you see what it illuminates, and without it, you would see nothing. (p. 46)

In the example, we can assume that the shared culture of the patient and the student gives considerable positive value to a wedding anniversary. A long and enduring marriage is viewed as a good thing, and an anniversary is an accomplishment that should be celebrated. Celebrations in most cultures have a component of eating, drinking, and socializing with friends and significant others.

Concern, the third attribute of self-interpreting beings, is tied to the notion that, because we are persons, things matter in a concernful way to us. We are in some way concerned with each context in which we find ourselves.

Concern is a key characteristic of the phenomenological view of the person. Although embodied intelligence and background meaning can account for how the person can be in the world and grasp meaning directly, concern accounts for why. Traditionally, the question of why people do things, make the choices they make, has been answered by mechanistic theories of motivation. (Benner & Wrubel, 1989, p. 48)

The authors challenge us to look beyond the mechanistic view of persons. Concern is specific to the person and his or her situation, not generically tied to a theory of motivation. Additionally, according to Benner and Wrubel, concern does not address motivation as a movement either toward or away from some object, person, or goal. Rather, as the authors remind us,

In the phenomenological view, the person does not move toward or away as subject to object; the person, through concern, is involved with the other. This involvement means that the world is understood in the light of the concern (e.g., what threatens the concern threatens the person). Furthermore, rather than having a subject-to-object relation or owner-to-possession relationship, the person is defined by his or her concerns. (Benner & Wrubel, 1989, p. 48)

In the example the patient is concerned that her anniversary date will slip away unnoticed. It can be assumed that most people do not have a deep concern about that particular calendar date, but she does because of the event of her marriage that is attached to it. She shares her distress with the student because of her concern. Concerned whether he is reading the patient correctly, the student confirms his perception of the situation with the patient's husband. The husband, also concerned about the patient's distress and the missed anniversary, concurs with the student that the anniversary cupcake might be a way to honor the symbolism of the occasion.

The situation is the fourth attribute cited by Benner and Wrubel (1989) related to humans as self-interpreting beings:

Because of concern, people are involved in a context. They inhabit the world, rather than live in an environment. Because of embodied intelligence, background meaning and concern, people grasp a situation directly in terms of its meaning for the self. This is what is meant by phenomenology. Furthermore, because of the direct apprehension of meaning, and because people do inhabit their worlds in an involved rather than subject-object way, people are constituted by their worlds and solicited by them. (p. 49)

In the story, the patient is hospitalized and restricted from eating or drinking because of her postoperative status. The patient and her husband are inexperienced with commemorating their significant date in the hospital environment. The student is in a situation that allows him time to reflect upon this patient and her situation. For example, we can speculate that he prioritized her tears and distress at least partly because he didn't have four or five other acutely ill people to care for. The patient's husband is also part of the situation. Had he not been there to affirm and support the student's idea, the student might not have acted on his plan. The student, patient, and patient's husband, with their shared background meaning and concern, interpret what is going on in this situation and begin to perceive or imagine possibilities, as yet unspoken or undone, for celebrating the anniversary in a new way.

This phenomenological view of persons differs markedly from mechanistic models of thought such as reductionism, cognitivism, or efficient causality. All such "scientific" models view persons as passive subjects acted upon by a number of forces. They all perceive people as coming into the world predefined (Benner & Wrubel, 1989, p. 29). By contrast, phenomenology asserts that people become defined in the course of living their individual lives.

A premise of this paper is that it is important to understand the uniqueness of each person cared for by the nurse. A way to understand the uniqueness of each person is to understand the story of one's lived experiences. Stories have the power to communicate what a patient or family member feels at home with (embodied intelligence), the background meaning that language and culture give to the person, the concern felt by the patient, and the perception of the unique situation. Hearing a patient's story may uncover the opportunity for patient and nurse to recognize the shared interpretation of their world at that time. This Heideggerian idea of *clearing* then sets up the possibilities for caring actions to emerge: "Because caring (concern) sets up what matters to a person, it also sets up what counts as stressful, and what options are available for coping. Caring creates possibility. This is the first way in which caring is primary" (Benner & Wrubel, 1989, p. 1). Indeed, the authors propose that nurses should "interpret" the patient's experience of illness, validating with the patient that the nurse's perceptions are accurate.

In the example we see the student nurse helping the patient and her husband cope with the stress of her illness through interpreting it accurately because the nurse understands the patient's story in the same way the patient intends him to hear it. He brings caring into the situation, hearing and witnessing the patient's story and understanding what the situation means to the patient. Her story, with its theme of sadness over the potential loss of an anniversary celebration, provides a bridge, linking the patient's concern to the student's imagination. Because of her story, the student is able to imagine her reality. When he imagines her reality, he begins to imagine possibilities for helping her gain some control over her situation.

Part 2. The Recollective Pathway

Can recollection of, reflection upon, or contemplation of a situation be taught to student nurses? It can be. Nurses who learn critically to reflect upon situations and relationships that they build with patients can learn a great deal about caring from the reflective process. Certainly, if reflection is to be used in clinical situations by nurses in order to discover individual and shared interpretation of the patient's world, nurses are to be encouraged to learn how to gather data through reflection. Only then can they begin to imagine possibilities for appropriate actions. But for reflection or recollection to be taught successfully, a different pedagogy from the conventional outcome-based model is needed.

The Recollective Pathway is proposed as such pedagogy. It builds on Nancy Diekelmann's (Diekelmann & Diekelmann, forthcoming) pioneering work with narrative pedagogy. Heavily influenced by interpretive phenomenology, the Recollective Pathway also serves as a learning environment in which conversations coming from shared narratives or stories can be gathered, listened to, and analyzed. In this way, individual and shared interpretations of being-in-the-world can emerge. The history and details of the pedagogy are presented next. Then, the learning that emerged from analyzing caring in this way is elaborated.

History and Development of the Recollective Pathway

In her work with narrative pedagogy in nursing education, Diekelmann states:

Narrative pedagogy is a good example of the nature of contemporary reform. Narrative pedagogy is not using storytelling as a strategy for learning. Nor is it pedagogy as such. It is a call for clinicians, students, and teachers to gather and attend to community practices in ways that hold everything open and problematic. The pedagogies that arise in this way are site specific and co-founded in all that already is. (Diekelmann & Diekelmann, forthcoming)

In the concernful practices of schooling, learning, and teaching cited as part of narrative pedagogy, Diekelmann focuses on three concepts: teaching and learning, holding everything problematic, and being open to the possibility of anything showing up.

The Recollective Pathway recognizes these concepts. Additionally, it explores the idea of story, specifically the idea of reflecting upon the story of the shared lived experience of patients, nurses, and teachers. It affirms the idea of reflection upon the story as useful in identifying the meaning of the experience for patient and student. Reflection can bring nurse, patient, and teacher to Heidegger's clearing. When the clearing occurs, the possibilities for uncovering caring interventions in that specific situation begin to emerge. Additionally, reflective activity, when shared with others in a class setting, represents learning for the entire class. For example, the student nurse and his classmates learned how attending to a symbolic loss for the patient might produce an analgesic effect in the patient.

Schon (1987) distinguishes between technical rationality and reflective practice because problems are often uncertain and unique instead of clear-cut and uniform, and because teachers and scholars "frame" the problems or "construct" the question to be answered. Schon states: "Although we sometimes think before acting, it is also true that much of the spontaneous behavior of skillful practice reveals a kind of knowing which does not stem from a prior intellectual operation" (p. 50). Schon also finds that "problem setting is a process in which, interactively, we name the things to which we will attend and frame the context in which we will attend to them" (p. 40).

As a further reminder, Schon (1987) indicates that when the process of reflection-in-action goes well, the practitioner interacts with the situation in such a way that it talks back to the practitioner. As the practitioner makes a move in the existing situation, it changes, such that each shapes the other.

This conversation with the situation is reflective. In answer to the situation's backtalk, the practitioner reflects-in-action on the construction of the problem, the strategies of action, or the model of the phenomenon, which have been implicit in his moves (p. 79).

In our previous example the student nurse begins to focus on the patient's sadness as explicated in her story. The patient is able to impress upon the student how important the anniversary date is. She effectively communicates to the student her interpretation of being-in-the-world in this place at this time. The student frames the context of the situation by paying more attention to the missed anniversary celebration than physiological explanations about the patient's increased pain. He sets the boundaries of his attention to the scenario in which the patient's pain may very well have a link to the sadness over the missed anniversary. He thinks that acknowledging the symbolic loss may improve the patient's condition by addressing her sadness. Armed with this intuition, the student approaches the patient's husband who enthusiastically concurs with his idea of a faked anniversary cake. This illustrates Schon's point of "talking back" or interacting with the situation. The student receives further confirmation from the patient's husband that he is on the right track. The husband's actions shape the situation and influence what the student does next; he purchases the cupcake and presents it to the patient.

The student in this situation is open to whatever might happen. He does not know that his reflective intervention will work. He works with the situation to discover what might happen. He is willing to let the situation change him through a shared understanding of the patient's reality.

The Recollective Pathway Course

The Recollective Pathway's task is to teach the process just illustrated by the story of the student nurse and the patient. This pathway was first utilized in an undergraduate elective course, Concepts of Caring, at the Washington State University College of Nursing in 1997.

Diagrammed, the Recollective Pathway looks like this:

1. Participants: voices of patients, clinicians, teachers, and students.
2. Community Building: actions focused toward guiding, respecting, listening/ witnessing.

3. Community-Centered Practices: recollective thinking by individuals, shared and transformed into community conversations.
4. Learning Emergence: what emerges as valuable to the practice of caring nursing. (Severtsen & Evans, 2000).

The Recollective Pathway Course provides an environment in which conversations that occur can be gathered, listened to, and analyzed by the group of learners. The story conversations allow caring embedded in various situations to come forth. Sharing these stories allows knowledge to emerge and to become explicit. The kind of insight provided by this learning does not come about through examination of a traditional concept of caring, the one-size-fits-all approach. Rather, it holds conventional academic ways of learning about caring problematic by questioning the assumption that the academic process of conceptualization or outcome assessment can teach everything that nurses need to know about caring. It therefore challenges the self-evident assumptions that conventional pedagogy makes about caring practice.

The Recollective Pathway diagram is now explored step by step. The differences between the teaching and learning that occurred in the Concepts of Caring course and the more traditional pedagogy of teaching caring in nursing programs is delineated.

Participants: Voices of Patients, Clinicians, Teachers, and Students

The Recollective Pathway presupposes that teaching and learning cannot be separated: "The concernful practices of teaching and learning are interwoven; they cannot be sundered. Teaching and learning belong together ineffably such that any attempt to separate them does violence to either or both" (Diekelmann, 1995, p. 195).

In the class the artificial hierarchy of teacher and student is ignored as much as possible; we foster the idea of the class as a community of learners in which all participants come together to learn about caring. Students understand that university policy dictates some external constraints on this idea. For instance, a syllabus is required with assignments, a bibliography, objectives, a course description, and grading criteria. But from the very beginning a concerted effort is made by the instructors to overcome the power of teacher over student and to develop a relationship of power sharing in a community of scholars. Students are invited to join the community of the course with the objective of exploring the topic of caring. They are assured that they know as much about caring as do the instructors. Learning about caring from reflecting upon caring or uncaring situations as told in stories is offered as a contrast to the conventional "concept package" idea of caring learned through lecture, testing, and cognitive gain.

The syllabus is presented as a guide to how reflective thinking might be focused around the topic. Three assignments are suggested. One is a series of questions to be answered after the course participants read and discuss *The Death of Ivan Ilych* (Tolstoy, 1960). This classic short story portrays many examples of caring and uncaring behaviors in the chief character and his associates as he struggles with a fatal illness. As the story is discussed, possible answers to the assigned questions are specifically addressed. When students realize that the questions in the assignment are going to be answered in the class discussion, they began to take fewer notes and to actually think about, reflect upon, and discuss what they think the answer might be to any specific question. They become familiar with the idea of thinking and talking about a story to discover caring or its lack.

Students are told specifically that lecturing or testing about the conventional idea or concept of caring will not occur. This decision was made, students are told, not because the conventional approach to the subject is flawed, but because developing an alternative way to learn about caring is the focus of the course. In the course the norm of thinking about what goes on in the story is more important than finding out what answer the teacher wants.

A second assignment promotes storytelling by requiring each student to write a story about a caring or uncaring occurrence that happened to him or her. Course participants (including the instructors) read their stories to the group, which functions as a supportive listening community by asking questions and clarifying meanings of the story. Instructors model writing stories and then discuss and listen supportively to the stories of others as they are shared. This strategy *calls out* stories of various experiences of the class participants: stories that are read in the course prompt students to remember and discuss other stories. The instructors make a deliberate attempt to establish the idea that stories reflect multiple perspectives and are embedded with layers of meaning. Stories, therefore, give nurses more information than can be obtained by asking a patient a question. The story becomes the key to understanding the reality of the patient's lived experience, the individual and shared interpretations of that situation, and, hence, the possibilities for caring. A third assignment asks students to read one of the stories about a patient's experience of illness in *The Patient's Voice* (Young-Mason, 1997) and answer the critical thinking questions at the end of the story.

After students are presented with the suggested assignments, as a group they chose all, some, or none of the assignments as a way to learn about caring. They are also asked to suggest other activities that might help them to think about and reflect upon the idea of caring as embedded within a phenomenon or story. The instructors make it clear that, for the purposes of the course, the phenomenon is the story. The ways that course members learn about caring are not completely random but emphasize learning about and understanding caring by teasing out the caring appearing in the story. To date, all students who have taken the course have opted to complete the three assignments, and they have suggested other activities as well. Their suggestions focus on sharing stories of family traditions, values, and cultural heritage as a way to know people better through observing common and diverse interpretations of an event. For example, watching a film in which the main character demonstrates love and gratitude toward her employers by preparing a lavish feast was used to demonstrate caring. Inviting a person struggling with a recurrence of breast cancer to come to class and tell her illness story was a way to actually listen to a patient and discuss with her the meaning of her illness.

Checking in with the course participants by sharing with other participants about how one's week has gone has become a classroom norm. The checking-in period has proved to be a way to socialize students to the process of calling out stories and also a way of letting important or urgent stories *tumble out*. The story that tumbles out, when discussed by the class, becomes a coherent account of something that has happened to the course participant in the past week as opposed to fragmentary snatches of the past week's activities. The idea of story as a chronicle with a beginning, an end, and a rhythm is introduced.

Grades for the course are contracted by completion of the three suggested assignments. If an assignment is deemed to be of poor quality, an instructor talks with the student outside of class to arrange for the student to satisfactorily complete the assignment. The instructors also reiterate that coming to class, talking, and interacting with other course community members is essential. To date, most students have earned an *A* grade, although grades of *B* or *C* have also been assigned.

In addition to the schooling aspect utilized by having both teacher and student experience or *live* the experience of writing an assignment, a specific attempt is made to include in the conversations about caring the voices of patients and of nurse clinicians. Many students and teachers have experienced personal health problems in which caring practice was either present or absent. Course members are asked to try to remember these incidents, as well as to recollect feedback they had received from coworkers or patients about caring practice in other situations.

One student wrote an *occurrence of caring* story about watching a baby boy being circumcised. She was disappointed in the lack of touching, cuddling, or any attempt to soothe the crying baby postoperatively, although she said that she "had nothing against circumcision." Other students disagreed, saying that circumcision is painful and that parents should have the right not to subject their male infants to this procedure. This led to a discussion about the rights of the incompetent, the place of culture and deeply held cultural beliefs in treatment protocols and options, and how caring nursing is often sacrificed in the name of efficiency (getting as many babies as possible circumcised at one time). Through the free give and take of stories and the lack of academic constraint to point students to the "right" story or answer, the course members became a community of scholars dedicated to delving into caring practice in all its complexity.

Story as a vehicle for making meaning in one's life is introduced by the book *Crow and Weasel* (Lopez, 1990). In response to a student telling her classmates how being read to as a child symbolized caring to her, one class participant brought *Crow and Weasel* to class and read the book aloud to the community. The book tells the story of two Indian braves who embark on a vision quest to learn how to live authentic, respectful, and fulfilled lives. In the story, one character cautions Weasel to "put your poem in order on the threshold of your tongue" (p. 45). As participants in the course told each other their stories, the instructors, through questioning and focused comments, tried in each case to fashion a coherent story with a beginning, middle, and end from the raw material of the original story. We practiced "putting our poems in order."

A character named Badger in *Crow and Weasel* states:

> I would ask you to remember only this one thing. . . . The stories people tell have a way of taking care of them. If stories come to you, care for them. And learn to give them away where they are needed. Sometimes a person needs a story more than food to stay alive. That is why we put these stories in each other's memory. This is how people care for themselves. One day you will be good storytellers. Never forget these obligations. (Lopez, p. 48)

In learning to listen to a variety of stories from literature and from other community participants, and in the discussions that followed the story-telling, the students practiced hearing diverse voices sharing stories. The strategy of listening to the stories of many enabled the students to increase their flexibility to hear and to consider multiple perspectives. Stories that were told in the class settings were always discussed in detail. Additionally, other perspectives about the meaning of the story, including respectful but frank disagreements, were encouraged in the discussion. The idea of thinking about the situation, hearing the story, reflecting upon it, and finally "talking back" to the situation was encouraged as a way to assist students to move out of a rigid view about what the patient might be experiencing.

Community Building: Guiding

The notion of story as a vehicle to discover caring is used extensively in the course. From assigned readings and in-class discussions, it is understood that a good way to know people is to hear and understand their authentic stories. As W. C. Williams said, "their story, yours, mine— it's what we carry with us on this trip we take, and we owe it to each other to respect our stories and learn from them" (as cited in Coles, 1989, p. 30). Instructors deliberately foster an attitude of openness to hearing each person's story and the idea that all present can learn from the stories.

A student in the course who had recently immigrated to the United States along with her mother and younger brother told her classmates about accompanying her mother to a physician's office for an appointment. The mother suffered from wrist and finger pain, probably as a result of working on an assembly line in a factory. The physician, after reviewing an x-ray of the mother's hand, told the student and her mother that "arthritis has dissolved the bones in your wrist and fingers." He stated that reconstructive surgery was the only option that he could offer the mother. When the student asked about other treatment options and pain relief for her mother, the impatient physician again told her that surgery was the only option and that if surgery were performed, the mother would not need pain medication.

The student, who up until that time had been perceived by the doctor as merely an interpreter for her mother, told him that she was a junior in a collegiate nursing program. She informed him that she had learned in school that the basis of informed consent was the patient being able to freely choose from various options. After she spoke to the doctor in this way, she told her classmates how his attitude suddenly changed: "He stopped treating us like dumb Vietnamese," she said. "Suddenly we could get a second opinion, he had pain medication for my mom, the arthritis had not really dissolved the bones, my mom could try wearing a splint, and on and on. He became interested in really helping us after I told him what I knew."

Other students were appalled at the behavior of the doctor. Many reiterated their belief that patients require a strong and capable advocate. Themes of powerlessness, discrimination, stereotyping, and anger poured from other community members. Students told their own stories of having witnessed similar situations. Then the discussion turned to why a physician would act in this way. Why was this behavior, suggesting burnout or even racism, so common in the healthcare industry, not only among doctors but also among nurses and other ancillary workers? Course participants explored the idea of involvement and its correlation to burnout. They discussed how a complex issue such as this cannot be satisfactorily addressed in a simplistic or dualistic way.

The convergence of stories illustrates again what Schon tells us about reflective practice—the ability to talk to the situation as it is unfolding. In this case, the situation is the student's story. As the story talks back to us, learning emerges. The conversations that unfold from the stories lead to an ever-widening circle of learning coming through the free-flowing interchange between participants and the situation (story).

Once the original story is constructed, it must be cultivated and revised until it accurately reflects the meaning it holds for the storyteller. Cultivating is analogous to Heidegger's clearing. It is the point at which the individual and the shared interpretation of being-in-the-world emerge for the storyteller and his or her listeners. As the story is told and retold, the voice of the storyteller usually becomes stronger and more focused. This happens because the important or significant issues or themes of the story become visible or explicit as the story continues to unfold. For example, the Vietnamese student learned to imagine a care worker's attitude through the questions or comments of her supportive community (the course participants) as she told her story.

The storyteller always learns from the story. What is learned has to do with knowing how and where the story is situated. What meaning does the story have in the storyteller's life? When the story becomes firmly settled or when the meaning of it is identified, the metaphorical *voice* of the storyteller becomes a powerful force, assisting in developing new goals or life direction relative to the situation that is giving rise to the story in the first place. An important way to strengthen the storyteller's voice through the work of cultivating and learning from the story is to connect themes in one's own story to similar themes in another's story. For example, themes of disrespect and powerlessness that were shared by the course participants in response to the student's story strengthened many voices within the course community. Course participants were vocal in declaring that the behavior of the physician in the story was unacceptable and that behavior like this must not be tolerated. They also came to a deeper understanding of organizational and technocratic constraints that might be identified as root causes of such behavior.

Community Building: Respecting

Thinking *with* stories, not about stories, was introduced as a way to empower class participants as they dealt with patient situations. The difference between thinking *with* stories and *about* stories is crucial. As one thinks *about* stories, one reduces them to content and then analyzes the content. As one thinks *with* stories, one treats the story as a complete entity. The story is not a piece of data from which to support or defend various propositions. Rather, it is the lived experience of the person telling it; it is the vehicle that allows the individual to identify meaning from the experience that gives rise to the story.

Stories we tell ourselves about what is happening to us are dangerous because they are powerful. Stories come to us from many sources; some we seek, many happen without our notice, others impose themselves on our lives. We have to choose carefully which stories to live with, which to use to answer the question of what is happening to us. (Frank, 1991, p. 81)

Respecting means calling out the authentic stories of others and then using those stories to think about those persons and their situations.

An authentic story has several criteria. First, it is an accurate story that correctly portrays the situation (Frank, 1995, p. 53). Yet one must resist the urge to think that, because a story is accurate, it is the whole or complete story. If a story does not correctly represent the worldview, the ethos, or the values of the person, family, or group that is its subject, it does not honestly represent reality for that individual or group, and it is not authentic. If patients feel their own reality has been ignored or unappreciated, they may ignore the healthcare provider and listen to advice from someone else who does incorporate their authentic story into their practice of healthcare.

Respecting also means holding in abeyance judgments that we often make about the person sharing their story. For example, a class member told of her anger at having to repeat a course because of a failing grade. The failed course was a medical–surgical theory course. The student had passed the companion clinical course. She shared her resentment at having to "put my life on hold" for another semester. She spoke of the unfairness of the poor grade in the theory course, stating that she missed a passing grade by only three points. "How could I fail a theory course and do so well on that same course's clinical application," she wondered aloud to her classmates.

As a teacher, I wanted to explain to her that failing a theory course and passing the clinical application course is a common occurrence. I also wanted to urge her to devote herself to learning all she could as she repeated the course, instead of continuing to feel resentful and angry. Had I chosen that option, as I responded to her story, I would have been ignoring or explaining away her authentic story with its themes of resentment and marginalization. Another way to hear her story could have been to draw conclusions about the unfairness of the tests in the course or the course instructor or about the entire academic or curricular framework in the school. Yet in whatever way the student's story might be judged, the consequence would remain the same: the authentic story would be devalued and lost. Instead of judging, the course participants focused on hearing the student's story. In this way, the course community supported the student as she reflected upon her experience of failing the course and being forced to repeat it. The participants also respected her attempt to formulate meaning out of this situation.

The students gradually came to understand that respecting the voice of the storyteller, as modeled in class, was a process that had the potential to occur in many nurse–patient interactions. They learned that true respecting means allowing the authentic story of the person a modicum of space and nurturance to grow and become the vehicle for meaning making in that person's life. One student expressed how the process works in this way:

Because sometimes they are not going to tell you straight out to your face. They're going to tell it through a story—you can gain insight on what they are trying to say. It's a much more comfortable way of people telling their true feelings—and more comfortable for the nurse.

Viktor Frankl, a Viennese psychiatrist who used the concept of story in his work with Nazi concentration camp inmates, first identified the meaning making that comes from the process described above. Frankl believed that a trained awareness of the significance in a situation reveals the meaning of the situation to a given individual and the free choice to be made in that situation (Frankl, 1985). A person can then make a responsible choice, and this choice is derived from discerning whether a given phenomenon is spiritual or instinctual. It should be noted that for Frankl *spiritual* does not have a religious meaning but refers to mental or immaterial processes as contrasted with the person's psychophysical self. Without the spiritual core as its essential ground, wholeness in an individual cannot exist. Authentic existence, according to Frankl, is present "when a self is deciding for himself, but not when an id is driving him" (Frankl, 1985, p. 27). For instance, should an individual respond to the loss of a body part by pure reaction or *instinct* (according to Frankl), the reaction precludes the ability of the person to make a free choice about the meaning of the loss. Conversely, if an individual, in the same situation, is able to reflect upon and consider the significance or meaning of the loss, a free choice can follow about how to respond to the situation.

In the above example the student in the situation responded, initially, with *instinctual* anger. She was angry at the teacher who failed her and at the school policy regarding remediation. In her anger, she had not yet been able to reflect upon what had happened to her. Frankl would say that she had not developed the "trained awareness" that would alert her to the fact that reflection on this situation was necessary. Her classmates helped her reflect as they allowed her to develop and tell her story.

Frankl found three elements rooted in the spiritual core of each person: intellectual knowing or realization, feelings the person experiences, and free choosing of values (Frankl, 1985). A response by a person in a situation such as significant loss could be used to illustrate these themes. The person knows, in an intellectual way, what happened to cause the loss. In this realm, the person deals with facts. Secondly, he or she feels a particular way about the loss experience. This feeling could be characterized as emotion. Finally, the person freely chooses a value or a set of values as a response to the loss. Frankl calls this free choosing of particular values "meaning" and states that the free choice of one value over another constitutes a kind of "ultimate freedom" (Frankl, 1984, p. 132). By becoming aware of the option of value or attitude choices, persons can formulate a response to the loss that enables them to decide what its specific meaning and implications for them might be. A potentially meaningful attitude becomes actualized through a person's free choosing of the attitude as a response.

As one compares the student's story about the failed course to Frankl's framework, it can be seen that the student knew, in an intellectual way, what had happened to cause the loss by failing the theory course. Secondly, the student felt disappointed, angry, and resentful about the failing grade. As the student told her story and reflected upon it, aided by the community of supportive listeners and their converging stories, the values that the student knew she must choose in order to make meaning out of the situation began to emerge. I do not mean to imply that there was a right or wrong set of values for the student to choose. Rather, the act of choosing any value, so long as it represents an authentic choice freely made, serves as the impetus for meaning making. Meaning making allows the person to move forward with whatever it is that the person needs to do next. It provides the next direction in the path that the person has chosen in relation to the particular event that called for meaning making in the first place. Although meaning making is intensely personal, the community was of substantial assistance to this particular student's experience of meaning.

In this case, the student decided that her attitude would be one of trying to learn as much as she could from repeating the failed course.

She reasoned that if she had passed the course the first time, she might not have been as confident or as certain of her practice as she might be if she repeated the course. "I think I can, maybe, put it all together this time," she said. She also found that her prospective employer was supportive of the necessity of her staying in school another semester. She told her employer of her changed plans when another course member told a converging story about notifying an employer about changed plans early and receiving positive feedback from the employer for having done so. This student was guided and supported as she made meaning out of the failed class and created a new destination and map for her career.

Community Building: Listening and Witnessing

Student nurses are quickly socialized by their program of study and clinical experiences into perceiving that their role in healthcare is to relieve suffering. The idea of actively doing something to relieve suffering becomes an ethical stance; in order to function as a compassionate nurse, the student thinks that he or she must be actively doing something. They are tremendously surprised to realize that helping a person to articulate his or her story, listening, and then bearing witness to that story is active helping and caring.

A crucial aspect of living with stories is listening to the stories. This seems self-evident, but students need to be reminded that if they are mentally leaping to diagnostic conclusions, they are no longer listening or witnessing. If a nurse pigeonholes a patient as being in denial, the nurse has stopped listening and started diagnosing or judging. Patients are very adept at watching their caregivers and determining if the caregivers can be trusted to listen and to bear witness to their stories. Frank reminds us,

Anyone who wants to be a caregiver, particularly a professional, must not only have real support to offer, but also must learn to convince the ill person that this support is there. My defenses have never been stronger than they were when I was ill. I have never watched others more closely or been more guarded around them. I needed others more than I ever have, and I was also more vulnerable to them. The behavior I worked to let others see was my most conservative estimate of what I thought they would support. (Frank, 1991, p. 70)

The stories that students told about their previous week provided a good way to practice nonjudgmental listening. Since each student and instructor had a story to tell about his or her week, the class perceived this activity as a fair way for everyone to practice telling a story. It was seen as important that all class members listen respectfully to the story that each participant told. The idea that we could all learn from each story, no matter how trite or commonplace the story seemed to be, was a new notion for students to consider. Some stories from participants were full of anecdotes about troubles with boyfriends or girlfriends. Others were chronicles of problems with school, with work, or with children and family relationships. Although students were always polite and respectful as the stories were told, it was evident from observing the class that some stories were perceived as being interesting, while others were viewed as "the same old stuff."

The instructors made a concerted attempt to comment on each story by specifically connecting it with another similar story. For example, one participant recounted a story of family turmoil because her teenage adopted child did not want to celebrate her birthday with her family. The participant spoke of feeling hurt by the behavior of the daughter, who had stated that birthday celebrations with her family were "boring" and that she would rather be with friends.

On the surface, this seems like a very ordinary story. Adolescent behavior typically places a higher value on friends than on family. A dramatic way to symbolically say "I'm sorry I was adopted" might be to state that one doesn't want a birthday celebration with one's adoptive family. But attempting any explanation of the behavior of the teen is, in a way, devaluing the mother's story. If the class had communicated to the mother that her teen's behavior was typical and that she should "get used to it," they would have been telling the mother how to react rather than letting her figure out how to freely choose to respond to her daughter. Instead, one of the instructors told a converging story about her feelings years earlier, when her teen angrily confronted her about being a "terrible parent" because she refused to cover for an unexcused absence at the child's school. The instructor spoke of her worry at that time over whether or not she was really being supportive of her child by making the child own up to the fact that she had cut several classes. "My child said that I was the only parent that she knew of who wouldn't cover for her kid," said the instructor. "I really wondered if that were true. I wanted more than anything to be a good mom," she added. "Was I doing the right thing?"

A student participant added her story about a time when, as a teen, she decided that birthdays with her family were "totally dull." After informing her parents that she'd rather not celebrate with them, she spoke of her surprise when her parents replied that if that were her wish, they would certainly honor it. She told the class that after her birthday came and went with no mention of it in the family, she realized that not celebrating a birthday was not much fun at all, and that she was very pleased to celebrate the birthday a year later. These examples related to the personal lives of the participants. But stories also converged on issues that the course participants faced in their clinical practice. Many of the stories were about the healthcare system, their attempts to practice within that system, and how other healthcare workers perceived them.

A class participant told a story about one of his patients. A young African American man, who came from a background of poverty and neglect, had relocated with his wife to the Pacific Northwest from Florida. They left behind family and associates to make a new life for themselves. Shortly after their arrival, the man was diagnosed with advanced esophageal cancer. The stress of the disease and treatment, the grim prognosis, the financial burden of treatment, and the lack of supportive friends and family pushed the wife to suicide. The student encountered a patient who was utterly alone, close to death, and in a completely unfamiliar place. The student stated:

After a while I realized that there were only so many backrubs, water sips and pillow fluffings that I could do. I began to see that sitting with him and listening to him tell me that all he wanted now was to be with his wife was the most therapeutic thing that I could do.

As the student told his story, he stated that he was "uncomfortable" telling his clinical instructor or other nurses on the unit about the great amount of time he spent "just sitting" with the patient. His story gave rise to a discussion about the healthcare system's focus on cure and doing, often to the exclusion of quality-of-life issues. The student reiterated his dilemma in the following way:

The problem was I felt kind of guilty that I was just like sitting down and talking with the patient because I felt like I needed to be doing something else. At the same time, I knew that listening to him tell his story to me was the only thing bringing some peace to this patient.

This statement caused another student to inform the class of her insight about the issue:

I try to perform those skills at the same time as I'm providing care and concern and a space for the patient to talk with me—but I don't think that the healthcare system as a whole appreciates that or gives credit to that and so it makes it really difficult for nurses to be able to actually have time to do that for clients.

The class discussion that took place regarding this issue of bearing witness to the patient's concern, questions, and story is another example of the conversations that occurred among patients, students, nurse clinicians, and the teachers of the course. As the participants reflected upon their various practice settings, caring practice became visible or revealed to the course members. In this way, these novice nurses were able to imagine an expanded repertoire of caring practices. But in contrast to outcome-based learning or conceptual teaching, the caring practices were identified by the students in response to the question of "What is caring practice in this situation?" rather than having caring outcomes taught to them by a pedagogical "expert."

Community-Centered Practices

Gradually, the norms, rules, and values of the community that comprised the caring course began to show themselves. Some norms became apparent very quickly. The community easily identified confidentiality as essential in the class sessions. The idea of "who gets the best grade" was early on judged not to be important in this class setting. Other norms or practices took longer to emerge. One was the community as a place where participants could feel safe. This happened because community members felt empowered to tell their stories in a confidential and supportive place. Additionally, the conventional hierarchy of "best answer" or "teacher's pet" disappeared as the community learned to withhold judgment on the stories being told by its members.

Perhaps the most profound community-centered practice to show itself was the idea that all individuals, but particularly those who struggle with health concerns, must face and must come to terms with the issues of control, desire, and relatedness. Frank (1995) identifies these issues as pivotal in his writing on story and illness (p. 27). It became apparent to the class members that serious illness destroys the destination and map that people use to navigate their lives. The issues of control, desire, and relatedness represent pivotal pieces of an individual's life that must be reworked as part of the formation of a new destination and map for life after illness or life coexisting with illness. To truly value ill persons, we need to understand how people can and should be protective of themselves.

These three issues represented to the course members fundamental and overarching concepts that have an impact on anyone who is ill. Members of the class community realized that competent, caring nursing practice is impossible unless the nurse considers the impact of altered control, body relatedness, desire, and cultural context on the person experiencing illness.

Altered Control. "Everyone must ask in any situation, can I reliably predict how my body will function; can I control its functioning?" (Frank, 1995, p. 30). People define themselves in terms of their body's varying capacity for control. So long as these capacities are predictable, control as an action does not require self-conscious monitoring. Frank (1995) asserts that persons live along a continuum in their bodies from predictability (certainty that their body will function in a specific way) to contingency (the body being subject to forces that it cannot control). When adults lose control over their bodies, they are expected to attempt to regain the control if possible, and if not, then they should at least conceal the loss. As an example, Frank offers the following illustration:

A man described to me the social problems he experienced when he lost bladder control following surgery for prostate cancer. He was expected to conceal the contingency of his bladder; stains and smells are stigmatizing. But he also found that sales people in home care stores were unwilling to discuss incontinence problems with him, in part, it seemed to him, because he was male (incontinence is, demographically, more a female problem) and perhaps also because he was younger than social stereotypes of incontinence allowed. (p. 30)

Body Relatedness. Body relatedness refers to how ill people relate to their bodies and also how they relate to others, both others who are ill and others who are well. People can intently regard their ill bodies by paying close attention to each symptom, or they may disregard their bodies, choosing to ignore symptoms. Modern medicine, as Frank (1995) points out, does much to discourage body association:

Robert Zussmann, in his study of intensive care units, quotes one physician who says, "I think you don't have to look at a patient here, basically. You don't have to examine a patient . . . the numbers, I feel, are more reliable." Such physicians then teach their patients that, with respect to how they feel, the numbers, or diagnostic images, or cardiac tracings are more reliable. Most of us, sooner or later, go to the doctor to find out how we feel, our distrust of subjective feelings being a form of dissociation. (p. 14)

This physician is an example of those who encourage people to prioritize what the diagnostic tests indicate over how they feel as inhabitants of their bodies. Patients may understand, after consulting with a physician, that it is better to ignore symptoms than to report them. Not reporting subjective symptoms, however, means that an important part of the data that make up a complete medical diagnosis may be missing.

Desire. Desire, the third issue, can be summed up as the ambivalence about what to wish for that people feel when they are ill. Many patients, of course, desire and often expect a complete cure of their illness and, thus, a happy ending to their story of illness. Indeed, as Frank (1991) points out, this is our societal expectation of the ill person:

Treatment in itself is not an expression that the individual is valued; it is an investment in the ill person's future productivity. The ill are regarded as healthy people inside broken down bodies that need fixing. The hard question is whether we can value the ill as people whose experience challenges the way the rest of us live. (p. 118)

Often, cure is not possible in the illnesses that people experience. The question then becomes one of desire—what is in the mind of the patient. Is it permissible to be both a "good patient" and to desire no more invasive treatment or treatment at all? Although most nurses and healthcare workers are quick to assert that patients have the right to make any choice of treatment that they care to, do we reward the behavior of the optimistic, cheerful patient who opts for aggressive treatment over the patient who decides to quit the fight? Frank (1995) cites the example of Stewart Alsop, suffering from leukemia, who writes of his approaching birthday by stating that "perhaps sixty is a good time to bow out" (p. 38).

Cultural Context. Humans can never be separated from the culture of which they are a part and from which their core values are formed. When considering the fact that people are self-interpreting beings, one is automatically forced to accommodate the place that culture and the cultural context of the individual makes in the self interpretive process.

Students in the caring course came to understand how closely intertwined cultural context and the stories of their clients were.

Learning Emergence

If illness represents a metaphorical loss of destination and map for patients, as Frank asserts, stories show us how a new destination and map is being formulated for each patient storyteller (Frank, 1995). In the course, the process by which the community learned about caring became uncovered. Students learned to see the power of stories in themselves and in others as storytellers. Two students comment on the process as it occurred in the course:

It's an amazing process, but the class really helped me, hearing people's stories and getting stories out of people and sharing stuff about myself, forms of stories, and it's a real way of communication between people. (Student, personal communication, September 1998)

I think life's experience is the best teacher and sharing those experiences with other people is one of the best ways of teaching the class. I'd love to take the class again and tell more stories and hear more. (Student, personal communication, March 1999)

The purpose of the course was to bring together students and teachers as a community of scholars who would learn collectively about caring, an important nursing concept. The truest test of learning is, of course, to observe after the fact the person who the learning influences or shapes. Accordingly, each student who completed the course was asked to participate in a private interview one year after the course was offered. Students were free to accept or decline the interview request. If they agreed to be interviewed, IRB-approved informed consent was obtained from them to tape-record and transcribe the interview and to use the material obtained without divulging their identities. Prior to the interview, students were alerted to the idea that they would be asked to tell a story. They were urged to begin to reflect on what that story might be. The private semi-structured interview began with the researcher's request:

Tell me a story that best illustrates how the course did or did not influence your nursing practice. The story should come from your own experience during the semester that the class was taught or from your experience since that time.

Probes were used judiciously to elicit data clarification. The student responses were tape-recorded and transcribed verbatim. All identifying
information was removed; participants were identified by pseudonym
only. A hermeneutic approach described by Benner, Tanner, and Chesla
(1996) was used to analyze and understand the data. A goal of the research was to study the phenomenon of an incident of nursing practice
of the participants. A second goal was to critically reflect how the course
content affected the participants' understanding of nursing practice. As
interpretive researchers, our priority was always to present accurately
the voice of the participants. As Benner (1994) states, "The ethical
stance of the interpretive researcher is one of respect for the voice and
experience described in the text" (p. 101).

Interviews were transcribed and rechecked for accuracy, and then
summaries of the interviews were written by each of the researchers.
Observational notes assisted in developing early themes. Exemplars
from the text were extracted to demonstrate similarity or contrast of
patterns of meaning, common situations, or embodied experience. They
were then coded and used to develop additional themes. Analysis identified nine areas of student response as shown in the list of themes. These
themes described learning that emerged during the class or that was
recognized later in clinical practice by the student participants.

Theme 1: Ways to Learn About Caring. Students noted that the focus of the course was to listen to the stories of the class participants.
Creating an environment of comfort and safety in the course allowed
the participants to focus on listening and reflecting upon what they
heard. They came to understand that stories have power and that listening to stories may be more important at a given time than doing a
particular nursing task. One participant stated, "And I never would have
gotten that [in other classes] to just listen, not try to judge, not try to
fix, at that moment, whatever it is, but just listen to their story" (student,
personal communication, 1998).

Theme 2: Barriers to Learning About Caring. Students identified
the lecture format in which caring is presented as a generic concept as
an important barrier to learning about caring. They cited the course as
teaching them to think about caring as a connected part of the life and
situation of each patient. They contrasted their behavior in clinical sites
with the behavior of students who had not taken the course: "And people
that weren't in the class, you know, I've noticed you know, them looking

more through the charts and stuff, whereas, we just kind of spend time sitting down and talking (with the patient) and finding out more information" (student, personal communication, 1999).

Theme 3: Providing Caring Nursing. Students reported that their nursing practice changed when they understood patients through their stories. Along with listening and calling out the story, students organized and tailored their care in a different way than the care they had previously provided, depending on the shared meaning of the illness experience as identified between themselves and the patient.

You just don't know, really know, how to react and stuff. And being able to sit down with her and have her describe to me what happened and everything, it just, it let me, I guess, kind of get inside of her and really understand what happened to her a little bit more than just reading it in the progress notes. (Student, personal communication, 1998)

I've really come to believe in my heart, that that's how you get people to do in the end what you want them to do, is first, you have to listen to them, you have to listen to their story, you have to find out their meaning and their understanding of where they're at and then you can start playing the role of the nurse and incorporating health habits, health care, health promotion. (Student, personal communication, 1998)

Theme 4: Effect to Caregiver of Providing Caring Nursing. An important learning that occurred for students involved the difference they perceived in how they felt about themselves as practicing nurses when they individualized caring nursing practice for each patient. "And I really found I felt a lot better when I left at the end of the day. Knowing I had had that time with those patients and took the time to make that much of a difference in their lives" (student, personal communication, 1998).

Theme 5: Barriers to Providing Caring Nursing; and Theme 6: Being Nonresponsive. Students remarked about the effects of working within the healthcare system. They identified as causes of burnout such factors as devaluing care, being nonresponsive to the concerns of patients, and focusing entirely on the cure paradigm.

I've always been aware, people become kind of lackadaisical and uncaring. They get, I don't know what the word is, they become flat, you know. It seems like after a while complaints to them get old and they just kinda don't want to hear it and they lose that caring feel about them. And that's one of the things I want to avoid. (Student, personal communication, 1998)

Theme 7: Providing Uncaring Nursing; and Theme 8: Detaching. Doing necessary tasks related to the cure paradigm without being emotionally present to listen to patient concerns was identified by students as a strategy used by many nurses to detach themselves from the sad stories that patients carry with them related to their illnesses.

One lady in particular, she told me, you know, she had a really rough life. How she had never married, she'd had guys off and on, she'd had a baby she had to give up. You know, all this stuff just by me taking the time, you know. I saw her as a person rather than this body in this bed dying from COPD. (Student, personal communication, 1998)

Theme 9: Facilitating Caring Nursing. Students identified that the key to facilitating caring in their practice was to allow the time and have the autonomy to listen to patients' stories. In this way the shared meaning of the illness experience emerged and enabled the nurse to individualize caring. This caring nursing practice also reaffirmed for the students that the ability to care is a major factor and motivator for them as members of the nursing profession. "The whole concept of listening to someone's life story and caring through that life story was just, for me, it was phenomenal" (student, personal communication, 1989).

Part 3: The Recollective Pathway as Explicated in the Culture of Illness and the Culture of Caring

Teaching and learning about caring was the goal of the course and of the class community. Narrative pedagogy characterized the class deliberations and became the course content. The Recollective Pathway provided the structure and the foundation upon which new knowledge about caring in nursing practice emerged.

A major focus of the course was thinking about caring within the culture of illness and understanding both the constraints to caring practice and ways to enhance caring from the cultural perspective. The Recollective Pathway provided structure and foundation to analyze the "human action of people making, defining, altering and transforming the means which they have to attain meaning" (Higgins, 1981, p. 93).

Students and instructors as course participants practiced using personal narratives to create an interpersonal bridge between the two cultures of illness and caring. Through focused listening, questioning, and respect for the stories told in the class, participants recognized the individual and shared meanings of being in both the world of illness and the world of care giving. Finally, the reflective process, when shared and interpreted, helped each student to identify and to depict both patients and nurses in everyday situations that were full of meaning and context. The class participants, by using reflection, were able to come to a new empathetic understanding of these two cultures.

The findings of this study are significant, both for nursing practice and for nursing pedagogy. Course participants indicated that caring nursing practice based on individual and shared meanings of illness can be demonstrated, modeled, and practiced in a classroom setting. They were then able to successfully transfer their knowledge of caring practice into clinical situations with their patients.

While affirming the contribution that scientific knowledge has provided to the discipline of nursing, we must also provide a place for reflection in nursing pedagogy. Through the Recollective Pathway, students in the course learned useful ways to make contact with patients, to provide patients with expert coaching, and to be with patients as a presence. These attributes, as exemplified both in the research presented here and in the paradigm cases cited by Benner and Wrubel (1989), inform caring nursing practice (p. 9). Students in the course were able, as a result of learning through narrative pedagogy and the Recollective Pathway, to build a bridge to the culture of illness and, for a time, to enter that culture. Through understanding individual and shared meanings of illness with their patients, they were able to introduce caring into patient situations and to identify themselves through their actions as members of the culture of caring. They were able to appreciate that "persons, in the phenomenological view, have not only a world in which things have significance and value but qualitatively different concerns based on their culture, language and individual situations" (Leonard, 1994, p. 50).

This work is offered in anticipation that it will add another pathway to our understanding of caring, both in the practice of nursing and the pedagogy of the profession. Caring can be looked at in an empirical, scientific manner, as a basic motivation, or as a way of being for nurses.

We have reached the paradoxical point that brings us both confusion and clarity in our phenomena and our methods. This paradoxical turn now invites an inclusion of all sources of data, both conventional and original sources. This is required if we are to move forward with meaningful forms of inquiry about the still largely unknown phenomena of caring, healing processes, and outcomes. (Watson, 2002, pp. 245–248)

For healthcare and nursing in the new millennium, it is crucial that nurses identify which elements of nursing practice are essential. To remain strong and viable, the nursing profession must utilize scientific knowledge but must also learn the art of reflection in order to truly understand the patient's meaning of being-in-the-world. Such reflection is particularly important in addressing the issue of caring. Only in this way can both expert and compassionate nursing care be practiced. Only in this way can it be taught and learned.

References

Baron, R. (1985). An introduction to medical phenomenology: I can't hear you while I'm listening. *Annals of Internal Medicine, 103*, 606–611.

Benner, P. (Ed.). (1994). *Interpretive phenomenology: Embodiment, caring and ethics in health and illness*. Thousand Oaks, CA: Sage.

Benner, P. E., Tanner, C. A., & Chesla, C. A. (1996). *Expertise in nursing practice: Caring, clinical judgment and ethics*. New York: Springer.

Benner, P. E., & Wrubel, J. (1989). *The primacy of caring: Stress and coping in health and illness*. Menlo Park, CA: Addison-Wesley.

Bevis, E. O., & Watson, J. (1989). *Toward a caring curriculum: A new pedagogy for nursing*. New York: National League for Nursing.

Bishop, A. H., & Scudder, J. R. (1991). *Nursing: The practice of caring*. New York: National League for Nursing.

Bishop, A. H., & Scudder, J. R., Jr. (1996). *Nursing ethics: Therapeutic caring presence*. Boston: Jones & Bartlett.

Boykin, A. (1995). *Power, politics and public policy: A matter of caring*. New York: National League for Nursing Press.

Coles, R. (1989). *The call of stories: Teaching and the moral imagination*. Boston: Houghton Mifflin.

Diekelmann, J., & Diekelmann, N. (forthcoming). *Schooling learning teaching: Toward a narrative pedagogy*.

Diekelmann, N. (1995). Reawakening thinking: Is traditional pedagogy nearing completion? *Journal of Nursing Education, 34*(5), 195–196.

Dreyfus, H. L. (1984). Beyond hermeneutics: Interpretations in late Heidegger and recent Foucault. In G. Shapiro & A. Sicca (Eds.), *Hermeneutics: Questions and prospects* (pp. 66–83). Amherst: University of Massachusetts Press.

Dunlop, M. J. (1994). Is a science of caring possible? In P. Benner (Ed.), *Interpretive phenomenology: Embodiment, caring and ethics in health and illness* (pp. 27–41). Thousand Oaks, CA: Sage.

Frank, A. W. (1991). *At the will of the body: Reflections on illness.* Boston: Houghton Mifflin.

Frank, A. W. (1995). *The wounded storyteller: Body, illness and ethics.* Chicago: University of Chicago Press.

Frankl, V. E. (1984). Man's search for meaning: An introduction to logotherapy. New York: Washington Square Press.

Frankl, V. E. (1985). *The unconscious god.* New York: Washington Square Press.

Gaut, D. A., & Boykin, A. (1994). *Caring as healing: Renewal through hope.* New York: National League for Nursing.

Heidegger, M. (1962). *Being and time* (J. Macquarrie & E. Robinson, Trans.). New York: Harper & Row. (Original work published 1927)

Higgins, M. (1981). Care, culture and praxis. In M. Leininger (Ed.), *Caring: An essential human need* (pp. 83–94). Thorofare, NJ: Charles Slack.

Leininger, M. (Ed.) (1981). *Caring: An essential human need: Proceedings of three national caring conferences.* Thorofare, NJ: Charles Slack.

Leonard, V. (1994). A Heideggerian phenomenological perspective on the concept of person. In P. Benner (Ed.), *Interpretive phenomenology: Embodiment, caring and ethics in health and illness.* Thousand Oaks, CA: Sage.

Lindeman, C. & McAthie, M. (1999). *Fundamentals of contemporary nursing practice.* Philadelphia: Saunders.

Lopez, B. (1990). *Crow and Weasel.* San Francisco: North Point Press.

Morley, P. (1981). Reflections on the biopolitics of human nature. *Caring: An essential human need: Proceedings of three national caring conferences.* (pp. 145–157). Thorofare, NJ: Charles Slack.

Neil, R. M., & Watts, R. (Eds). (1991). *Caring and nursing: Explorations in feminist perspectives.* New York: National League for Nursing.

Paterson, B., & Crawford, M. (1994). Caring in nursing education: An analysis. *Journal of Advanced Nursing, 19*(1), 164–173.

Phillips, S. S., & Benner, P. (1994). *The crisis of care: Affirming and restoring caring practices in the helping professions.* Washington, DC: Georgetown University Press.

Schon, D. A. (1987). *Educating the reflective practitioner: Toward a new design for teaching and learning in the professions.* San Francisco: Jossey-Bass.

Severtsen, B. M., & Evans, B. C. (2000). Education for caring practice. *Nursing and Health Care Perspectives, 21,* 172–177.

Tolstoy, L. (1960). The Death of Ivan Ilych. In *The Death of Ivan Ilych and other stories* (A. Maud, Trans., pp. 95–156). New York, Signet (original work published 1886).

Travelbee, J. (1966). *Interpersonal aspects of nursing.* Philadelphia: F. A. Davis.

Watson. J. (1979). *Nursing: The philosophy and science of caring.* Boston: Little, Brown.

Watson, J. (2002). *Assessing and measuring caring in nursing and health science.* New York: Springer.

Watson, J., & Ray, M. A. (1988). *The ethics of care and the ethics of cure: Synthesis in chronicity.* New York: National League for Nursing.

Young-Mason, J. (1997). *The patient's voice: Experiences of illness.* Philadelphia: F. A. Davis.

6

Preceptors as the Champions of the New Nurse

The Context in Which Student Nurses Learn the Culture of Caring

Louise G. Rummel

Introduction

Caring is what nurses do. Everyone knows it. But can work related to being preceptors to undergraduate student nurses be explicated within a theme of caring and culture in health, healthcare, and healing? I believe that registered nurses (RNs) who experience *being as* preceptors are the culture bearers to the professional nurse. Preceptors transmit the dominant values of the nursing profession to the novice entrant. These values are caught rather than taught.

There is a crisis in relation to recruitment and retention of nurses throughout the world, including in New Zealand (Cobden-Grainge & Walker, 2002; Walker & Bailey, 1999). Questions are raised as to why nurses leave nursing. New nurses report that they will remain in nursing after graduation one year at the most (Gower & Finlayson, 2002). Morieson (2002) reported that in Victoria, Australia, the problem is now understood as a shortage of nurses "willing to nurse." One reason is that student nurses, as they are acculturated into the culture of nursing, do not feel welcomed into the caring community that they wish to enter. Nursing students expect to be welcomed into the profession but instead often find that they are an imposition on an already overburdened staff. This chapter addresses a dilemma: how do we teach nurses to care in a culture that is not always conducive to caring (Rummel, 2002)? Over-burdened RNs who accept the challenge of being preceptors do not fail to recognize the importance of preparing new nurses to understand the centrality of caring to healing and health. They cope with teaching students, as well as simultaneously providing nursing services, and purveying the culture of nursing.

Background

The prime purpose of this study (Rummel, 2002) carried out in New Zealand was to understand the experiences of RNs who act as preceptors to undergraduate student nurses in acute care settings and to uncover the meaning they derive from these experiences. With increasing demand for skilled beginning nurses who are entering practice in an increasingly complex healthcare environment, the contribution that RNs as preceptors make to nursing education should be made explicit.

In recent years, the distance between theoretical teaching and clinical learning experiences has been blamed for widening gaps in education (Crookes, 2000). The debate was fueled by the Ministerial Taskforce on Nursing claiming that "currently, [nursing education] programs are not producing graduates of a consistent standard, . . . teaching Resources are spread too thinly and students are not always receiving appropriate clinical placements" (New Zealand Ministry of Health, 1998, p. 60).

In previous research (Rummel, 1993), student nurses heralded their learning in clinical practice through the efforts of RN preceptors as greatly significant. What was missing from this early work was the voice of the preceptors and how they experienced teaching student nurses. The research reported here addresses that deficit. Further, due to government reforms in both the health and education sectors throughout the 1990s, major changes took place in nursing education and nursing practice. Those changes affected how clinical lecturers carried out their clinical teaching roles and how student nurses experienced their clinical placements. Most significant was the fact that the clinical lecturer was no longer closely aligned to student nurses in their clinical placement, and RNs as preceptors became clinical teachers for students. My interest is in how RNs managed this new responsibility in addition to their normal patient care assignments. I was also mindful that, although historically student nurses learned from their more senior counterparts on the wards, academic advancement of the profession now requires nurses to hold a bachelor's degree to practice in New Zealand.

Research Approach

An interpretive approach using Heideggerian hermeneutics was chosen as a way of uncovering the experience of being a preceptor. The experience of *being* requires a human science approach to understand how being acts in and on a world (Taylor, 1989). Heideggerian hermeneutic phenomenology is especially suited to understanding human concerns, which include meaning, experiential learning, and practical everyday activity. The interpretive approach also offered an opportunity to move beyond traditional ways of knowing concerning preceptoring, ways that are strongly influenced by the explanatory and predictive methods of natural science (Benner, 1994).

Significance of the Study

The background literature reviewed for the study revealed that the term *preceptor* was derived from the noun *precept*, from the Latin *praeceptum*, referring to a maxim or command (Onions, 1955). The first located use of the word *precept* is in Psalm 119 (Holy Bible, King James Version). The literature points to the concept of preceptorship rather than "being a preceptor." The term *preceptor* first appeared in the general nursing indices in 1975 as a classification indicator (Shamian & Inhaber, 1985). Most studies related to being precepted, and preceptorship programs assumed that preceptorship was beneficial. One American study on a preceptor model of clinical instruction included the experiences of students, preceptors, and clinical instructors (Nehls, Rather, & Guyette, 1997). Inquiry revealed that most of the literature originated in the United States, with a paucity of empirical literature related to the topic of the *experience* of being a preceptor. There were no studies in New Zealand related to the human science perspective of preceptoring undergraduate student nurses. Additionally, little is known about how RNs manage their dual role of teaching students and caring for patients. Formalization of preceptorship programs for undergraduate student nurses was still in its infancy in New Zealand, although the need for such programs had been identified.

As an educator, I believe understanding the preceptor experience is crucial to the quality of future nursing education and to the quality of care delivered to people cared for by nurses. It is only through student nurses learning the practice of nursing by immersion in the culture of the professional community in which preceptors play a central part that these powerful learning experiences can be transmitted. The research explored and made visible what preceptors found most meaningful and significant in *being as* preceptor.

Key Terms and Concepts

Preceptor. A preceptor is a RN who works in a one-to-one relationship with an undergraduate student nurse who is learning the practice of nursing in a clinical placement in an acute care setting.

Culture. Culture in this context is defined as the dynamic everyday tensions, values, and norms with which we live that bring meaning to the everyday world of nursing practice. It includes the history of nursing in context: the beliefs, customs, and practices that are part of nursing. Nightingale (1859/1946) believed strongly that nurses should work to initiate an environment that was conducive to healing. A century and a half later, this value for nurses is still central to the practice of nursing.

Caring. The generic values of the nursing profession are that nurses learn and promote values of caring (McCance, McKenna, & Boore, 1999; Watson, 1988). Benner and Wrubel (1989) claim that caring is primary to healing. The *Code of Ethics* of the New Zealand Nurses' Organization (2001) states that caring is the moral foundation of nursing:

It is a professional and societal expectation that nurses' work requires caring, an involvement of self and a real concern for the well-being of another. Caring as a philosophical base for practice . . . encompasses the concepts of compassion, commitment, competence, congruence, confidence, conscience, culture, collaboration, communication and consultation amongst others. (p. 10)

There is a danger, however, that caring as a professional and personal value is being obscured by the corporate lens of cost cutting and the restructuring of healthcare delivery systems in which nurses simply try to survive each day (Irving & Snider, 2002). New Zealand is not different from the rest of the world. It too has healthcare systems under siege by cost cutting at a time when an aging and diverse population requires more healthcare rather than less. Such a healthcare context inevitably affects preceptors and student nurses learning the practice of nursing.

Cultural Conditioning. Cultural conditioning in nursing has taken place over a long history of hospital-based education for nurses in which nurses were trained to deliver nursing care to meet service needs of the healthcare agency. Education was purported to be taking place, but the daily round of clinical demands upon nurses meant that education happened surreptitiously, rather than following a well-defined curriculum model. In such a model, ideally, classroom teaching would be complemented by clinical experience to embed the knowledge of the practice of nursing. The cultural conditioning that established nursing education within hospital wards has continued, either overtly or covertly, to be a major cornerstone of nursing education. It is still believed by many nurses, especially those who are employed in clinical agencies, that a hospital is the only place where nursing practice can and does take place. Yet in the 21st century, the traditional work of nurses is undergoing major reshaping; caring is taking on new dimensions.

Care has moved from a focus upon meeting the health needs of the individual to meeting the health needs of population groups. Further, the practices of nursing are moving from hospital walls to hospitals without walls and into communities. Today's nurses are educated much more broadly within tertiary education settings. Nurses are educated to think of caring in a global perspective. Health is viewed holistically with sensitivity to individual and group interpretations of health as those are perceived within differing cultural contexts. In particular, traditional healing practices often complement orthodox medical care, and nurses are conversant in a number of complementary health practices such as massage, aromatherapy, and reflexology (Taylor, Lillis, & Le Mone, 1997).

For nurses working with informed populations of differing peoples, the ability to communicate effectively and the ability to negotiate healthcare to include specific cultural beliefs, customs, and practices are essential skills required within a consumer- and technology-driven environment. The ability of consumers to direct their own healthcare requires nurses not only to be skilled communicators but also to practice cross culturally in a culturally safe manner. The development of these skills begins in nursing education programs as student nurses learn the practices of nursing.

Additionally, nurses are educated to be politically aware in order to advocate sensitively for disadvantaged groups in society. On a societal level, this advocacy includes safe housing and care for the disabled, the chronically mentally ill, the elderly, and minority groups who are too few in number and who lack power to speak for themselves. Nurses are being educated to become primary healthcare leaders in the 21st century (KPMG Consulting, 2001). Yet, this broad context for contemporary nursing (rather than the historical hospital environment) requires core skills that are learned in the practice of nursing. The preceptor plays a key role in the inculcation of these practices.

In interpretive research, because meaning is always situated, context refers to the historical, political, social, cultural, and, in this instance, professional nursing background in which the experience of the preceptor is lived and interpreted. Context relates to the ways persons are connected in the world and always implies temporality (Benner & Wrubel, 1989). Heideggerian hermeneutics understands *being* as situated within a specific temporal context where human concerns and actions are afforded meaning and significance. Therefore, in this study, for *being-as* preceptor, the immediate day-to-day preceptor–preceptee activities within the acute care setting constitute the temporal world of preceptor practice.

The Study

A phenomenological hermeneutic study was conducted to understand the meaning of being a preceptor to undergraduate student nurses in an acute care setting (Rummel, 2002). The question asked was, "What is the experience of being a preceptor to undergraduate student nurses in the acute care setting?"

Research Method

Following approval granted through two ethics committees, fifteen volunteer RN preceptors were interviewed twice. The preceptors' experience ranged from 10 months to 32 years in nursing. Each interview was one hour in length and was tape-recorded. The resulting transcripts were reviewed by the participants and formed the basis for the data analysis. The hermeneutic analytic process was conducted according to seven steps of reading and rereading transcripts, identifying themes that emerged from each transcript, and looking across transcripts to see what common themes emerged. Common themes were conceptualized in search of relational themes and identifying a constitutive pattern that was either directly overt or inferred in all the transcripts. It is important to recognize that the hermeneutic process does not move forward linearly but rather moves backward and forward in a questioning spiral *of* the data and *from* the data in order to identify the thematic patterns within it. The final work is in writing and rewriting the research report, which explicates the themes supported by narratives from the research data.

Phenomenology seeks to reveal human perceptions and subjectivity in order to understand what it is like to experience a phenomenon first-hand. Because little is known about preceptors' firsthand experiences of *being as* preceptors, in this instance phenomenology is used to reveal what it is like to *be as* a preceptor from the preceptors' own experience or, in other words, what preceptorship means or signifies to them (van Manen, 1990). An inherent concept in phenomenology is *lived experience*. Coming to know what it means to be a preceptor is best understood by the people who live the experience in their everyday world. The preceptors' stories of *being as* preceptors to undergraduate student nurses show that they immerse their practice as preceptors in their everyday practice of nursing. It is from the insights gained from these stories that we may increase our understanding of what it is like to be a preceptor to undergraduate student nurses.

Hermeneutics and the Philosophical Works of Heidegger

Hermeneutics illuminated both the conduct and the interpretations of the interviews that formed the substantive data for the study. The interpretive process was based upon the works of Martin Heidegger, particularly *Being and Time* (1962) and his later essays. A particular nursing focus was gained through work by notable nurse scholars Nancy Diekelmann (1990) and Patricia Benner (1984, 1994), which provided invaluable insights into analysis and the interpretive process.

In *Being and Time* Heidegger (1962) focused on the fundamental question of the meaning of Being. "Being-what-it-is" is understood in terms of its Being, that is, what it means to be a person (p. 27). Moreover, "Being-in-the-world" he terms *Dasein* or "being there," which is our normal mode of existence (p. 27). Contained in this idea is the notion that the physical world is saturated with meaning that is captured in language, embodiment, temporality, and space. Heidegger describes all this as the "lifeworld," which is the real world of our everyday living that we normally take for granted. For preceptors in the context of the study, the real world was the world of patients, students, and other health professionals.

Heidegger gives three characteristics of Dasein: *existentiality, facticity,* and *verfallen* (1962, p. 237). Heidegger claims that all three characteristics are unified in his notion of "care," which is our basic way of being in the world. *Existentiality* refers to our humanity in time that is "being ahead of oneself" and living into possibility. *Facticity* or being "already-in-a-world," refers to living in the present. *Verfallen* is about "being alongside" others in the world, being caught up in the everyday world about us without giving too much thought to what is going on around us. In the state of *verfallen*, Dasein does not take responsibility for what it does (Guignon, 1993, p. 30; Heidegger, 1962, p. 165). All three constituents of Dasein have a relationship to time or temporality that is essentially future, past, and present, which is constitutive of *being* ontologically. If one is living into possibility that is ahead of oneself, one is always becoming what one already is.

World

For Heidegger, "being-in-the-world" means being human. "World" here refers to a relational world where we participate in a world with other human beings within cultural, social, and historical contexts (Diekelmann, Allen, & Tanner, 1989). In the Heideggerian view, persons live as self-interpreting beings in a world where meaning is created for us directly from a background of pre-understandings passed down in language and cultural practices. This background is never completely clear to us, but we cannot divorce ourselves from it nor can we ever be free of its influence. Consequently, we cannot withhold ourselves from our background; it is pervasive. We interpret our everyday experiences through a veil of background meaning. Both preceptors and preceptees are caught up in the way they interpret their experiences of *being-in-the-world* of nursing practice, an interpretation that has been passed down in the language and the cultural practices of nursing.

The Preceptors' World

RNs, who became "participating preceptors" in the study, were already "thrown" (Heidegger, 1962, p. 174) into the world of nursing practice. This throwness is an unspoken, unaware way of experiencing the everyday world. The familiar world for the RNs of the study was the context of caring for patients in the acute care setting. This "everydayness," according to Heidegger (1962, p. 38), is a pre-reflective, uncritical mode of "being-in-the-world." In the ward context, to be called upon to be a preceptor often meant a sudden change of plans and a sense of losing touch with the familiar or well-known ways of being a practitioner. It involved a change in focus to one that is in between worlds. The preceptor's attention must consciously be directed toward the student, who brings an educational and cultural orientation with him or her in learning to be a nurse, whereas the preceptor brings to the situation his or her orientation that is grounded in the practice and culture of healthcare delivery.

Meaning and Language

Taylor (1985) drew attention to the nature of language and its importance as part of being human. In his view, only the human being has the capability of creating meaning, because to be human is to be part of a social world where language gains its inherent meaning. For Heidegger, "meaning is that from which something is understandable as the thing it is within a world of human existence" (King, 1964, p. 7). Knowledge emanates from persons who are already in the world. The situation includes the "relevant concerns, issues, information, constraints and resources at a given span of time or place as experienced by particular persons" (Benner & Wrubel, 1989, p. 412). Meaning structures are public and also locally circumscribed. Local culture comes in a variety of forms. These forms shape the way we assign meaning and respond to things. For this work, the local culture is the lifeworld of preceptors and student nurses in the acute care setting.

Heidegger (1962) employed hermeneutics to understand and interpret Dasein or *Being-in-the-world* (Palmer, 1969). Dasein seeks to understand itself and its world in order to see the possibilities available to it. Dasein uses language to show something beyond just words: namely, being. Gadamer (as cited in Palmer, 1969) claimed that hermeneutics is a meeting with Being through language. Hermeneutics focuses upon philosophical questions of the "relationship of language to being, understanding, history, existence, and reality" (p. 42). It brings to light or into the *clearing* the hidden meaning language evokes. Hermeneutics does not have rules for undertaking interpretations of text; rather, it has a circle of interpretation and understanding (Leonard, 1994).

Heidegger (1962) states that in all interpretations there is always a fore-structure of understanding and an "as" structure of interpretation (p. 193). He claimed that being "as" something appropriates meaning to a certain way of being-in-the-world. In this research that "certain way" relates to *being as* preceptor. The "as" gets its structure from a fore-having, a fore-sight, and a fore-conception. The fore-having is something we have in advance of what will constitute the totality of the experience. That is our taken-for-granted background understanding of the phenomenon of interest, which makes interpretation possible. It is an interpretive point from which we have a definite conception of the phenomenon under discussion. "Fore-sight" according to Heidegger is something we see in advance and is directed by our "fore-having." Fore-conception however, is something we grasp in advance and can direct our interpretation of what is to be understood. Heidegger (1962, p. 191) explains that we do not approach an interpretation without presuppositions and assumptions. It is the becoming aware of these pre-conceived understandings that is important if we are to interpret text authentically.

Heideggerian Work Employed in the Interpretive Process of the Research

In the interpretation of transcripts from the participating preceptors, I have drawn upon Heidegger's (1971) essay "Building, Dwelling, Thinking." He claimed that there is a kind of thinking that results from attention to the relationship between *building, dwelling,* and *thinking*. In his essay, Heidegger used the word *dwell* to describe how we, as human beings, are on the earth. He believed that we must first "build" before we can "dwell" (p. 148).

He also identified the notion of the *fourfold* in this essay by referring to the unified presence of the earth, sky, divinities, and mortals—in the "thing." The "thing" gathers the world. After reading many commentaries (Edwards, 1998; Guignon, 1993; Inwood, 1999; Kolb, 1986; Krell in Heidegger, 1993), I find that Heidegger depicts the *fourfold* as sources of energy and influence. He identifies the four influences as a style of unifying where all essences share equal expanse and no one "thing" dominates. Here, I have interpreted Heidegger to mean the unity or the holism of the world. Each element requires the others to complete the whole. Where all forces meet, there is a gathering. We experience this gathering place as subjectivity, as lived time and space, and as "being" (Kolb, 1986, p. 138). "Being" in this case refers to being a community of relationships.

To put this notion into the context of *being-in-the-world* as a preceptor, and *being with* others within the nursing context, it is difficult to make explicit the complexity of the influences that gather all those involved in healthcare services. Nevertheless, these influences are the background to the practice of both preceptors and students within the world of nursing practice. It must be remembered, however, that normally, we as humans are in the world without an awareness of our background influences. These are simply taken for granted (Benner, 1984, 1994; Benner & Wrubel, 1989).

Since *being-in-the-world* is temporal and situated, the particular era of history for the preceptors as they precepted undergraduate student nurses is significant. There is a circle of interpretation for the preceptor and the student that brings together the historical, sociopolitical, cultural, and personal influences of their own lives as they practice as self-interpreting beings within the world of nursing practice. As well, there are the organizational culture, the local nursing culture, the concerns and needs of the related educational structures, multiple patients, the demands of a linear time frame, and the calling forth of relevant knowledge and skills in the provision of nursing services. Preceptors must first weigh their own practice requirements for their primary roles as RNs and, secondarily, as teachers, guides, supporters, and assistants to student nurses. In an interpretation of the *fourfold* for this research, I see that all the influences that are background to the practice of both the preceptor and the student come together to influence the space in which the preceptor dwells in his or her world of nursing practice.

Dwelling takes place through cultivation and construction. Heidegger (1962) took us back to the original word from which the idea of dwelling comes. In the original translation from the German, *Bauen* is used to mean that we stay in place or remain. Further, the Gothic word *wunian* says more distinctly how this remaining is experienced. *Wunian* is a related word to the idea of dwelling and means to be at peace. If we relate this idea to the preceptors, one could say that the preceptors are assisting the student to be "at peace" or comfortable with the reality of the world of nursing. Preceptors are guiding students to fit well into the world of nursing. Additionally, *friede* (peace) means to free. Epitomized in the derivation of the word *friede* is also the idea of preserving from harm or danger, or safeguarding. Likewise, a related meaning of *friede* is the idea of *sparing*. *Sparing* means that we do not harm the one we preserve. The fundamental character of dwelling is sparing. Undergraduate student nurses learn to dwell in the world of nursing practice by way of journeying within it. The unity of dwelling and journeying appears to be the unity of space and time (Pöggeler, 1989).

Ready to Hand-Unready to Hand

Another Heideggerian concept adopted in the interpretive process was the term "ready to hand-unready to hand." This concept is used by Heidegger to relate to equipment. In the case of a hammer, he argued, knowledge of the hammer comes about in its use. He used this example to illustrate the different properties related to theoretical and practical activity. We can know about equipment in a theoretical way (unready to hand), but it is in the use of equipment that we discover its manipulability. This manipulability has the kind of Being that belongs to equipment. Its purpose is to achieve an outcome. With familiarity, equipment becomes ready-to-hand. Practical understanding has its own kind of insight (Heidegger, 1962, p. 98).

Thinking

Fundamentally, Heidegger proposed a way of thinking about the things that we usually take for granted. Thinking does not have to be linear, systematic, logical, or calculative; rather, thinking is dwelling in the world and never separated from "Being." "Thinking is the engagement of being-in-the-world" (Heidegger, 1993, p. 219). Thinking is captured in the hermeneutic language of stories from the preceptors' practice as they journey with students in the world of nursing practice. This thinking *is* nursing (Rather, 1990). The stories reveal the *how* of the thinking of the preceptors. Heidegger placed importance on thinking *Being* first prior to "the distinction between theory and practice, or contemplation or deed" (Heidegger, 1993, p. 215). Heidegger calls attention to the inseparability of being and thinking. This research calls attention to how *being as* preceptors is revealed in the preceptors' own words as they disclose their fundamental way of *being-in-the-world*.

Findings of the Study

The findings of the study were summarized in the constitutive pattern of *Safeguarding the practices of nursing* as the central theme revealed through intensive hermeneutic analysis of all data. This central theme of *Safeguarding the practices of nursing* comprised four relational themes: *Becoming attuned, Emerging identity of* being as *preceptor, Assessing where the student is*, and *Preceptors as builders of nursing practice through teaching reality nursing.*

Becoming attuned—The call related to how RNs responded to the call for *being as* preceptors to students in their clinical placement. What was evident in this relational theme was that, while many preceptors precepted unwillingly, others appreciated that someone had to *dwell* with students in order for them to learn the practices of nursing. Preceptors safeguarded nursing practice as they "cultivated" students by encouraging, fostering, helping, and nurturing them in the real life world of practice. They also learned to "grow" students, to extend and stretch them as they worked alongside them. In this way they transmitted the culture of caring to them as the nurses of tomorrow, as well as ensuring that they met the standards required for quality client care.

Emerging identity of being as *preceptor—Keeping the student in mind* related to preceptors cultivating their own identity of *being as* preceptors as they worked with students meaningfully in the world of nursing practice. The relational theme revealed how the preceptors constantly keep the student in mind as they themselves deliver nursing care. They are conscious of teaching students through role modeling, as well as keeping a watchful eye on the student as the student practices. The preceptors revealed that even when the student was not on duty, they were thinking of how they could assist the student to learn.

Assessing where the student is—The preceptor and preceptee working and growing together revealed how preceptors constantly assessed where students' learning needs lay in order to evaluate their safety to be left to practice on their own and their readiness to advance their knowledge of practice.

Preceptors as builders of nursing practice through teaching reality nursing focused entirely on the practices of precepting students engaged in direct patient care.

The research also revealed through the preceptors' narratives an awareness that they walked in an in-between space between the world of nursing practice and the world of nursing education. This in-between space was a difficult one for *being as* preceptors because in reality they were torn between three masters. First, as RNs, preceptors are professionally accountable for caring for patients. Second, they are responsible to their employers to uphold the organizational standards of quality of practice. Third, as preceptors, they were now responsible for student teaching and learning.

Interested readers are now invited to join the hermeneutic process of experiencing and interpreting for themselves particular narratives that comprised the constitutive pattern of *Safeguarding the Practices of Nursing: The lived experience of being-as preceptor to undergraduate student nurses in an acute care setting.*

Relational Theme—Becoming Attuned to the Call to Be a Preceptor

RNs who became preceptors responded to the "call" of precepting simply because the students were "there." They projected themselves into a place where they no longer experienced an easy, or unthinking, everydayness in their familiar world. They moved or were thrown into a place where they became aware that they were bridging two worlds: caring for patients as a practitioner and being a preceptor to an undergraduate student nurse by acting as a teacher and a guide. Behind the attunement lies self-consciousness. Heidegger (1962) suggests that as part of the pursuit of self-understanding for Dasein "the call reaches the they-self of concernful being with others" (p. 317). As a result, "being" becomes self-conscious, an inauthentic self (p. 169). The "call" refers to the partly open field of possibilities and the way this is unveiled for preceptors (Kolb, 1986). Preceptors respond to the call to be a preceptor out of their caring about new students and about the survival of the profession of nursing. For some this meant an entry into a new world that brings with it some "unsettledness."

Unsettledness is an interesting concept. Dreyfus (1991) in his commentary on Heidegger's *Being and Time* refers to *Unheimlich*, which is translated as "uncanny," but Dreyfus prefers to translate it as "unsettledness" (p. xii). Both translations refer to a feeling of "anxiety." "Anxiety," as employed by Heidegger, reveals the nature of Dasein and its world. Preceptors experienced some "anxiety" related to a sense of not being at home in this new world of precepting. Participants disclosed their concerns about the restless movement between the two worlds of teaching and practice. Precepting often began with little warning. The student arrived as the staff nurses came on shift duty. Suddenly, a student was "there." It was often left to the RNs to volunteer to precept students.

Offers to help came from those who were listening to the call, those who were willing. When the RNs came "on shift," a general enquiry would be made as to who would be willing to take a student for the day. "Dale" discloses how he came to be a preceptor under these conditions:

It always seems to be the case when we have students, "who wants to take this student?" [Dale laughs.] You have a bit of sympathy for them, and you think, well, you know, rather than just land with somebody who doesn't really want to take the student you say, "well, okay, I'll take the student and maybe they'll have a better experience." So that's pretty much it. When I see the students turn up I think, yeah, okay, I'll give them a break. (Dale, interview 1, p. 1)

In Dale's interview, there was an implicit recognition of the literal meaning of being thrown rather than the Heideggerian sense of the thrownness of being with others in an unreflective mode of everydayness. Dale shows that students are thrown into the practice setting, and they may "land with somebody who doesn't really want" to precept them. He discloses a state of mind toward precepting students that appears open and welcoming, born out of caring about students. But what is the nature of Dale's laugh? Could it imply that Dale sees the whole process as being perhaps embarrassing or uncomfortable? Is this discomfort born out of a memory of living those tense moments when Dale himself was the student waiting to see which RN would be willing to be a preceptor? His statement that he will give students "a break" suggests that he, too, remembers what it was like to be a student and not welcomed in the clinical placement.

The culture of nursing in acute care settings is all about relationships with patients and their families, with medical practitioners, with colleagues, and essentially with students learning to be nurses. In the context of the research, wards were often understaffed or staffed with a variety of auxiliary staff. There were often very few RNs who were familiar with the ward. This often meant that student nurses were an added burden to the staff present and therefore were not particularly welcomed. Dale responds to the call out of his caring about students learning under these conditions.

Subtheme—Being Thrown. One preceptor ("Jessie") remembered all too well what it was like to be "thrown on to the wards." Despite the difference in surface meaning, this feeling of "being thrown in" is indeed similar to Heidegger's idea of "thrownness," as Jessie has no control over the situation; her feeling is dissimilar in so far as she is conscious of her uncomfortable feeling related to "being thrown in." In order to prevent students feeling like she did, she showed her concern for the students by responding to the call:

I actually look back on my student days with some horror because I was just literally thrown onto the wards. I was never seen as supernumerary. I was a pair of hands and—and for me that's an experience I'll never forget. . . . And I thought, "God! These poor students!" They used to come on in the morning shift—there'd be five of them—and they'd stand there and they were just . . . "Oh! We've got students today! Do you want to take one?" And then they'd have another person the next day. And another person the next day, and there was no continuation for them. I was quite horrified. (Jessie, interview 1, p. 1)

In everyday use, "being thrown into" something means a sudden thrusting into a situation for which one does not feel prepared. The person experiences feelings of insecurity, of not being in control, and finds distress in the unexpectedness of the situation and feelings. For some, this would be discouraging, while others would find it challenging. To be "thrown onto" the wards as Jessie was is not the (by comparison) easy experience of the relational everyday world of nursing practice as Heidegger's idea of "being-in-the-world" implies. Jessie recalls an historical past and senses "enduring" (Heidegger, 1977) practices that would best be overturned. She is concerned that students still have the same experience in the present. She remembers that feeling of being a student and being abandoned. It is an uncomfortable feeling and not forgotten. The listener gains an impression that the students are placed in a lottery situation while the RNs in the setting decide who will take a student for the day.

Jessie paints a picture of the students coming onto a morning shift and just standing "there." Heidegger addresses "being there" in his discussion on the word *Dasein* (Heidegger, 1962, p. 26). Dasein's "there" refers to a shared world. The shared situation is known as the "clearing." In the clearing, the "Being" is unconcealed. For "Being" to come to understand itself depends upon shared practices. For both preceptors and students, Heidegger's use of "the clearing" portrays the "centered" way of a particular Dasein or *being-in-the-world*. Dasein also brings its "there" along with it. That is, the preceptors bring whatever experiences they have had to date into the new situation. In particular, preceptors bring a wealth of nursing experience that comes from "being there" in the world of nursing practice and being immersed in the culture of nursing. Students seek to learn the practice of nursing and expect to draw on this experience. As one preceptor put it:

When you're a student you look at this RN and you think—[they] know so much, I know so little. . . . And yet, as an RN looking back, . . . I think, yes, that is right. But now is the opportunity to tap into that person that knows so much and have the person that knows so much teach the one that knows so little. (Lee, interview 1, p. 3)

Relational Theme: The Emerging Identity of Being-as Preceptor—Keeping the Student in Mind

Subtheme: Precepting as "Nursing" the Student. Because nursing is a practice that claims to have care as its focus, there are times when whoever needs care calls out a response from a nurse to "be there" for that person. In a paradigm narrative, a preceptor gives an account of a student in whom she recognizes unresolved grief expressed by the student following the death of a patient. The preceptor shares her experience:

She was a fairly junior student, probably in her first year. In fact I think it would have been her first year. She had worked out in the community. And it was quite strange, we were talking about death, and at that stage we had a lot of very ill patients and quite a few had died, just prior to her coming. And she was looking after a male patient, probably in about his 60s or 70s. I can remember talking to her,—we'll call her June. I was talking to June and she just sort of very flippantly said, 'Oh, my father died six weeks ago.' And I thought that's quite strange. And she didn't seem to show any emotion or—you know, anything—and I felt that it was a little bit flippant, and I just sort of held that in the back of my mind. Anyway, she was doing very well, looking after this patient, and then she changed to afternoon shift, and I happened to be on that day. And she wasn't under my care or anything, but she walked into the room, just to say hello, because she had built up quite a rapport with this gentleman. The relatives were sitting round the bed, and the patient had died. And she got such a shock that she went hysterical. Went absolutely hysterical. I've never seen anyone behave in that way in my life. She actually crawled under the bed. And she sobbed her heart out. And she kept saying, 'Oh, I'm sorry I wasn't there, I'm sorry I wasn't there.' And I knew that she had reverted back to her father's death . . . the man that she was nursing was probably about the same age as her father, and it was like a—a replay. (Bernie, interview 1, pp. 7, 8)

In this narrative, the preceptor reveals her engagement in the world of nursing practice and her involvement in being a preceptor to the student nurse. She implies that the student and she have an established relationship, and within this she has background knowledge of the student's prior experience of her father's death. It is because of this background knowledge that she is able to relate to the student's reaction to the patient's death. Coping with death is a very human experience, with each person coming to it from his or her own perspective. For student nurses, death is something not yet experienced and generally feared; they are not sure how it will be for them on their first encounter. They are not sure what to expect to see, and they are not sure of themselves and how they will respond in the situation. The preceptor makes the statement that the student "was not under my care." This is an interesting statement in so far as it shows that the preceptor considers the student to be part of her caring role as a nurse.

The preceptor does not say whether the student was anticipating her patient's death. With family sitting around the bed, it is highly likely that the student would recognize the nursing practice, grounded in the culture of caring, of family surrounding the dying person. Nurses recognize the healing powers in family support and their presence at the bedside (Benner, Hooper-Kyriakidis, & Stannard, 2001). What the preceptor reveals is that the student is devastated and becomes hysterical with the event. The preceptor then recalls a conversation that reveals the likely explanation for the student's distress.

The preceptor shows that she is engaged in the world of her student and sees the immediate need of the student is to be cared for. The preceptor, as an expert nurse first and foremost in the situation, is able to understand immediately the important issues and responds to the needs of the student, who for her, in this instance, takes precedence over the patient and the patient's family. Benner, Tanner, and Chesla (1996) state that the hallmark of the expert nurse is to home in immediately on the salient issues that are occurring in the situation and respond appropriately. The preceptor relates to the student as if she is the patient as her continuing narrative reveals: "And anyway, I couldn't get her out from under the bed, and it was really not appropriate that she was behaving in that way."

The preceptor reveals that she is mindful of the patient's family, the death of the patient, and the student. Mindfulness is described here as "focused thinking"—a form of thinking that is thoughtful, attentive, and watchful. The preceptor is attuned to the feelings, emotions, and events in the situation, since the experience of dealing with death and caring for the dying is a cultural practice with which she is familiar. She continues:

And I got her out of the room, and she was almost frozen, like her legs wouldn't move. And the Charge nurse at the time didn't understand the situation and she said, get her out of there! And that wasn't really appropriate either, but fortunately I could understand what was going on, and I pieced it together with my memory of her saying her father had died six weeks before. (Bernie, interview 1, p. 8)

The charge nurse's reaction to the student's behavior could have compounded the situation, but the preceptor maintains a moral agency within the situation (Benner, Tanner, & Chesla, 1996) and continues "to be there" for the student. She continues:

And so I took her outside . . . we were on the ground floor, and—there was a chair out where people would go and sit in the sun. There was only one chair so I grabbed another one quickly and we sat outside, and I really just had to hold her until she'd stopped sobbing. And eventually she stopped her sobbing and quieted down. And I asked her, 'Is this something to do with your dad dying?' And so we sat there for, it must have been an hour. (Bernie, interview 1, p. 8)

The preceptor reveals how she comforts the student and allows the student to express the grief that, she believes, had not been expressed when her father had died. The student's response, in the preceptor's words, allowed for her "catharsis." The preceptor, motivated out of the student's need, provides the caring that will allow the possibility for emotional healing for the student.

One could wonder how the preceptor has the time to spend "one hour" with the student when her primary focus should be on the patient. However, in her expert way of dealing with the situation, she also makes provision for her patients. She continues: "And in that time I had to go back and explain what I was doing, and make sure my patients were all right." The preceptor is mindful that she must still care for her patients. One of the difficulties for preceptors was the "double accountability" they felt being both a preceptor and a practicing practitioner. This preceptor continues:

And I made her a cup of tea, and we sat out there in the sun, and it was quite pleasant, the birds were singing in this little tree, and—I could listen to her. And she wasn't there when her father died; she got there too late. And that was—what triggered it off, and not being there for this patient. So she talked about her father's illness and it was expected, the death, but it was still quite sudden. . . . And it got to the point where she'd calmed down, she'd gone through the catharsis, she'd cried and expressed that. And she'd got to a reasonable state, but she was in no state to actually go back onto the ward. And we were walking together, and I didn't quite know what to do with her then, because I didn't have the time to spend—and then her tutor walked around the corner at exactly the most perfect moment, so I could hand her over. And it was really lovely, and I said, "She needs to be taken right off the ward and she probably hasn't got energy to walk or anything, but she just needs to, maybe have something to eat and another drink, and just be nurtured." And so off they went, and they must have talked things through; I don't know all the details. They came back to the ward, probably about an hour and a half later. By that time the relatives of the patient had left, and the patient then had to be washed, and readied to be taken to the morgue. And the nurse then came back and she said she would like to help me. And I thought that was quite brave, and I said, "You know, you've really been through a lot today, you don't need to do this." But she really wanted to. She'd talked it through with her tutor, and she assured me that she wanted to do it as well. So—we did it together. And it was a very lovely experience. And we washed the patient, and we dressed the patient. And everything went very smoothly. And it was like she was following something major through to complete her own grief. And—you know, we put flowers in the room, and we did everything just—perfectly, by the book. And then it was time for her to go. So it was a very nice way of completing something.

Diekelmann (1990) identified the importance of knowing the student in the teaching and learning process in nursing education. Because the preceptor knows the student and the student's background, she is able to understand immediately what is happening to her student with the advent of the death of her patient. The patient's death initiates the student's hysteria. The preceptor understands that because of the recent loss of the student's father, the death of the patient when the student isn't present triggers feelings of guilt in the student for not being present for the death of both her father and the patient.

The preceptor, by "being there" with the student, helped her to grieve in a way that was therapeutic and provided the student with a sense of closure and healing. What is most noticeable here is the way the preceptor cared for the student. The student experienced firsthand what it is like to be cared for by both her preceptor and her tutor. The tutor was wonderful for the student and for the preceptor, who then experienced a sense of release. That the preceptor took so much care of her student is an outstanding example of how preceptors take care to nurture developing nurses. Her student is a privileged student. The preceptor embodies caring, enabling the student to experience firsthand what it is that nurses do. The student now knows how to care for others, for she herself has been cared for and has experienced emotional healing that will free her to care for others.

Subtheme: Gifting Time to Share. "Rebecca" illustrates the practice of preceptors keeping students in mind regardless of the business of their own practice. She relates the following narrative:

I had a great experience with a second-year student who I had for about four or five weeks and she was a student I knew from the beginning because our clinical nurse educator talked to me about her, that she has not achieved in her previous clinical experience. She was someone, when I first met her, very anxious . . . very nervous about the whole experience. . . . She'd sort of babble away, trying to impress me with her knowledge [laughs], sounding very confused about what she was talking about. And I'd sometimes just look at her in absolute astonishment; I mean her stress levels must have been enormous. So I was very aware of that, and wanting her to relax. And my personal belief about education—you can't learn unless you're feeling good about yourself and I like to give lots of positive reinforcement for things I see they're doing well, and like to really try and help them feel good about themselves early on. Because I think when you're feeling confident and good, you do well. (Rebecca, interview 1, p. 2)

Rebecca's background understanding is that her student has not achieved to date, and she recognizes that her student's past is likely to affect how she will "be" in her clinical placement. Her way of *being as* preceptor to her student is that she is concerned about the way her student is experiencing being in the world as a nursing student in the world of nursing practice. At the same time she compares herself with colleagues who seem not to be so caring toward their students. She continues:

I see other nurses being quite hard on their students and being very judgmental—they can't believe how much they don't know and—you know, 'Surely I wasn't like that.' There's this real perception that tech. students [those student nurses receiving their education in a polytechnic setting] are so dumb these days. There's this real thing, they still don't have enough clinical experience . . . I don't see that myself. And I also believe . . . that I see other nurses being quite hard and their students don't succeed as much as they could, I'm sure, because they're in this total stress state. (Rebecca, interview 1, p. 2)

Horizontal violence is a concept that has been used extensively to apply to the nursing culture when nurses oppress fellow nurses (Farrell, 1999, 2001). The preceptor draws attention to an environment that is not conducive to learning because there is a lack of caring toward how nursing students are experiencing being in the world of nursing practice. Students who have preceptors who are "hard" on them do not experience a caring environment in which they could best have freedom for learning. Rebecca outlines the perceptions that lie behind the expression of horizontal violence, that is, that the students are "dumb" and do not have sufficient clinical experience. Students have equal amounts of time, in a metaphysical sense, for theoretical learning in an educational institute and clinical learning through their practice. Nurses as teachers who think this way are contributing to the problem rather than finding a solution.

Relational Theme: Assessing Where the Student Is At—
The Preceptor and Preceptee Working and Growing Together

Subtheme: Preceptor as Being Vigilant. Preceptors safeguarded the patient by being vigilant with students and at the same time safeguarded students as they learned the practices of nursing. This vigilance is born out of the need to be accountable for their patients (their prime responsibility) and for student learning. The following narrative shows this double accountability. The preceptor reveals that she has a strong recollection of a situation from which both preceptor and preceptee learned a great deal:

We were in a six-bed room and on an afternoon shift, and she had gone around and done all the five o'clock obs. [vital sign observations] for all these women. There was one woman that she'd taken a temperature of, and her temperature was 37.7 [99.9F] at five o'clock. And she didn't tell me that. And I didn't check—I made the assumption that at her level as a second year nurse she would know norms and would know when something's out of the norm to let me know.

But in this instance, when it came round to nine o'clock before the next lot of four hourly observations were due, this particular woman started rigoring.

I mean, I immediately started obviously cooling her down. We got some fluid therapy for her and the student was watching all of this. And in the midst of getting the house surgeon and getting this done, getting blood cultures taken and a fan and getting Panadol into her—found out that her temp had been up at five o'clock and the student hadn't told me. And so later on that evening, once we'd sorted it out, the rigoring stopped and sorted out the situation, talking to the student I said that I'd assumed she would tell me things that were out of the norm. So that was a learning experience for me. She learnt that with a temperature of that nature, I could have given Panadol and assessed the person to see where that temp was coming from . . . I was talking to the student about— if I'd known, that I would have looked into that and probably would have seen that [infected IV] site and got something done about it, because she actually still had fluids going into it. And so that was a big learning experience for both of us. So now I guess I'm more vigilant about assessing where they're at before we start. You really do need to trust that they know . . . before you allow them to go off doing things on their own. (Rebecca, interview 1, p. 3)

Preceptors identified the need to trust the student. This trust was developed through a host of behaviors witnessed by the preceptors that required them to keep noticing and attending to what the students were doing. The preceptors' vigilance required energy and commitment born out of caring for the safety of both patients and students. Both of these factors took their toll on the preceptor.

Preceptors spoke of the stress that they felt as they tried to balance the needs of students and the needs of patients. Stress, according to Benner (1984), is a disruption in meaning. The meaning for preceptors as practitioners is first to provide care for their clients but, as well, to teach student nurses. Coping is the re-creation of meaning within the situation. For preceptors, coping strategies included allowing students to observe them in their practice, explaining their actions to their students, and, when time permitted, talking about what had transpired in any given situation. Rebecca here ensures that her student learns from the situation, but she also learns herself about the meaning of being a preceptor.

Relational Theme: The Preceptor as Builder of Nursing Practice— Teaching Reality Nursing

Subtheme: Engaging the Patient in Student Learning. A practice of preceptors is to involve the patient in the student's learning. The culture of nursing practice includes first and foremost patients who require nursing services. Engaging the patient in the learning process requires the preceptor to manage the learning situation skillfully and ethically because the patient is inevitably present. Preceptors whose main focus is with the patient and their health outcomes engage patients in such a way that they feel part of the student learning process. Gaining the patient's permission to allow students to undertake a procedure or to observe surgery or diagnostic tests is part of students' routine surgical learning experiences. Preceptors set out to make students' experiences as interesting and informative as possible, which includes negotiating with the patient, surgeon, physician, and theater staff and gaining written consent so that students can attend procedures as observers. Such observations provide students with a familiarity and a fuller understanding of the depth of the patient experience and increased awareness of the extent of trauma to the body and the effect this may have on patient recovery. Learning about these complex issues assists students to care empathetically for patients after surgery.

Gaining the patient's permission to allow students to practice procedures requires an approach that engenders confidence between the patient and the student. The preceptor teaching reality nursing is the person who prepares the ground in order for this to occur. "Emma," in caring for a patient postoperatively, tells how she involves both the patient and the student in the learning context while caring for a patient:

We recently had a man who needed his bag to be changed—his stoma bag, he had a rod in his. So that was a little bit more unique than just a bag change. He needed his readyvac removed . . . I gave her some education with that and then I talked her through removing the readyvac. And then putting the bag onto the patient's stomach to catch the flow through the hole we had left. Of course the patient was involved. We had to get his permission. The student had never pulled out the readyvac before so we had to make sure it was alright with him and he was right there. (Emma, interview 1, p. 2)

Emma reveals another common practice of preceptors: "talking through," which was identified first by Blazey (1995). "Talking through" takes place at many points throughout the day-to-day practice of the preceptor. It is an intrinsic part of involving the patient because it occurs prior to procedures and during procedures. The practice of talking through allowed students to build practical knowledge by practicing skills in a safe and supervised situation that engenders confidence.

Talking through also allows preceptors to develop confidence in their ability to successfully teach students.

Often, talking through preceded procedures in a process of questioning and answering. The practice focuses upon a particular patient and procedure and involves the preceptor and the student working together. The practice also takes time and will usually occur in the preparation room of a ward. The preceptor will question the student as to why a procedure such as catheterization would be undertaken in order to check the student's knowledge. Students can either answer well or require "prompting." Talking through allows the preceptor to pass on practical tips that empower the student in the real situation. This engenders camaraderie between the preceptor and the student and also safeguards the patient and the student in the lifeworld of clinical practice. "Florence" presents an exemplar of how practical tips are communicated to the student in the practice of talking through as a student undertakes the catheterization of a female patient:

And I said [to the patient], "This is [the student]. She's working with me today. Either she or I will be able to help attend to your needs today." And she asked the patient really well. She said, "Look, I'm a nursing student. I'm learning. Would it be okay if I catheterize you?" And she explained what it meant and what it was for and she was good. She said why the doctors wanted it, or why we nurses wanted it in, and it was a nursing decision, to put it in, and how she would benefit, and that sort of thing. And the patient was quite happy for her to do it. That was really good, because sometimes they just absolutely don't want to know.

I said to her, "What we tend to do is we just bring a whole pile [of catheters]. We bring like four. Because once we're all sterile we don't want to have to go—if you're by yourself especially, you get very annoyed." . . . I said it was up to her which way she did [it]. And we talked through her rationale for choosing which way that she did [it], and she gave me a good rationale, and she did use the double glove one, which is actually the ward protocol now. (Florence, interview 1, p. 5)

There were many instances in which preceptors shared similar situations of talking through procedures away from the patient. Talking through also occurred between the preceptor and the preceptee with the patient as they worked together in a shared practice world.

Subtheme: Being as *Preceptor as Letting Students Grow.* Preceptors are mindful of the need to prepare students to be competent when they enter the workforce as beginning practitioners. When learning experiences emerge unexpectedly from practice situations, preceptors grasp opportunities to let students grow. "Jane" describes how she works alongside a student to let her "grow" as a practitioner.

My third-year student did a dressing on a lady who had a right hemicolectomy. And about six–seven days down the track her wound dehisced, completely open. Like we get little wounds that just sort of break down a bit, but this was completely open, bowel exposed and what not. And we worked through it together really. She had all the tools and was gloved up and it was just basically doing the wound assessment, what products you need to pack it with and how to dress it. The only time she got into difficulty was when she had to probe the kaltostat right up underneath some sutures that were left in. So that was where I jumped in and had to take over. I tried to talk her through it but she couldn't—she had to see it done . . . and she had a feel as well. (Jane, interview 2, p. 1)

Jane paints a graphic portrait here of a student who felt confident in doing a complicated dressing when given a learning opportunity to grow in her practice while supported by her preceptor. The student is able to manage the wound assessment, choosing the products and dressing the wound for what she could see. As soon as she is required to "pack" the wound where she could not see, her courage fails her. But Jane provides the backup and takes over, showing the student how to explore the sinus so that she can "feel" the length and width of what she could not see. Much of nursing is an embodied experience. The students' feeling will complement her visualizing the sinus and will help her dress the wound next time. In fact, Jane later states, "She feels now that she could probably do it by herself" (Jane, interview 2, p. 2).

Continuing the subtheme of letting students grow their practice, other preceptors made a conscious decision to challenge students. This challenge occurs only if the preceptor thinks the student is capable of further growth and development. Florence shows how she challenges a second year student to care for a client who has complex nursing care requirements:

Now we've been together for about two days and I'd shown her the ward and that sort of thing. I said you can either have an IDC [indwelling catheter] patient that isn't too much work, or you can have the one that's a challenge. And I will help you with the challenge, but you can have the choice. I was really quite impressed, and I thought okay, I've got to watch this. This patient had an IDC, a blood transfusion, IV fluid transfusion, fecal catheter. She had five lines anyway. And the student—she walked into the room, and she sort of scratched her head, and she looked at everything and she looked at me and said, "Okay, I can do this." And she was good. She did chunk it down in each machine, which is what we do too. She did ignore the patient too, a bit, but hey! She took the challenge . . . Some people will just walk in the room, especially students, because they're allowed to and they go, "Oh! I can't do this! I'll take the easy patient!" even though we as nurses can't say, "Oh! I don't want that patient." (Florence, interview 1, p. 10)

Florence shows how the student assesses her patient and the nursing responsibility and claims, "Okay, I can do this." Florence elaborates how the student assessed the situation by breaking down the machinery into one machine at a time. Florence observes that the student did not "talk" to the patient. Benner (1984) notes that novice nurses can focus on only part of practice at any one time, as this occupies their full attention. Later, as novices become more familiar, they shift their gaze to take in more of what is going on in the situation. The student no doubt was concentrating so much on the machinery that she could not talk to or take in the patient much at all.

In Heideggerian terms, the student in this situation first experienced the unready-to-hand mode of being in the world of nursing practice (Heidegger, 1962, p. 103). As time progressed, the student was able to focus more on the patient than the machines. It could be said that the student eventually experienced the machinery being ready-to-hand (Heidegger, 1962, p. 105) and became more comfortable with it. She could then appreciate her patient. Heidegger (1962) felt that technology would objectify the person, thus reducing Dasein or their *being-in-the-world* as a subjective experiencing person.

In modern-day healthcare, technology is a reality for the very ill person. Nurses know the meaning for the person living with the machinery. It can become the focus of professional attention at the expense of the patient. Familiarity with the machinery takes time for an RN and takes even longer for a student nurse. As time progresses the student becomes more comfortable caring for the person and the machines, as Florence relates.

As the week progressed she talked more to the patient and was less worried about the machines. Initially she was quite worried about pulling something out. Which, okay, is a worry for all of us. We tend to be a bit more careful when people have lines everywhere. So, yeah, she was a lot more careful on her first day than she was on her last day. Not to say that she wasn't careful on her last, she was just more realistically careful. (Florence, interview 1, p. 11)

The complexity of the patient's health status and the nursing care required for the patient by the student is illustrated in Florence's story. Florence describes the dual responsibility of teaching the student and caring for very sick patients. She again reveals the vigilance of preceptors to keep a close eye on their students. Preceptors who let students grow into the reality of practice must constantly weigh students' ability to manage a challenging situation safely for the patient and themselves. Their judgment is critical to ensure the patient's safety, but also for the development of competent practitioners. The preceptor tries to meet both demands: safe care of the client and effective learning for the student. Satisfaction comes when both are realized.

Being as Preceptor—Working with Students "Hitting Reality"

As the preceptors worked with preceptees, they were conscious of preparing the nurses of the future. To move this process forward, another practice of preceptors was ensuring that the students understood the reality of nursing. Some students did not always take their professional responsibility as seriously as they might. Preceptors grasped opportunities to hit students with the reality of nursing, which was difficult for some students to accept. "Sarah" reveals one such situation:

When the reality of practice actually makes demands that you may be not prepared for, with a student who is going off at half past nine and came up with a big smile to say she was off, and I said, "Have you written your report?" No she hadn't. And I said, "Well you actually need to because you've been doing the care of that patient." And she said, "But it's half past nine." And I said, "Yes, I know, but you've been doing the care of that patient, so you actually need to write up what you've been doing." Her face was a picture, because she didn't want to be there. You know, half past nine was her finishing time and she was out of there, and it was a real struggle for her to actually stay. And I must say, she didn't do it very graciously [laughs]. But then . . . a couple of times I've been ungracious too! But I could see for the first time there had been that real conflict. You know everything was lovely, but for the first time there was the conflict of reality hitting, and that she actually had to do something she didn't particularly want to do. And I think we all have to come to a place with that . . . you actually can't go off. And that's what I think that nursing is about. And it's the unexpectedness of it, I think. She wasn't prepared for it [Laughs]. (Sarah, interview 1, p. 14)

There is unexpectedness about nursing practice that holds the potential to interfere with the best-laid plans. In the narrative, Sarah states that the "student's face was a picture." For the first time in "hitting reality," the student recognized that she carried responsibilities for documenting nursing activities in relation to patient care, and if she had not done it in the previous eight hours she needed to stay later to follow through. This professional responsibility is a legal requirement. Students often think that their student status gives them freedom that is not reality oriented. Sarah teaches her student that reality nursing is accountability-based. While preceptors are engaged in teaching, students do not learn the reality of nursing practice until something happens to bring the lesson home. Such was the case in Sarah's exemplar.

Subtheme: The Fishbowl Room—Preceptor as Taking "Time Out to Put In." There were moments in preceptors' practice when they needed to take time out with students to reflect and explain situations when they felt that the students had been left out. In these circumstances, the preceptor would work with the patient and the patient's family through a crisis of a sensitive nature in which the student was not as involved. However, in the working partnership between preceptor and preceptee, the preceptee was aware of the patient and the family's experience. In these situations, the preceptors would keep the students involved at a distance and felt a responsibility to pass on to preceptees how they had managed a crisis situation. When there was time, the preceptor found space for teaching. Jane reveals this practice:

I introduced the student and myself [to the patient and the family] and said that the student will be back to "just do your care." They were a Maori family and so I felt that they didn't really need our support as such; we just needed to do what we had to do because they were supporting each other . . . The day before, when she went in to care for this patient, she also knew when to just leave them alone. And when I walked past, I could hear her talking to him. . . . She had made a connection with him as well. And then the rest of the family turned up. She left them well alone. Because the grandson had died in a car accident, they were going to see him. She [the student] came to me and said, "The family's all there, it's not appropriate to try and take him to the shower," and I said, "That's fine." She recognized that. And when the family had gone she went back in and said, "What do you want to do now?" And he [the patient] was all keen to get up because he knew that if he got up, got mobilizing, that he may make the tangi [Maori burial ceremony] in time. And after it was all over I spoke to her in our fishbowl room and I said to her, "I'm sorry if you felt left out today," and she said, "No, I didn't." She knew that it was something that only my charge nurse and myself could do . . . but she'd seen it all happening and she'd learnt quite a bit on the side as well. (Jane, interview 1, pp. 8, 9)

Jane, the preceptor, shows how she respects the cultural safety of her patient and his family by providing a context in which they could grieve in a culturally appropriate manner without the intrusion of staff. Her student is drawn into the situation but is also aware of the cultural practices appropriate for the patient and family at this very sensitive time of loss.

The concept of cultural safety relates to the government principle of safety for the consumer of healthcare and is therefore of importance to nursing service providers in institutions. The Cultural Safety Model (Ramsden, 1990, 1993) formed the basis of establishing culturally safe practice for nurses. A government objective to acknowledge and give effect to the Treaty of Waitangi (1840/1975) as a founding document for New Zealand society establishes a bicultural context for all healthcare services and reflects the unique nature of New Zealand culture.

The Treaty of Waitangi incorporates a Maori perspective on health that is holistic. It recognizes that health includes Te Taha Wairua (the spiritual dimension, to have faith and to experience communion with past and present), Te Taha Tinana (the growth and development of the physical dimension of the body throughout life), Te Taha Hinengaro (the emotional dimension, the ability to think and feel and communicate emotions), and Te Taha Whanau (the family dimension, to know what it is to care, to be cared for, and to belong) (Durie, 1994). All components must be satisfied for Maori to experience holistic health in an environment of care and healing. To establish understanding among nurses of the importance of culturally safe nursing practice, the Nursing Council of New Zealand (1999, 2002) published cultural safety guidelines for nursing practice.

The student had learned vicariously by listening and watching her preceptor and her preceptor's charge nurse. She was able to act in a culturally appropriate manner because she was aware that there were certain protocols that needed to be observed. Jane, her preceptor, took a mental note not to leave her student out, so she arranged for "time out to put in" explanations in order that her student could also share in the special moments that occur in the practice of nursing. This well illustrates that, although students are assigned to preceptors, students can and do learn in many other ways, from different people, patients, and families that they encounter in the healthcare context.

Being as Preceptor—Feeling Alone in the World of Nursing Education

As pointed out, government reforms have altered the way nursing education and healthcare agency function. Both lecturers and nursing staff within hospitals have experienced the change in that they are expected to do more with less. What is of significance is that the changes have occurred stealthily, leaving both preceptors and lecturers to work out new ways of managing nursing education in clinical placements. New partnerships are emerging, but many, as yet, are still seeking ways to facilitate student learning. Rebecca discloses the burden of responsibility:

And these days where the tech tutor isn't around, and it's, you know, it's you as the RN doing so much of the teaching in the clinical situation. Yeah, you're it really. [You're the one who has to] make sure that they get what they need to learn out of the situation and often it is stressful. And often it adds to the stress of my day. (Rebecca, interview 1, p. 1)

Jane concurs that it is stressful *being as* a preceptor by reiterating the theme of isolation and the uncertainty of not knowing whether preceptors are providing what is needed for the student.

So a lot of it—it's all left up to us really. Especially if some people don't want to precept. But the way staffing is, they've had to, especially second year students. And I think that makes it more difficult, because if you're not willing to have a student there and willing to teach them, or if you don't know if you're teaching them properly, then I think that can add more stress and it also impinges on their whole experience. So from that point of view, we don't have much support. (Jane, interview 2, p. 3)

Jane and Rebecca express feelings of being left alone and being uncertain. Clearly, precepting is stressful. Preceptors experience a *way* of working with lecturers from the Polytechnic/University that is different from their own experience of being a student. Instead of finding help from clinical lecturers, they feel that "it's left up to us." This lack of educational support for precepting is a reason for concern, and the question arises: how can this situation be addressed?

Even though a number of the preceptors spoke of their isolation from the lecturers from the educational institute, and despite the challenging, changeable, chaotic nature of the practice reality, they still maintained that they enjoyed their experience of *being as* a preceptor to undergraduate students. Yet, many felt that if they received more support, the experience would be more worthwhile. Jane comments:

As staff nurses we're supporting the students all the way, but there's very little support for us in the role. Nothing. That probably makes this more . . . well, [it] makes me more angry anyway. [It's to do with] the fact that all the work that we put in is not actually being recognized. The students say, "Oh thanks, see ya." And that's the last that you really hear from them, or see of them, and then along comes another one. So I think it's a bit sad that there's not that support there for us. People like me are expected to have answers just like that all the time. (Jane, interview 2, p. 3)

Jane and Rebecca show the dual burden of responsibility that preceptors carry. Jane continues:

It's a big responsibility. Because you sort of [hope that] your workload eases up a bit but it doesn't. You're actually constantly watching and making sure that they're all okay and things that take you half the time have taken longer and . . . But you've still got to make sure that you're out the door on time, and that you've handed over and that everything's documented, and . . . I find that quite difficult sometimes. (Jane, interview 2, p. 3)

Lee continues the theme of being busy, short staffed, but still accountable for patient care and student learning.

Particularly when we are busy and if we're short staffed, you know. I'm carrying a full patient workload as it is, plus a student and plus trying to give the student direction and guidance. [That means] getting them to think about where they are at their practice, trying to fit in practical skills they need to get involved in, as well as overseeing their patients. And making sure that they are providing appropriate care to the patient needs. So it is very time consuming. (Lee, interview 2, p. 3)

Lee, Rebecca, and Jane illustrate the demanding but uncertain nature of *being as* preceptor. There were feelings of being undervalued for the efforts made in the interests of student learning. Precepting was viewed as being physically and intellectually draining and very time consuming. Preceptors also found themselves in an uncertain place in that they found it difficult to know if they were providing a suitable clinical experience for students.

Subtheme: Experiencing Preceptoring as Being as *"Doubly Accountable."* The theme of being doubly accountable pervaded the research. Florence disclosed that preceptors felt that they were doubly accountable as they were accountable for the student as well as the patient. Florence illustrates the reality of practice:

It's resting on our shoulders and that's bad—well, that's our job and we do it. But when we have to be responsible for a student on top of looking after our patient, then we're doubly accountable, because we're accountable for that student's actions as well. [For example], around giving medication sometimes . . . they all want to do the IV medications and whatever the tech rules are—I can never figure them out, they keep changing—but if it's under our direct supervision and it's okay with us for them to do it, I think they are allowed to do it. So we did it one day, and I did the same thing as we do when we're precepting a new grad, you have to know what the drug is and what you're giving. And that was okay. She gave the drug and that was fine. And then I came back, I don't know where I'd gone to, and she said, "Oh, I've flushed that drug." And I said to her, "You're not actually supposed to do that without me there because I've got to know what you flushed it with. Well, what did you flush it with?" And she'd connected him back up to the fluids that he was on and flushed him with dextrose/saline, which is not usually recommended for a lot of medication. So we checked out the medication and it was actually okay. It wasn't recommended but it wasn't detrimental either, and I said to her, "It's really good that you want to learn this stuff, but this is actually over and above what you have to do to be registered. You also have to sit another exam to do this. And I do really need to be here when you're doing that." She was trying to help . . . Sometimes we have to explain that to them, that we are responsible for these patients. And it's quite hard to do. It's not easy. Especially when you're having a really busy day, and the student wants to do something, and you want the student to do something, and we all know what it was like when we were students. (Florence, interview 1, pp. 2–3)

Florence identifies the tension in preparing competent nurses of the future. In teaching reality nursing, preceptors acknowledged that students needed to learn specific skills, but they also needed to be safe.

Florence states that students try to help but are unaware of the "give and take" that prevails as they learn the practice of nursing. The in-betweenness, that ever-pervading "restless to and fro between yes and no" (Heidegger, 1966, p. 75) in decision making; the disease in managing patients' safety and giving students practice to prepare them to be competent nurses coexists. Despite this, preceptors concede what is expected of them, as we see when Florence continues her dialogue:

And all of a sudden when she's registered she's expected to be able to know how to do it, no sort of hand holding, nothing, unless you've got very supportive staff on your ward, you're just expected to know how to do it and go in and do it, bang! (Florence, interview 1, pp. 2–3)

Dale continues the theme of what students need to learn and identifies a need for movement in nursing education to prepare students for the 21st century:

[There is a] hospital policy which allows students under the supervision of [an RN] to give intravenous therapy or intravenous medication whilst they're in their second or third year. There's not a lot of focus on intravenous medications or therapy for students. [That] is a real shame because it's only a couple of years down the track and they're going to be using those tools in therapy of a patient and if they don't start getting it from the very start, they're on the back foot once they get out there.

[It's about] focusing on the gap between what the students are getting and what they need. And I guess there's a whole bunch of stuff. And it's really—it's really [being] caught between a rock and a hard place . . . I find I tend to focus on going over those sort of things if I notice [problems] when I'm working. You know, I was really lucky with the student that I had that she was very proficient with those basic skills, which just made it—it was marvelous, absolutely brilliant. And like I was saying before, the more confident you are, the more confident you're going to be in going that step further and learning something new. And as she was confident with those skills I could think, well, what else can I go on with? Yeah, we didn't get as far as I would have liked to if we'd had, say, two or three weeks together . . . So the practical experience does get left behind a wee bit. It's really easy to demonstrate to a different clinical tutor, every time you're out in a clinical placement, the same thing. So I don't know—I tend to have this assumption . . . I almost let the student lead the way. (Dale, interview 1, p. 2)

Dale continues exploring a theme about the student's readiness to practice and implies that there is a gap between nursing education and their nursing practice. It is true of today's healthcare system that technology is dominant in healthcare and is a predominant part of contemporary nurses' practice. Students need to be prepared for the possibilities inherent in the future.

Preceptors are all too aware of the need for the student to be given every opportunity to "practice your practice" (Sarah, interview 2, p. 1) in the reality context. Sarah once again draws attention to the inbetweenness, the tension between theory and practice:

I think [students need] a little bit of theory and then jumping into some practice . . . I mean practice sometimes means exactly what it says, practicing—*Practicing your practice.* And communication skills, all those sort of things, I mean they can only be practiced and I think they're quite different in hospital as a nurse . . . I think knowledge without some practice hooks to hang it on is actually very hard to retain. (Sarah, interview 2, p. 1)

Sarah discloses her belief that, if knowledge is not linked to practice, it is hard to retain. When knowledge and practice come together, practice is transformed. Later, Dale reiterates this thought:

I think there's that real comfort zone when there's somebody there with you all the time. You can turn to [your RN] and say, "Am I doing this right? What do we do now?" Then there isn't a hang of a lot of anxiety going on for you because you're not holding the baby, so to speak. Your patient is the main focus. (Dale, interview 1, pp. 2–3)

Students are cushioned from the reality of carrying the responsibility for their actions when the preceptors are keeping them safe in practice. Eventually, however, the reality of being "the nurse" and the accountability that accompanies that existence will have to be claimed as "mine." A student's eventual authenticity as *being-as-a-nurse* on graduation is reliant upon Dasein (the student) claiming mineness, that is, choosing to embody the professional nurse (Heidegger, 1962, p. 68).

A question remains for nursing education and nursing service agencies about how to develop students' practice as safe and competent new practitioners, while meeting the challenges of continual change in healthcare. At present, the preceptors are the ones who carry this burden. But who cares for the preceptors?

A Mantle of Care

Nurses take on the mantle of care. In Bishop and Scudder's (1990) view, the moral and personal are closely intertwined in nursing practice. The authors make a compelling argument that nursing practice has a moral foundation based upon care, that it is a practice founded on moral principles steeped in a moral tradition founded in the human sciences. It is secondary to the technological practices that are derived from the natural sciences. In this perspective, nursing differs from medicine in that medicine is now principally based upon a curative regime immersed in the natural sciences. Similarly, Watson (1988) perceives that nursing has a moral imperative to care. Human sciences have the capacity to articulate both the social institution with its inherent culture, policies, and standards of practice and the actual practice carried out by practitioners in the interests of client care. Bishop and Scudder cite Tymieniecka's 1983 work, in which she states:

Health care can be articulated professionally in terms of concrete practice, such as assessing monitoring and intervening, etc. But it also can be articulated in terms of the moral sense in that such care is articulated as concrete benevolence. The moral sense places the good of the other over our own but also allows us to understand "the 'good' of the Other," as "our own good or the Good in general." (p. 90)

Heidegger (1971) discusses what it is like for us to undergo an experience with something: this "means that this something befalls us, strikes us, comes over us, overwhelms and transforms us" (p. 57). In considering this statement in relation to the statement made by Tymieniecka (as cited in Bishop & Scudder, 1990, p. 90), what strikes us and overwhelms us is that preceptors reveal that they are constantly caring about the "good" of the other (that is, their students and their patients) over their own good in order for good—in the general sense of the services that nursing offers to patients—prevail. They accomplish this by being in constant dialogue with their preceptees, observing them in their practice, teaching them the practices of nursing, and teaching them generally how to live in the world of nursing practice. They accomplish all of this while they primarily care for patients.

Nursing students experience a "lived" curriculum that transforms them through experiences that make isolated pieces of information learned in a classroom meaningful. The person who facilitates that process is the preceptor. Preceptors and students are both immersed in a particular communal culture, the culture of nursing. The values and beliefs of the nursing profession pervade the lived world of nursing practice. That preceptors care for students and about student learning at the same time as not compromising the care of their patients is a measure of their commitment to safeguarding the practices of nursing.

Conclusions from the Study

Adopting the Heideggerian notion of "authenticity" or mine-ness (Heidegger 1962, p. 68) to refer to the ways preceptors are in their world, the study showed that preceptors could not be wholly in either the world of nursing practice or the world of nursing education. Rather, they were caught in between both worlds. Heidegger claims that for Dasein to be wholly authentic, people must choose their way of being in their world. Dasein is essentially one's own possibility. For preceptors, the choice was not always present. Many preceptors find the role imposed upon them out of need. However, preceptors who responded to the call accepted that they were the transmitters of the culture of nursing and cared about the preparation of new nurses. They enjoyed the experience of *being as* preceptor but found it challenging.

The preceptors in this study believed that they were insufficiently prepared to be preceptors. This feeling came in the light of uncertainty that they were teaching students the correct knowledge because of lack of familiarity with contemporary degree education for nurses entering the profession. Additionally, *being as* preceptors and serving as teachers, guides, and supporters of student nurses became secondary to their primary function of *being as* nurses and providing nursing services to patients. Preceptors are the bridge between the worlds of nursing practice and nursing education and require appropriate support to walk strongly in both worlds.

Students value RNs' reality-oriented practice, for it is with patients that student nurses learn best the practice of nursing. The strength of the study was the many exemplars of preceptors' practice. Examples of these included the preceptors' practice of "keeping the student in mind" and "keeping an eye on" students when they were engaged in other activities; the practice of "talking through" procedures and then withdrawing students for reflection upon practice to identify learning from it; and the need to "assess where the student is" to ensure their safety for practice and their learning needs. Preceptors are in the best position to teach reality nursing to student nurses, but they also require educational preparation for the role as teachers. The emphasis in New Zealand remains on the technical aspects of nursing, however, rather than on an integrated academic and practice approach in developing new nurses.

Preceptors who are RNs primarily employed to care for patients now take a greater role in nursing education than they did in earlier decades. Conversely, close contact and support of preceptors by clinical lecturers has decreased. A change is required in the way nursing education is managed within the profession to incorporate cooperation and collaboration between the sectors. This change will necessitate addressing how preceptors and clinical lecturers *are* in their worlds of nursing practice and nursing education. Each partner must have the freedom to choose to *be*, in Heideggerian terms, their authentic self and own their place in both worlds. In between stand the new nurses who are reliant upon both partners to prepare them appropriately for tomorrow's world of nursing practice.

Implications for Education

The study demonstrated the lack of preparation of preceptors to precept undergraduate student nurses. As a minimum, preceptors should hold a bachelor's degree, but a master's degree should be a requirement to be aspired to within a nationally achievable time frame. The study highlighted the difficulty for preceptors having the dual responsibilities of patient care and precepting student nurses. Preceptors require a reduced patient assignment from their employing agencies in order to focus some of their energies on precepting. A joint working arrangement between clinical agencies and educational institutes will facilitate student nurses' learning. Preceptors require being conversant with degree program learning outcomes, what these mean for student nurses in their clinical placement, and the outcomes expected of undergraduate student nurses at the conclusion of their nursing education program (Nursing Council of New Zealand, 1999).

Education and service sectors that collaborate to understand the curriculum requirements of the bachelor's degree program will work collaboratively to reach mutually satisfying outcomes for both. The two sectors dialoguing effectively with each other and listening to each other's concerns will enhance patient safety and student learning and will develop a will to work cooperatively to reach mutually satisfying outcomes for both.

Preceptors who undertake an adult learning instruction course would be able to teach adult students in an educationally sound manner. This could be arranged as a partial payment for preceptor services between the clinical agency and educational institutes. In particular, it is important that preceptors understand assessment processes and are able to assess students' learning in an educationally sound manner to ensure that developing nurses are safe in their practice of nursing. Nursing education schools are accountable for their graduates (New Zealand Education Act, 1989), and it is essential that preceptors, who now take an active role in the assessing of students' safety to practice, be fully cognizant of what this accountability entails.

Implications for Practice

The historical way students have been absorbed into the practice culture requires review. A changed and changing sociopolitical and cultural health and educational context demands different preparation for students if they are to fit the practice world of the future. A commitment is required from clinical agencies to identify and prepare preceptors educationally and practically. This can be seen as a joint investment between education and service settings. A way of budgeting for this need could be worked out at leadership levels across institutions. An environment that supports "thinking out loud" so that students feel confident in sharing their thinking, accessing relevant research related to patient care, and being encouraged to take part in the team culture of discussion related to patient care would foster an environment in which academic advancements made in healthcare are brought to life within the ward environment. Shared decision making will promote a moral community in which all professionals value each other's contribution to the patients' health outcomes.

The establishment of a joint taskforce to address how preceptors and clinical lecturers can form effective joint partnerships in nursing education supported by their respective institutions is a feasible way to move forward. This would involve recognizing that each institution will be required to work out arrangements at a local level as to how a collaborative partnership will work between sectors. An important adjunct to the research is that nursing education and nursing practice are in a constant spiral of change. Cooperation and collaboration are required. Nurse leaders must seize the moment to enact a collaborative partnership between the sectors to ensure that future nurses can provide quality care to people.

Implications for Research

Action research is a tool used to explore and develop a way for clinical agencies and educational institutions to work together. For the profession of nursing to realize its potential as a major player in health reforms worldwide, preceptors must play a key role as the teachers of clinical practice in the acute care setting. But preceptors require students to see "the big picture." There is an increasing need to promote health rather than to focus intensely on the care of the sick. People suffer episodes of illness but return to their communities to convalesce. Nurses can and are poised to extend their scope of practice to take on new roles focused on health outcomes for people (Nursing Council of New Zealand, 1999).

Future hermeneutic research could explore the effect on preceptors' practice once they are engaged or have been engaged in the preceptor role. The impact on experienced RNs' lives of *being as* preceptors to undergraduate student nurses should be investigated in order to understand what influences their satisfaction with and performance in the role. A better understanding of what clinical teaching means for RNs would assist nursing education and nursing service to more fully meet the needs of RNs employed as clinical teachers.

Summary

This chapter has shown the diversity and the flexibility of preceptors as they teach and learn from undergraduate student nurses. Many issues arise from the accounts of the preceptors to show the tiring and responsible nature of precepting practice. Uncovering the world of the preceptor raises many questions, and we are left wondering how they manage to meet the many demands placed upon them. Demands of safe practice from the patients' point of view always take priority, but providing quality care from an organizational point of view is important as well. Both are an inescapable part of the preceptors' role. Added to this is the additional responsibility of students learning the practice of nursing. All of this "for-the-sake-of-which" (Heidegger, 1962, p. 232) is for students attaining their chosen career and engaging in ongoing solicitude for the profession of nursing.

What is equally shown is that preceptors must still maintain their primordial way of being in the world of nursing as an RN. The way participating preceptors uncover the challenge they face daily to balance their many responsibilities provokes thinking of what we need to do if the profession of nursing is to sustain the practice of nursing.

Preceptors are concerned about students as people and as students, caring for and about them both personally and professionally. Preceptors reveal the importance they place on ensuring that students learn the precepts of nursing. In this way they safeguard student nurses as developing professionals and equally safeguard the profession from students who may have not made the best career choice.

In the culture of healthcare there are many practices that portray the skill of those engaged in providing services to people who need healthcare. None are more important than those of the preceptor. As preceptors work with students, they recognize that there is an inherent need to challenge students in the learning context in order for them to prepare new nurses for the reality of day-to-day work as a nurse and for the accountability that accompanies professional practice. The practice of safeguarding both the student and the patient is paramount and a constant vigil for the preceptor. It is the preceptor who prepares the nurse of tomorrow to be a competent and caring nurse. However, the pressures of the organizational culture where healthcare is delivered militate against the altruistic values that are central to nurses and nursing.

All the while, preceptors as builders of nursing practice continue to carry on and spend their time teaching reality nursing to students as well as nursing their patients. The narratives shared in this chapter reveal that *being as* preceptor requires RNs to be willing, flexible, versatile, energetic, knowledgeable, highly organized, and a sensitive communicator. Their dual accountability to patients and students requires that they walk in between two worlds, each with its own cultural norms, customs, beliefs, and practices. Each world brings tensions to preceptors' day-to-day practice that require negotiation and working through. That RNs who respond to the call of *being as* preceptor continue to feel the burden of responsibility and accountability to the next generation of nurses is a privilege and a gift that all too often is taken for granted.

References

Benner, P. (1984). *From novice to expert: Excellence and power in clinical nursing practice.* Menlo Park, CA: Addison-Wesley.

Benner, P. E. (Ed.). (1994). *Interpretive phenomenology: Embodiment, caring and ethics in health and illness.* Thousand Oaks, CA: Sage.

Benner, P., Hooper-Kyriakidis, P., & Stannard, D. (2001). *Clinical wisdom and interventions in critical care: A thinking-in-action approach.* Philadelphia: W. B. Saunders.

Benner, P. E., Tanner, C. A., & Chesla, C. A. (1996). *Expertise in nursing practice: Caring, clinical judgment, and ethics.* New York: Springer.

Benner, P., & Wrubel, J. (1989). *The primacy of caring: Stress and coping in health and illness.* Menlo Park, CA: Addison-Wesley.

Bible. (1611). Authorized version [cumprivilegio]. London: Oxford University Press.

Bishop, A. H., & Scudder, J. R. (1990). *The practical, moral, and personal sense of nursing: A phenomenological philosophy of practice.* Albany: State University of New York Press.

Blazey, M. E. (1995). *An interpretive analysis of the teaching and learning aspects of the practice of precepting.* Unpublished doctoral dissertation, University of Florida, Gainesville, Florida.

Cobden-Grainge, F., & Walker, J. (2002, April 26–27). Nursing—A career in crisis. Paper presented at the Nursing Research Section New Nurses Organization Conference titled *Research: Contributing to the Future of Nursing.* Bryant Education Centre, Hamilton, NZ.

Crookes, P. A. (2000). Commentary: Critique of the graduate nurse: An international perspective: A response to Jennifer Greenwood. *Nurse Education Today, 20*(1), 26–27.

Diekelmann, N. L. (1990). Nursing education: Caring, dialogue and practice. *Journal of Nursing Education, 29*(7), 300–305.

Diekelmann, N. L., Allen, D., & Tanner, C. A. (1989). *The National League for Nursing criteria for appraisal of baccalaureate programs: A critical hermeneutic analysis.* New York: National League for Nursing.

Dreyfus, H. L. (1991).*Being-in-the-world: A commentary on Heidegger's being and time, Division 1.* Cambridge, MA: MIT Press.

Durie, M. (1994). *Whairoa: Maori health development.* Auckland, NZ: Oxford University Press.

Edwards, S. D. (Ed.). (1998). *Philosophical issues in nursing.* Basingstoke, UK: Macmillan.

Farrell, G. A. (1999). Aggression in clinical settings: Nurses' views—A follow-up study. *Journal of Advanced Nursing, 29*(3), 532–541.

Farrell, G. A. (2001). From tall poppies to squashed weeds: Why don't nurses pull together more? *Journal of Advanced Nursing, 35*(1), 26–33.

Gower, S. E., & Finlayson, M. P. (2002, September 19–20). We are able and artful, but we're tired: Results from the survey of New Zealand hospital nurses. Paper presented at the College of Nurses, Aotearoa, conference titled *We Are Able and Artful Nurses.* Nelson, NZ.

Guignon, C. B. (Ed.). (1993). *The Cambridge companion to Heidegger.* Cambridge, UK: Cambridge University Press.

Heidegger, M. (1962). *Being and time* (J. Macquarrie & E. Robinson, Trans.). New York: Harper & Row. (Original work published 1927)

Heidegger, M. (1966). *Discourse on thinking* (A translation of *Gellasenheit* by John M. Anderson and E. Hans Freund with an introduction by John M. Anderson) New York: Harper & Row.

Heidegger, M. (1971). Building, dwelling and thinking. In *Poetry, language and thought* (A. Hofstadter, Trans., pp. 143–161). New York: Harper & Row.

Heidegger, M. (1977). *The question concerning technology and other essays* (W. Lovitt, Trans.). New York: Harper & Row.

Heidegger, M. (1993). *Basic writings: From Being and time (1927) to The task of thinking (1964)* (D. F. Krell, Ed.; rev. and expanded ed.). San Francisco: HarperCollins.

Inwood, M. (1999). *A Heidegger dictionary.* Oxford: Blackwell.

Irving, J. O., & Snider, J. (2002). Legal and ethical issues: Preserving professional values. *Journal of Professional Nursing, 18*(1), 5.

King, M. (1964). *Heidegger's philosophy: A guide to his basic thought.* Oxford, UK: Basil Blackwell.

Kolb, D. (1986). *The critique of pure modernity: Hegel, Heidegger and after.* Chicago: University of Chicago Press.

KPMG Consulting (2001). *Strategic review of undergraduate nursing education: Report to the Nursing Council.* Wellington, NZ: Author.

Leonard, V. W. (1994). A Heideggerian phenomenological perspective on the concept of the person. In P. E. Benner (Ed.), *Interpretive phenomenology: Embodiment, caring and ethics in health and illness* (pp. 43–64). Thousand Oaks, CA: Sage.

McCance, T. V., McKenna, H. P., & Boore, J. R. P. (1999). Caring: Theoretical perspectives of relevance to nursing. *Journal of Advanced Nursing, 30*(6), 1388–1395.

Morieson, B. (2002, September 18–19). Keynote address: *Nursing the system back to health. Results: Australian Nursing Federation (Victorian Branch). Nurse/Patient ratio implementation.* New Zealand Nurses Organization Annual General Meeting. Rotorua Convention Centre, Rotorua, NZ.

Nehls, H., Rather, M., & Guyette, M. (1997). The preceptor model of clinical instruction: The lived experiences of students, preceptors, and clinical instructors. *Journal of Nursing Education, 36*(5), 220–227.

New Zealand Education Act 1989, Section 162 (ii) and (iii). (RS). Vol. 34.

New Zealand Ministry of Health. (1998). *Report of the Ministerial Taskforce on Nursing: Releasing the potential of nursing.* Wellington, NZ: Author.

New Zealand Nurses' Organization. (2001). *Code of Ethics.* Wellington, NZ: Author.

Nightingale, F. (1946). *Notes on nursing.* Philadelphia: Edward Stern. (Original work published in 1859)

Nurses Act. (1977). [New Zealand]. (RS). Vol. 33.

Nursing Council of New Zealand. (1999). *Standards for registration of comprehensive nurses.* Wellington, NZ: Author.

Nursing Council of New Zealand (2002). *Guidelines for cultural safety, the Treaty of Waitangi, and Maori health in nursing and midwifery education and practice*. Wellington, NZ: Author.

Onions, C. T. (Ed.). (1955). *The shorter Oxford English Dictionary on historical principles* (3rd ed.). Oxford, UK: Clarendon Press.

Palmer, R. E. (Ed.). (1969). *Hermeneutics: Interpretation theory in Schleiermacher, Dilthey, Heidegger, and Gadamer*. Evanston, IL: Northwestern University Press.

Pöggeler, O. (1989). *Martin Heidegger's path of thinking* (D. Magurshak & S. Barber, Trans.). Atlantic Highlands, NJ: Humanities Press International.

Ramsden, I. (1990). *Kawa Whakaruruhau: Cultural safety in nursing education in Aotearoa*. Wellington, NZ: Ministry of Education.

Ramsden, I. (1993). Kawa Whakaruruhau: Cultural safety in nursing education in Aotearoa (New Zealand). *Nursing Praxis in New Zealand, 8*(3), 4–10.

Rather, M. L. (1990). *The lived experience of returning RN students: A Heideggerian hermeneutical analysis*. Unpublished doctoral dissertation, University of Wisconsin–Madison.

Rummel, L. G. (1993). *The proving ground: The lived world of nursing students in their pre-registration clinical experience*. Unpublished master's thesis, Massey University, Palmerston North, NZ.

Rummel, L. G. (2002). *Safeguarding the practices of nursing: The lived experience of being-as preceptor to undergraduate student nurses in acute care settings*. Unpublished dissertation, Massey University, Albany Campus, Auckland, NZ.

Shamian, J., & Inhaber, R. (1985). The concept and practice of preceptorships in contemporary nursing: A review of pertinent literature. *International Journal of Nursing Studies, 22*(2), 79–88.

Taylor, C. (1985). Language and human nature. *Human agency and language: Philosophical papers* (pp. 248–292). Cambridge, UK: Cambridge University Press.

Taylor, C. (1989). *Sources of the self: The making of the modern identity*. Cambridge, MA: Harvard University Press.

Taylor, C., Lillis, C., & LeMone, P. (1997). *Fundamentals of nursing: The art and science of nursing care* (3rd ed.). Philadelphia: Lippincott.

Treaty of Waitangi Act. (1975). [New Zealand]. (RS). Vol. 33.

Van Manen, M. (1990). *Researching lived experience: Human science for an action sensitive pedagogy*. London: Althouse Press.

Walker, J., & Bailey, S. (1999). The clinical performance of new degree graduates. *Nursing Praxis in New Zealand, 14*(2), 31–42.

Watson, J. (1988). *Nursing: Human science and human care: A theory of nursing*. New York: National League for Nursing.

Contributors

Nancy L. Diekelmann is Helen Denne Schulte Professor at the University of Wisconsin–Madison School of Nursing, a fellow in the American Academy of Nursing, past president of the Society for Research in Nursing Education, and chair of the University of Wisconsin–Madison Teaching Academy. A noted authority for her work in nursing education and primary healthcare, Dr. Diekelmann has received two Book of the Year awards from the *American Journal of Nursing* for her textbooks *Primary Health Care of the Well Adult* and *Transforming RN Education: Dialogue and Debate* (coauthored with Martha L. Rather). Her current research uses interpretive phenomenology to explicate the narratives of teachers, students, and clinicians in nursing education. Dr. Diekelmann has described an alternative approach for nursing education—narrative pedagogy. She is coauthor with J. Diekelmann of a forthcoming book, *Schooling Learning Teaching: Toward a Narrative Pedagogy.*

Joanna Basuray, BSc, MSc, PhD, is Associate Professor of Nursing and director of the campus Multicultural Institute at Towson University, Maryland. In addition to working as an ICU, emergency, and pediatric nurse, she has taught in nursing for 23 years. Her foci in teaching and clinical practice are child and family health and cultural diversity. From the beginning of her nursing career and professional growth, Joanna had cultivated a deep interest in the impact of cultural diversity on healthcare and vice versa. Initially, she pursued a self-initiated approach to integrating cultural diversity into the healthcare practice. In 1986, she developed a course on multicultural healthcare at the University of North Dakota. Later, at Towson University, she developed a diversity-focused course that is now required in the nursing curriculum. In addition to directing the campus Multicultural Center, she works with several professional and community organizations toward diversity-related goals. Joanna has presented numerous invited papers at healthcare conferences in the United States and abroad. Her most recent publication is a chapter on healthcare in India in Madeleine Leininger and Marilyn McFarland's third edition of *Transcultural Nursing: Concepts, Theories, Research and Practice* (McGraw-Hill, 2002).

Andrew Estefan, RN, BN, DNSc, MN, CertAWT, is an academic and registered mental health nurse, lecturing at Griffith University in Brisbane, Australia. Andrew has a background both in clinical practice and as a vocational educator. Clinically, his interests lie in acute psychiatry, Borderline Personality Disorder, and trauma. Andrew's interests in education relate to mental health nursing, therapeutic communication skills, diversity, and marginalization. His methodological interests include post-structuralism, Queer Theory, and narrative, and his current research investigates the nature of self-injury in gay men. Andrew has published in the areas of self-injury and developing therapeutic response skills in undergraduate and postgraduate nursing students.

Kathryn Hopkins Kavanagh, BSN, MS, MA, PhD, is a medical anthropologist. Prepared as a psychiatric and mental health clinical nurse specialist, she has taught for many years with the University of Maryland System and also for Northern Arizona University, for which she directed a baccalaureate program on the Navajo and Hopi Reservations. Her interest in cross-cultural aspects of healthcare led her to conduct a series of summer field schools on the Pine Ridge Reservation in South Dakota, where students worked with Oglala Lakota health initiatives. Identifying as one of the growing genre of independent (and often itinerant) scholars, she currently teaches courses in medical anthropology, indigenous healing traditions, and American Indian cultures for the University of Maryland on its Baltimore County campus. Widely published in cultural aspects of healthcare, she coauthored *Promoting Cultural Diversity: Strategies for Health Care Professionals* with Patricia Kennedy. She continues to write on various diversity-related topics.

Jacqui Kess-Gardner, BSN, BA (Corporate Communications), is a registered nurse, special educator, motivational speaker, aerobics instructor, makeup artist, and hairstylist—in addition to managing the career of a son who is a concert pianist. Specializing in gerontological care, Jacqui is Nurse Manager at a long-term facility, Keswick MultiCare Center, in Baltimore. She has been published in *Guideposts* and is author of *The Incredible Journey*. She has recently completed a book of poems called *Straight from the Heart*. Jacqui is an advocate of the blind and works closely with the National Federation of the

Blind to fight for equality and opportunities for the blind and visually impaired. She married her high school sweetheart, and she and James have two sons.

Virginia Knowlden, RN, BA, MEd, MA, EdD, is Professor Emerita, Saint Joseph College, West Hartford, Connecticut, and Adjunct Professor, Southern Connecticut State University, New Haven. Noted for her work about caring in nursing, Dr. Knowlden authored *The Communication of Caring in Nursing*, a text derived from two studies concerning nurse caring in community and high-technology settings. The latter study was funded by the Charles A. and Anne Morrow Lindbergh Foundation; Dr. Knowlden is the only nurse to have been funded by the foundation. She is also the author of published articles. Her current research utilizes hermeneutics to explicate the narratives from nurses concerning the shunning of patients.

Margaret McAllister, RN, RPN, BA, MEd, EdD, FANZCMHN, MAARE, is Senior Lecturer in Nursing at Griffith University in Brisbane, Australia and has a background in nursing, mental health, and education. Margaret has 10 years teaching experience, currently coordinates the Master of Mental Health Nursing and the Graduate Certificate in Mental Health, and takes an active role in curriculum development within the Bachelor of Nursing Program. She has completed educational and clinical research projects in qualitative and quantitative methods. A fellow of the Australian and New Zealand College of Mental Health Nurses and a member of the Australia Association for Research in Education, Margaret serves on a number of editorial and research boards, as well as reviewing for numerous health and education journals. In 2002, she was a visiting scholar at Flinders University and the University of Adelaide, where she addressed clinical groups on research, education, and practice issues related to her recent research and publications in education, qualitative research, and deliberate self-injury.

Jennifer Rowe, RN, BA, DipEd, GradDipEd(Nurs), MPhil, PhD, lectures in the School of Nursing at Griffith University in Brisbane, Australia. She teaches in both undergraduate and graduate programs. She has a clinical nursing background in children's nursing. With considerable experience in utilizing interpretive and critical methodologies, she researches social aspects of child and family health, well-being and nursing care.

Louise G. Rummel, RGON, BA (Soc Sc), MA (Hons, Nursing), PhD, is the Research and Academic Development Leader in the Department of Nursing and Health Studies, Manukau Institute of Technology (MIT), New Zealand, where she works with staff and students nurturing a research culture. She is a member of the MIT Research and Ethics Committee and works part-time as a research and ethics adviser for this committee. Louise completed her PhD in Nursing in 2002 at Massey University. She has been involved in nursing education for two decades and is passionate about processes of student teaching and learning, particularly clinical teaching. She is a member of the New Zealand Nurses Organisation Nursing and Midwifery Advisory Committee and the NZNO National Nursing Research Committee. She has been an intrepid visitor to the Advanced Heideggerian Institute and is indebted to Dr. Nancy Diekelmann and her husband, John, for their teaching and knowledge in interpretive phenomenology.

Billie M. Severtsen, PhD, RN, is Associate Professor at the Washington State University College of Nursing in Spokane. She has taught at that college since 1975. Her areas of teaching expertise include professional role development for nurses and ethical issues in healthcare. She has been instrumental in curriculum reform and revision at the College of Nursing. Her research and publication efforts are focused in the areas of narrative pedagogy and storytelling. She developed the Recollective Pathway, a teaching and learning methodology designed to create a community of learners in the classroom. Dr. Severtsen is a member of the Hastings Center, a scholarly organization dedicated to analysis of ethical issues.

Deb Spence, RGON, RM, Certificate in Accident and Emergency Nursing, BA (Education), PG Certificate in Adult Tertiary Education, PG Diploma in Social Sciences with Distinction, PhD (Nursing), is principal lecturer in the School of Nursing and Midwifery at the Auckland University of Technology in New Zealand. She has a strong practice background in acute care nursing. Her interests in relation to teaching include relationships of theory, practice, and research in nursing, cross-cultural practice, hermeneutic methodology, working collaboratively with clinicians to advance nursing practice at the postgraduate level, and supporting the development of clinically focused research. Her doctoral thesis, completed in 1999, bears the same title as her chapter in this volume. She is currently undertaking funded research that focuses on articulating the contribution of education to advanced nursing practice.

Index

abandonment, 24; of being, distress of, 65
Abbott, M., 150
ability: meaning of, 100; to teach, 242
Aboriginal culture, 37
abortion, 167, 168
Absalom, K., 15
abstracting, 106
abuse, 24; childhood, 24; physical, 24; to-
    ward client, 163; verbal, 24
academic: advancement, nursing's, 220; com-
    petence, 150; constraint, teaching and,
    198; culture, 107, 120; exercise, 125; inte-
    gration of practice and, 255; learning,
    195; multiculturalism in, 133; story, 136;
    work, 106
acceptance, 54, 88, 96, 99, 112, 160; social,
    26
accountability, 161, 256, 259; for caring,
    230; for learning needs, 230; and nursing,
    246; for patients and students, 250; pre-
    cepting as double, 236, 239, 245, 249,
    250, 252, 258; professional, 230, 258; vigi-
    lance and, 239
acculturation: into nursing, 218; to Western
    culture, 118, 128, 129
acting out, 24, 27
action(s): care as belief-in-, 121; care as
    emerging through, 122; concrete, 106;
    meanings and, 144; of New Zealand
    nurses, 145; observing caring, 119;
    reflection-in-, 193; responsibility for, 252;
    strategizing, 194; striving as, 160; waiting
    and, 50

activity(ies): caring, 123; daily, 121; docu-
    menting, 246; of living, 65; missionary,
    109; practical, everyday, 220, 229;
    preceptor-preceptee, 223; reflective, 147,
    193; self-interpreting, 187, 188, 189, 190;
    taken for granted, 187; theoretical, 229
acute care settings, 219, 221, 223, 226, 231,
    232
adaptability, 109; human, 3
adapting, 130, 162; cultural, 113, 129
administrator(s), 112; hospital, 10; school,
    93, 118, 123
adolescence: behavior of, 206; self-harm
    and, 4
adoption, 111, 128; attitude toward, 206;
    child, 206; of values, 108
adult education, 108, 256
advocacy, 8, 9, 13, 16, 92, 93, 97, 222;
    across cultures, 158; of patients, 200
aesthetics of engagement, 173
affect, self-harm and, 26
Afghanistan, 108; mountains of, 110
Africa, 114, 118
African American(s), 73, 96, 141; and black-
    ness, 99; blind child, 99; clients, 87,
    120; culture, 122; families, 68, 100; fe-
    male, 100; nursing students, 120; patients,
    207
age(s), 141, 143, 151; posthumanist, 55;
    self-harm and, 24; of students, 118
agency(ies), 16; clinical, 222, 256, 257;
    healthcare, 248; moral, 236; questions for,
    252

agenda: caring, 32, 123; diversity-related, 115; of dominant culture, 26; hospital, 22; of managing client, 33; of teachers and students, 53, 123; religious, 110
aggressive treatment, 11
aging populations, 221
Agra, India, 112
Ahuja, A., 27
Albrecht, G. L., 98
Alexander, L., 35, 36
Alice, 165
Allen, D., xv, 225
Allen, D. G., 164
aloneness, 248
Alsop, Stewart, 210
Alston, M., 27
alternative and complementary healthcare practices, 135
altruism: human reciprocal, 184
Amanda, 153, 154, 161, 162, 163
ambiguity: role, 31
ambivalence about people who are ill, 210
America: Central, 114; middle-class, 136; South, 114
American: Chinese, 129; culture, race and racism and, 118; Indians (Native Americans), history and status of, 115, 134; minority groups, 125; society, 10
American Indians (Native Americans): 198; history and status of, 115, 134; study of preceptorship, 220
Americanizing, 118
Americans, 113
analysis, 35; of caring, 192; data, 144, 148, 212; discourse, 22; as part of nursing role, 164; of stories, 192
analytic process: hermeneutic, 223
Andrews, C., xv
Andrews, M. M., xv, 8, 10, 14, 15
anecdotes. See story
anger, 200, 202; instinctual, 203
Anglican British missionaries, 112
angst of unfamiliarity, 98
Anne, 159, 160, 162
anniversary missed, 186, 187, 188, 189, 192, 194
anomie, 65
anonymity, 148
answering: process of questioning and, 242
anthropologists, 84, 183, 184

anthropology, 117, 118, 150; reflective, 105
anticipating prejudgments, 4
Antonovsky, A., 51, 55
anxiety, 7, 10, 12, 158, 159, 174, 176, 238, 252; feeling of not being at home, 231; teaching, 115
Aotearoa (New Zealand), 152, 176
apology, 98
appearance: to blind people, 84; normal, 83
Appleton, C., 122
applied disciplines, 12
approach(es): "back-door," 116; behavioral, xi, 42; biomedical, xii; chameleon, 162; client-focused, 48; cognitive behaviorist, 120; critical, 51, 56; cultural, 161; diversity and multicultural, 115; eclectic, 135; ethical, 212; ethical-moral, 118; exclusionary, xii, 121; fundamentalist, 111; hermeneutic, 212; holistic, 247; human science, 220; inclusive, 118; interpretive, 141, 220; mechanistic, 190, 191; of nurse educators, 123; one-size-fits-all, 195; phenomenological, 191, 214, 215; post-modern, 55; post-structural, xi, xii, 36; problem-centered, 54, 55, 56; problem-solving, 28; rational, 45, 47, 54; religious, 121; scientific, 191; solution-focused, 55, 56; spiritual, 121; system-focused, 48; to caring, 183; to difference, 126; to teaching caring, 120; unreflective, 48; women's studies, 116, 133. See also paradigm
Arabic, 129
Arabs: policies toward, 134
Aranda, S., 162
Armstrong, J. D., 10
Arnetz, B., 31
aromatherapy, 222
Aroni, R., 35, 36
art: caring as moral, 185; of engagement, 173; New Zealand, 143; and spirit, 65
arthritis, 199, 200
articulating, 143, 159; healthcare, 253; story, 205
Asia, 114; arrivals from, 129; language, 129
Asians, 153; appearance of, 129
Aspen Reference Group, 135
assertiveness, 98, 125, 154
assessment: of caring action, 119; cultural, 14; culturally sensitive, 14; fearing, 127;

in healthcare, 253; outcome-based, 184; of outcomes, 195; of patients by students, 244; process, 256; of student progress, 239, 255; self, 14

assimilation of immigrants, 118

association: of body, 209; dis-, 209

assumption(s), 64, 97, 116, 144, 175, 251; about caring, 121, 183; about culture, 165, about thinking, 127; assessing, 195; challenging, 195; interpretation and, 227; of pedagogy, 187; of student knowledge, 239

asylum: seekers of, 135

Atkinson, P., 105, 106, 107, 135

attending: conscious, 188; to, 12, 193

attentiveness, 12; challenges to, 244; professional, 244

attitude(s), 4; of care workers, 201; choices and, 204; of educators, 120; meaningful, 204; of New Zealand nurses, 145, 146, 163; nursing practices and, 29; of openness, 199; public, 28; taken-for-granted, 161; of teens, 207; toward adoption, 206; toward birthday, 207; toward clients of different cultures, 174; toward family, 207; toward ill persons, 210; toward parents, 206

attunement, 231, 236; assessing students', 230

Auckland, 149

Australia, 36, 218; nurses, 22, 162; psychiatry, 26

authentic: existence, 203; self, 115, 130

authenticity, 26, 198, 252, 254; as *being-as-a* nurse, 252; of meaning, 64; of narrative, 64; ontological, 64; in perspective, 227; of voice, 108

author(s): autobiography and, 63; Western, 130

authority, 10, 11, 13; competence and, 14; distributing, 53; of experience, 45, 48; harnessing, 53; of nurses, 158; positions of, 53; of tradition, 4; using, 54

autobiographical ethnography, 63

autobiography, 63, 100, 105; ethnographic, 63; feminist, 63

autoethnography, xi, xii, 105, 106, 108, 135

autonomy: of nurses, 38; of practice, 113

"Autumn leaves," 89

avoidance, 29; of strangers, 147

awakening, 133

awareness, 168; of background influences, 228; critical, 64; cultural, 150, 161; of patient experience, 241; political, 222; of reality, 99; self-, 115, 161; of significance of situation, 203; trained, 203, 204

Ayurvedic medicine, 126, 135

baby(ies), 7, 8, 12, 15, 16, 65, 69, 98; circumcised, 198; delivery of, 113; as metaphor, 252; "perfect," 66, 71

baccalaureate program: nursing, 120

Bach, 91

bachelor's degree, 220, 255, 256

background(s), 14; cultural, 223; different, 173; diverse, 145; elite, 128; historical, 223; meaning, 189, 191; nursing, 223; political, 223; of poverty and neglect, 207; self and, 225; shared, 191; social, 223; of students, 118; taken-for-granted, 227; temporal, 223

Badger, 199

Baer, H. A., 9, 10, 135

Bailey, S., 218

balance, 7, 15; between caring for and caring about, 16

Ballinger, C., 34

Baltimore, 91, 92; School for the Arts, 95, 96

Banner, L. W., 65

Baptists, 128

Barker, P., 32

Barks, C., 108

barriers: educational, 114; to learning, 212

Bartlett, H., 31

Basuray, J., xii, 105, 110, 111, 119, 132, 263

Bateson, M. C., 105, 130

Bauen, 228

beauty, 173; ontological function of, 173

Becker, H. S., 62

becoming, 133; attuned, 230, 231; more, 172; more like patient, 162; what one is, 225

Beethoven, 64, 89, 90, 91

befriending, 3

Behar, R., 63, 64, 100, 105

behavior(s), 128; abnormal, 28; acting out, 24, 27; adolescent, 206; associated with learning disabilities, 23; Bengali, 131; caring, 120; caring as learned, 122; changing, 54; culturally sensitive, 109; culture and,

behavior(s) *(continued)*
182; learned, 23; pathological, 28; patterns of, 3; of physician, 200, 201; practical, 15; self-harm, 22, 23; valuing of, 210; witnessing by preceptors, 240
behavioral: model, 26; theories, 23
behaviorist: approach, xii; cognitive, 120
Beil, W., 15
being-already-in-a-world, 225
Being and Time, 224
being(s) (Being), 62, 65, 97, 98, 99, 229, 259; abandonment of, 65; alongside, 225; a student, 248; *in between*, 158; biological, 3; care, Dasein and, 5, 14, 15; caring as way of being in the world, 185; a chameleon, 162; as community of relations, 228; complexity of, 107; concernful, 231; cultural, 3, 187; and doing, 168; essentialness of, 99; estrangement with, 65; existence and, 99; experience of, 220; face-to-face, 160; for, 133; fully present, 9; harmonious, 99; -at-home, 98, 231; -at-home, not, 98; human, 11, 32, 141; human, caring and, 32; human, meaning of, 187; language and, 226; learned, 23; left alone, 248; meaning of, 98, 224; mode of, 175; negative, 97; as a nurse, 252; oneness of, 136; one self, 176; ontologically, 225; -open, 11, 13; order of, 107; -possible, 5, 11; potential for, 6, 12; as preceptor(s), 220, 221, 223, 224, 227, 230, 231, 234, 238, 245, 248, 249, 254, 257, 258; present, 160; present and particular, 116; self-interpretation of, 210; sensory, 64; situated, 223; social, 3, 98; in society, 187; of striving, 161; -there, 5, 11, 159, 224, 234, 237; thinking and, 229; thrown, into precepting, 232; unconcealment of, 99, 233; understanding of, 99; vigilant, 239; ways of, 44; *-what-it-is*, 224; wholeness of, 64; with, 5, 11, 13, 17, 32, 33, 207; with client, 42, 45; with others, 228, 231
being-in-the-world (Being-in-the-World), 5, 6, 8, 14, 62, 99, 141, 185, 187, 194, 200, 216, 226, 227, 228, 229, 233, 258; caring as, 185; choosing, 254; meaning of, 216; of nursing practice, 238, 244, 258
beliefs, 4, 15, 17, 110, 150, 169, 221, 259; about caring, 120, 122, 123, 150; about rights, 160; cultural, 198; Eastern, 113;

human, 106; of nursing profession, 254; religious, 110; respect of, 140; spiritual, 123, 140; systems, student-teacher, 121; uncertain, 248; values and, 64
Bell, D., 126
belonging, 64, 247
Ben-Ari, A. T., 63
benevolence: care as, 253
Bengali: appearing, 131; becoming, 131; being, 126; community, 132; name, 126
Benhabib, S., 65
benign neglect, 110
Benner, P., xv, 13, 15–17, 32, 124, 145, 147, 158, 172, 182, 185, 186, 188–191, 212, 215, 220, 223, 224, 226, 228, 235, 236, 244
Bennett, M. J., 10
Bennun, I., 23
Berman, L., 168
Bernie, 234, 236
Beverly, 154, 161
Bevis, E. O., 184
Bible, 220
biculturalism, 143, 161, 247
biography: cultural, 63; history and, 62
biological: beings, 3; dimension, teaching about, 118; fact, 97; perspective, 25
biomedical perspective, xii
biomedicine, 9, 10; culture and, 9; curative regime of, 9, 253; orthodox, 9; power of, 10; practice of, 134; scientific philosophy of, 9; Western culture and, 134
biosocial: disorder, 25; perspective, 25
birth, 62, 65–66; giving, 63, 65
birthdays: attitudes toward, 207
Bishop, A. H., 155, 158, 185, 253
bishop: Lutheran, 111
Black. *See* African American
black and white, 129
black liberal arts college: teachers in, 122
blackness, 99
"Black thing:" 90
blame, 98
Blazey, M. E., 241
blindness, 67, 68, 70, 72, 73, 76, 92, 95, 97, 98, 100; and appearance, 84; culture of, 98, 100
blood products, 8, 9, 10
Board of Education, 75
Bochner, A. P., 62, 63, 100, 105, 106, 107
Bock, P. K., 98

body(ies): attitudes toward, 210; broken and ill, 23, 210; dying, 214; experience of, 25; fragility of, 41, 98; fragmented, 98; growth and development of, 247; intelligence of, 188; physical, 41; predictability of function of, 209; relatedness, as issue in healthcare, 209; as socially influenced object, 25; whole, 98

bonding, 70

Bonner, G., 30

book(s), 75, 76, 80; on tape, 95; writing a, 96

Boore, J. R. P., 221

Borderline Personality Disorder, 42

Boss, M., 5

Bottorff, J., 6, 119

boundaries: ethnic, 171; of self and other, knower and known, 126

Bowers, L., 29

Boykin, A., 185

Boyle, J. S., 10, 15

bracketing, 144

Braille, 80, 93; Olympics, 93; reading, 93

Brandes, S., 63

Braun, B., 51

breakdown, 16

breathing: consciousness of, 107; meaning of, 100

bridge: between worlds, preceptors as, 254

Briere, J., 23

Brisbane, 36

British, 113; colonialism, 109, 110, 111; Crown, 176; missionaries, 110, 112; novels, 128; Raj (rule), 110

Brody, H., 63

brothers, brotherhood, 75, 110, 172, 199

Brown, D., 31, 32

Buber, M., 116, 117, 129

Buddha, Buddhism, 135; *as-it-is-ness*, 64; Zen, 109

building: community, 205; nursing practice through precepting, 230

Buller, S., 32

burn-out, 17, 27, 31, 200, 213

Burns, K., 28

Busfield, J., 30

Butterworth, T., 32

Byrne, M. W., 122

Caillois, R., 25

California, 93

call: listening to, 232; responding to, 233; to be preceptor, 231

calling out: stories, 196, 213

Calof, D., 23, 51

camaraderie: engendering, 242

campus multicultural institute, 115

cancer: breast, 197; esophageal, 207; struggle with, 197

Cant, S., 135

Capitol Hill, 92

"carative factors:" 184

care, 3, 5, 7, 8, 15, 17, 88, 119, 140, 141, 159, 166, 167, 171, 191, 208, 257; acute, 157, 173; automatic, 49; as belief-in-action, 121; challenge of complex, 244; client, 253; comfort measures, 8; community-based, ix; concentrated, 170; constant, 17; constraints on, 21, 30; control of, 27; for critically ill, 17; cultural congruence and, 114, 162; culture, 8, 150; culture-based, ix; culture-specific, 10; delivering, 54; devaluing, 213; for disabled, 222; discourse of, 28; domination and, 6; and dying patient, 237; of elderly, 223; empathetic, 241; experience of, 151; family, 247; focus on delivery of, 222; global perspective, 222; Heidegger's ideas of, 225; holistic, 9–10; individualized, 22; intensive, 17; intimacy and, 156; journey, 134; locus of, 222; machines and, 6, 7; mantle of, 253; of mentally ill, 223; of minority groups, 223; by missionaries, 111; moral imperative to, 253; need to, 166; negotiating, 54; nursing, 21, 27, 95, 141, 166, 245; objectification of, 16; and patients, 226, 241, 246, 249, 254; paradigm, 213; practices, 55, 140; for preceptors, 252; quality of, 257; safe, 151; for self, 6, 18; self, by nurses, 31; shaping, 213; silence of, x; standards of, 17; stimulation and, 7; stories of, 181; structure of, 6; for students, 254; teaching, 218; TLC, 8; traditional viewpoints and, 135; transcultural, 150; unrealistic demands of, 27; vulnerability in, 29

care-based foundation of practice, 253

caregiver(s), 213; ability of to listen and witness, 205

caring, ix, x, 3, 6, 38, 65, 96, 106, 119, 120, 121, 130, 143, 172, 173, 174, 185, 191, 215, 218, 258; about, 15, 258; and

caring *(continued)*
academic culture, 123; agenda, 32; appearance of, 31; approximations of, 8; behaviors, 120; and being human, 32; beliefs
about, 123; and change, 126; competence
and, 45; comportment, x; concept of, 182;
concern for, ix, x, 124, 125; connecting,
105; construction of, xii; co-occurrence of
with culture, xii; constructs, 184; cost of,
17; course in, 194, 195, 208, 211, 214,
215, 230, 235; as culture, 120; culture
and, ix, x, 3, 7, 18, 105, 107, 108, 125,
126, 135; culture conducive to, 219;
definitions of, 125, 181; discourse, 32, 29;
diversity-sensitive, 122, 184, 116; and
early socialization, 121; effect of, 123;
efficiency and, 198; embedded in situation, 185, 186; emotional responses and,
31; enculturation to, 120; ethic of, 184;
ethnographic study of, 105, 119, 120;
examples of, 196; exclusionary, 121;
expression of, 17, 122, 123; as female
activity, 183; food and, 197; for, 16, 247,
258; *for* and *about*, 133, 172; generic,
185, 186; in health care, 96; human, 107;
humanistic expression of, 122; humans as,
107; ideology, 122, 124; intentions in, x;
interpersonal, 183; interpretation of, 136;
issue of, 216; lack of, 239; language and,
32; learning about, 95, 212; learning from
reflection on, 196, 197, 198; literacy, 49,
50; literature, xi; making visible, 208;
meaning of, 108, 115, 119, 122, 124, 159,
160; as moral art, 185; nature of, 21;
need for, 64, 162; nursing and, 32, 119,
151, 195, 197, 213, 214; nurturing of, 99;
observing, 119; occurrence of, 198;
outcomes, 208; patient-centered, 10;
perception of, 117; philosophy of, 120,
147; possibility and, 191, 197; practice,
21, 22, 32, 33, 47, 50, 56, 208; practices
of preceptors, 235, 253; praxis and, 136;
as primary, 191; promoting, 120;
reading and, 198; recognition of, 181;
reflective, 185; relationships, 50, 116,
165; responsibility, 160; rhetoric, 56;
for safety, 240; scholarship and, 125;
science of, 184; search for, 125; for self,
117, 123; significance of, x; skills, 21, 52,
56; spiritual, 121, 123; for stories, 199;
as story, 205; for students, 121, 232, 238;
study of, 21; and Taoism, 136; teaching,
105, 123, 181, 194; as therapeutic intervention, 6; traditional views and 135;
transcultural aspects of, 181; transhistorical aspects of, 181; un-, 196, 213; unconditional, 133; uncovering, 193; understanding of, 125, 197; universality of, 107;
values, 49, 56, 120, 221; valuing, 124;
ways of, 136; as way of being, 214, 215;
as worrying, 160
Carlson, G., 23
Carper, B. A., 46
Carson, J., 31, 32
case studies, 50, 118
caste(s): lowest, 110; system, 110
cast out, 112
catharsis, 236, 237
Catholic church: immigrant services program of, 115
Catholicism, 122
celebration(s), 187, 188; attitudes toward,
206; missed, 194
celebrity, 88
Cesara, M., 63
challenge(s), 65, 100, 119, 146, 154; assumptions, 195; of being preceptors, 219, 254;
of complex care, 244; of cultural safety,
141; to immigrants, 114; of learning, 173;
of nursing school, 95; of *other*, 160, 166;
of school, 205; situational, 245; of socializing students, 123; to understanding, 170
chameleon: being a, 162
change(s), 10, 55, 56, 109, 130, 162; and behavior, 54; focus on, 150; in focus, with
precepting, 226; in healthcare, 31, 248,
252; institutional, 257; needed, 255;
nurses' power to instigate, 124; personal,
109, 133; positive, 99; possibilities for, 33;
of rules, 129; societal, 148; spiral of, 257;
in student preparation, 256; time and,
126; tradition and, 126; "turning around"
as, 15; in understandings, 146, 169, 170
characters: in stories, 62
charitable causes: support of, 129
Charles A. and Anne Morrow Lindbergh
Foundation, 18
Charmaz, K., 97, 99
chastity, 131
Chatterjee, P., 110
Chávez, R. C., 63
checking in, 197

Cherryholmes, C., 27

Chesla, C. A., 13, 16, 147, 212, 235, 236

child, children, 62, 95, 112, 113, 114, 157, 167; adopted, 206; Black, 88, 99; blind, 76, 77, 78, 82, 88, 99; care about, 119; Chinese, 167; disabled, xii, 96; giving away, 68; grown, 108; handicapped, 81, 92; holding dear, 62, 68, 100; "perfect," 63; Samoan, 159; second, 66; stories and, 127; teenage, 206

childbirth, 62, 63, 65, 66

childhood, 113, 122, 132; abuse, 24; early experiences, 120

Childress, H., 63

Childs, A., 30

China, 167, 168

Chinese, 167; American nurse, 129; appearance of, 129; medicine, 135

Chladenius, J. M., 106, 119

choice(s), 106, 109, 112, 114, 115, 168, 170; to embody, 252; Faustian, 98; free, 203; of husband, 112; question of, 190; responsible, 203; in situation, 203; of treatment/no treatment, 210; of values, 204; of way of being-in-the-world, 254

Chopin, 91

Christian: born individuals, 109; brotherhood, 110; catechism, 127; evangelical, 121; love doctrine, 121; name, 114; Nurses Fellowship, 121; promises of missionaries, 109; religion, 121, 136; student, 121; way of life, 121

Christian and Western culture, 113; religion, 121; values, 120

Christianity, 108, 111, 114; conversion to, 112; evangelical, 123; Gnostic, 135; promises of, 109

Christmas, 79; eve, 127

chronicity: caring and, 185

church, 112, 127; Baptist, 128; Catholic, 115; community, 122, 171; Episcopalian, 128; and state, 112; work organizations of, 133

circle: of interpretation, 226, 228; of interpretive understanding, 226; of learning, 200

circumcision, 198

circumspection, 15

citizenship, 129

city, 154

civil servants, 111, 112

civilization: levels of, 150

Clampitt, A., 64, 65

class(es), 10, 128, 151, 153; confusion with race, 126; discussing, 116; generalizations about, 118; lower, 110; upper, 108; working with different, 163

classification, 34; by color, 129; fearing, 127

classism, 116, 128, 136

classroom: settings, 199; teaching, 222

clearing, 62, 99, 188, 191, 193, 200, 233; language and, 226

Cleary, M., 28

client(s): as body and behavior, 43; care of, practitioners of, 253; context, clinician and, 22; defining "cultural safety," 141; detachment from nurses, 32; discontented, 119; diverse, 57; invalidation of needs of, 32; line between healthcare provider and, 117; management of, 33; objectification of, 32; power and, 53, 54; problems and solutions and, 55; recovery of, 21; risk from, 29; silence and, 53; supervision of, 30; as unique, 45; vulnerability of, 146; well-being of, 50; who self-harm, 36, 40, 41, 45, 47, 48, 50, 54; working with, 54. *See also* consumers; patients

clinical: agencies, 222, 257; colleagues, 146; communication, 16; competence, 150; context, 28, 256; demands, 222; environment, 30; experiences, 205, 222, 238, 239; instruction, 220; instructors, 220; interaction, 16; knowledge, 13; language in practice, 166; learning, 239; learning experiences, 219; lecturers, 219, 249, 255, 256; nurse educator, 238; nursing practice, value of, 124; paths, 29, 30, 51; placement, 219, 232; placement(s), populations, 52; practice, 13, 124, 207, 219, 242; practice, culture of, 124; precepting in, 230, 248, 251; reasoning, 16, 55; reflection in, 192; roles, 131; setting, stories and, 53; skill, 15; teaching roles, 219, 257; teaching sites, 122; tutors, 251; wisdom, 15

clinically mentally ill: care for, 223

clinicians: clients, context and, 22; consumers and, 10; experienced, 124; interaction with students, patients, teachers, 208; nurse, 198, 208; pedagogy and, 193;

clinicians *(continued)*
practice and, 56; voice and, 52; voices of, 195, 198; white, 122
clinics: ante-natal, 158; posters in, 159; practice in, 113; women's health, 167
Clinton, M., 31, 32
closure, 237
Clough, P., 105
coaching, 47, 48, 124
Cobden-Grainge, F., 218
Code of Ethics, 221
Code of Nursing Ethics, 140
codes: analytical, 212; ethical, 141; moral, 110
coercion. *See* hegemony
coexistence: human, 140
cognition: theoretical, 15
cognitive: behaviorist approach, 120; gain, 196
coherence, 63, 64
Coles, R., 199
collaboration, 256, 257; need for, 255; nursing and, 221
colleague(s), xv, 238; conversations with, 146; intermediary, 148; learning from, 116
collecting cultural histories, 115
College of Nursing, Washington State University, 194
colonialism, 108, 151; British, 109, 110; economy and, 110; education and, 110; European, 109; healthcare and, 110; post-, 108
colonial oppression, 114; affect on nursing education in India, 115; writing about, 115
colony: India as British, 111
color, 141, 143; people of, 126; skin, 129, 153
comfort, 30, 252; with controversial discourse, 116; level, 188; with machinery, 244
coming to know, 167, 169
commitment, 221, 240; to respect, openness, concern, 174; to safeguarding practices, 254
communication, 4, 7, 12, 13, 14, 15, 25, 42, 44, 47, 48, 49, 54, 55, 98, 154, 191, 258; clinical, 16, 158; with colleagues, 146; cross-cultural, 159; difference and, 125; effective, 154, 222; of emotions, 247; with God, 98; human, 105, 164; interpersonal, 174; need for, 125; nursing and, 221;

opportunities for, 115; preceptor to student, 242; silence and, 53; skills, 222, 252; stories as, 211; teaching, 52; therapeutic, 51; verbal and nonverbal, 116; written, 147
community, 10, 11, 28, 98, 108, 135, 142, 156, 173, 199, 200, 257; through apology, 98; attachment to, 131; Bengali, 132, 133; building, 194, 199, 205; care in, ix; celebration, 129; church, 122; classmates as, 201; conversations about, 195; daily life in, 97; healthcare, 108; Indian, 131; learning, 195, 198, 209, 211; meeting, 154; moral, 256; nurses and, 164; organizations, diversity in, 115, 135; practices, 193, 195, 208; of relationships, 228; religious, 127; Samoan, 171; of scholars, 198, 211; schooling and, 209; supportive, 201, 204; university, 135; work in, 234
compassion, 17, 32, 88, 96, 122, 161, 172, 221; expression of, 98, 161; nurse and, 205
competence, 14, 45, 56, 123, 140, 221; academic, clinical and culture, 10, 150; and development of practitioner, 245, 251, 252; in practice, 14; social, 26
complementary healthcare practices, 135, 222
compliance, 12
comportment: caring, x
compromise, 146, 162
compulsions, 24
concealment, 62
concentration, 244
concepts: of caring course, 194, 195; of integrating, self, cultures, meanings, understandings of caring, 129
conceptualization, 195
conceptual teaching, 208
concern, ix, xi, 6, 13, 15, 17, 33, 159, 168, 174, 190, 191, 192, 208, 249; for caring, 124, 125; and imagination, 192; and phenomenological view, 190; problems as main, 55
concernful: being with others, 231; practices, 193, 195
conditioning: cultural, in nursing, 222; operant, 23
"confessional tales," 63
confidence, 99, 221; engendering, 241; gaining, 116, 125; in identity, 174; lost,

129; nursing and, 221; with procedures, 243

confidentiality, 208, 211

conflict: agreement and, 166; between educators' need and academic culture, 123; hermeneutics of, 166; between horizons, 166; intrapersonal, 174; marital, role, 113, 127; potential for, 127; in teaching, 242; among values, 168

confusion, 165, 166

Congress, 92

connecting, connections, 98, 114, 117, 162, 214; caring, 105; cultural/personal, 105; meanings and action, 144; nurturing, 9; social, 22, 51; text, 100

conscience, nursing and, 221

consciousness, 63; layers of, 106; of breath, 107; self-, 63, 106, 231

consent: informed, 200, 211

conservatism, 131

Conservatory (Peabody Institute), 66, 96

considerateness, 6

constitutive pattern, 223, 231

constraints: organizational, 201; technocratic, 201

consultation: nursing and, 221

consumer(s), 50, 54; and clinicians, 10; driving environment, 222; voice and, 52. *See also* clients

contact, 214

containing risk: role of, 31

context(s), xii, 3, 21, 22, 26, 33, 36, 52, 99, 106, 125, 190, 256; acute care, 157; altering behavior with, 128; changing, 256; clinical, 28, 53; clinician-client, 22, 53, 56; cultural, xii, 25, 105, 109, 133, 163, 175, 182, 209, 210, 211, 221, 223, 225; culturally safe, 247; educational, 256; embodied, 65; framing, 194; healthcare, 22, 221, 248, 256; historical, 221, 223, 225; of human existence, 141; interpretation and, 143, 149; learning, 258; of life histories, 63; meanings in, 142, 146; mental health nursing, 32; New Zealand, 141; nursing, 223, 228; of patient care, 226; pedagogical, 122; political, 223; of practice, 22, 27; of preceptor, 228; problem-centered, 54; reality, 252; research, 232; of school and hospital, 123; of self-harm study, 52; social, 223, 225; sociopolitical, 174, 256; study, 225; temporal, 223; variables and, 184, 185

contextualized lives, 64, 149

continuum: space-time, 117

control, xi; altered, 209; gaining, 192; in hospital, 191; as issue, 209; loss of, 54; magical, 26; need for, 29, 54; nurses as "social policemen," 29; over practice, 38, 39, 54; sense of, 25; thrownness and, 232

convalescence, 257

convergence: of stories, 200, 204, 206, 207

conversation(s): analyzing, 195; about caring, 198; community-centered, 195; converging, ix, xiii, 99; gathering, 195; listening to, 195; overlapping, 13; with situation, 192, 193; story, 195; between teachers and students, 186; telephone, 149; unfolding, from stories, 200

conversion, 112, 114; to Christianity, 108, 111, 112; conviction of, 109; ideological, 118; models of, 112; of Muslims, 110; targets for, 110

Cookie, 68, 75, 78, 79, 80, 84, 85, 86, 91, 92, 94

Coon, T., 28

cooperation: need for, 255, 256, 257

co-participation: in dialogue, 136

COPD, 214

coping, 25, 37, 44, 235; prayer and, 80; as recreation of meaning, 240; self-harm and, 24; with students, 219; with uncaring bureaucracy, 123

corporate interests in healthcare, 158

corporeality, 25, 97, 98

corporeal world, 98

cosmos: personal, 134; sacralized, 134

cost-containment, 30, 158; framework of, 29

Council of Nursing and Anthropology, 150

counseling, 3

county human relations commission, 115

courage: failure of, 243

course(s): administrators and, 118; in caring, 194, 195; on caring, 208; clinical, 202; in nursing, 108; Recollective Pathways, 195; on spirituality, 123; theory, 202; transcultural nursing, 115, 117, 118

craniofacial malformation, 98; reconstruction, 92

Crawfold, L., 63

Crawford, M., 184

creativity, 51, 55, 110; story and, 62

creed, 141

Creedy, D., 27

crimes against humanity, 134
crises, 40, 41, 167, 185; management of, 246; nursing, 218
Cristofori, Bartolomeo, 86
critical: awareness, 64; illness, 17; listening, 143; pedagogy, 57; perspective, 14, 33; racial theory, 126; reflection, 21; thinking, 51
critique: nurses and, 164
Crookes, P. A., 219
Crow and Weasel, 198, 199
Crowe, M., 25, 32, 41
crying, 68, 94
cultivating students, 230
cultural: adaptation, 113; awareness, 14, 150; backgrounds, 149, 150; beings, 3; beliefs, in treatment protocols, 198; biography, 63; competence, 10; conditioning, in nursing, 222; congruence in care, learning about, 114; congruence in nursing, 140; congruent intervention, 10, 162; context, 25, 105, 109, 209, 210, 211; differences, 136, 151, 166, 173, 174, 248; discourse, 32; disorder, 25; gestures, 98; groups, 10, 113; health beliefs, 174, 256; histories, collecting, 115; horizons, 149; imposition, 11; influences, 117, 228; inhibition, 108; interactions, 14; invasion, 109; issues, media and, 145; issues, nursing and, 150; landscapes, 106; meanings, 26, 100; norms, 112, 259; nursing, 145, 146, 153, 160; oppression, 108, 127; orientation, 108; origins, 114; practices, 236, 247; relationships, 26; safety (Kawa Whakaruruhau), 141, 143, 144, 145, 149, 150, 151, 176, 222, 247; satisfaction of communication, 176; self, 105; sensitivity, 51, 109, 123, 146, 150; shaping, 157; suppression, 108; texture, 97; theory, 26; tradition, 133; transcending differences in, 173–174; understanding, x, 165; values, 17, 108, 130
culture(s), ix, 8, 106, 114, 130, 154, 163, 176, 215; Aboriginal, 37; academic, 120, 123; advocating across, 158; African American, 122; American, 118; being-in-the-world of, 187; biomedicine and, 9; of blindness, 100; blood, 240; and care, 8, 135, 140, 150; care based in, ix; of caregivers, 182; and caring, ix, x, 3, 7, 18, 105, 107, 108, 125, 181, 214, 218, 230,

235; as caring, 120, 123; Christian, 113; of clinical practice, 123; communal, immersion in, 254; conduciveness to caring, 219; connection, person and, 105; construction of, xii; context and, xii, 64; co-occurrence of with caring, xii; cross, 145; and death, 236; definitions of, 151, 152, 182, 221; dialectics of, 141; of disability, 100; and discourse, xii; discussion of, 131; dominant, 26; Eastern and Western, 108; embracing, 128; and experience, xii; of family, 65; of healthcare, 26, 258; of healthcare delivery, 226; history as, 98; of hospital, 187; of illness, 214; of ill persons, 182; indigenous, 113, 149; integrating, 129; interaction across, 147, 159, 160, 161, 175, 176; and interpretation, xi, 136, 149; intervention and, 9; language and, 4; learned, 3, 4, 108; local, 226, 228; meaning of, 108; Middle Eastern, 113; minority, 51; Muslim,114; of New Zealand, 149, 247; of NICU, 8; nurse, 187; nursing and, 115, 159, 218, 219, 221, 224, 232, 240, 254; of nursing school, 123; organizational, 122, 123, 228, 258; orientation to, 6; other than own, xii, 149, 151, 156, 159, 162, 170, 175, 176; of patient, 187; of personal narrative, 63; policy and, 8; and political context, xii; praxis and, 136; preunderstanding and, 225; of professional community, 221; resistance to, 49; self and, 107; shaping experience and, 63, 119; shared, 97, 98, 189; shock, 129; significance of, x; of social institutions, 253; sociopolitical definition of, 151; and teaching, 125; transmission of, 254; values and, 187; of violence in nursing, 239; web of, 25; Western, 6, 108, 113, 118; workplace, 49
Culture Care: theory of, 140
cupcake: as symbol, 186, 194
curative biomedicine, 9, 10
cure, 112; desire for, 210; expectation of, 210; focus on, 207; nursing and, 234
curing: healing and, 9; as male activity, 183
curriculum(a), 149, 183, 184; caring in nursing, 183, 184; change in, 51; design of, 117; development of, 50; Eastern, 134; general education, 115; "lived," 253; marginalization of diversity, 115; model, 222; for nursing people from culture other

than own, 140, 141, 142, 151, 153, 156, 158, 159, 162, 174, 175, 176; as powerful, 117; self-harm as topic in, 51; traditions and interpretation of, 142; transformative, 117; variations in, 130; Western, 134, 140
Curry, D., 25
customs, 5, 221, 259; respect of, 140

Daddy, 80
Dahlberg, K., xv
Dale, 232, 251, 252
Dallas, Texas, 83, 86, 87, 89, 91
Dallender, J., 31
Danaher, G., 34, 35
danger, 29
Danish missionaries, 110; Lutheran, 111
Darbyshire, P., xv
darshan: sense of, 121
Dasein, 6, 11, 12, 14, 17, 99, 224, 225, 226, 231, 233, 244; care as *Being of*, 5, 15; as own possibility, 254
Das Man, 5
data, 47, 146; analysis of, 148, 212; collecting, 35, 144, 148, 192, 212; dialogue with, 143, 147; spiral *of* and *from*, 224; substantive, 224
daughter, 206; father's, 130
daughter-in-law, 130
David, M., 99
day-to-day practice, 241, 259
death, 172; coping with, 235, 237; father's, 35; feared, 235; meaning of, 234; near, 111; of patients, 234, 235, 237; as unfamiliar, 235
Death of Ivan Illych, The, 196
de Boer, G. M., 153
decision making, 251; shared, 256
deconstruction of generalizations, 118
defining: understanding and, 142
definitions: of caring, 125
degree: bachelors, 220, 255
dehumanization, 126
Delgado, R., 126
Delhi, 112
delivery: healthcare, 31, 157, 158; labor and, 7
demands of safe practice, 258
demographics, 99
denial: judging as, 205
Denmark, 111
Denzin, N., 64, 145, 148

Department of Education, 150
depersonalization, 126
descent. *See* heritage
desire: as issue, 208
desolation: sense of, 26
destruction: history of, 134
detachment: emotional, 31, 32
determination, 100; self-, 13
deterministic: framework, 127
development: faculty, 108; personal, 117; spiritual, 121
deviant: identity as, 98
DeVita, P. R., 10
D'hoore, W., 31
diagnosis, 26; images of, 210; listening and, 205; medical, 210
dialectic(s), 4, 7, 11, 14, 21, 22, 63, 107, 109, 175; between cherished and tension, 159; critique, 51; of history, culture and language, 141; between identity and difference, 166; between part and whole, 12; part-whole, 142; in practice, 41; between risk and trust, 29; between security and danger, 29; of risk, 29
dialogue, 16, 21, 44–45, 53, 106, 117, 125, 144, 145, 256; in clinical setting, outcomes of, 53, 116; co-participation in, 136; with data, 143; dialectic and professional, 176; of difference, 125; goals of, 106; knowledge and, 147; personal, 105; between preceptors and preceptees, 253; relationships as, 116; social, 148; storytelling and, 53; subject-to-object dialogue, 116; teaching and, 53
diaries: ethnographic, 63
dichotomies, 29, 50, 108, 123; social-philosophical, 136
Diekelmann, J., 192, 193
Diekelmann, N., xv, 192, 193, 195, 224, 225, 237, 263
difference(s)/*difference*, xii, 14, 17, 21, 22, 97, 126, 140, 153–156, 159, 160, 162, 170, 172; babies that are, 97; care and, 140; celebrate, 109; between clinicians and consumers, 10; critical, 158; cultural, 136, 140, 152–154, 159–161, 166, 173; denying, 141; deviance and, 98; dialogue of, 125; as difficult, 154; distance and, 153; dramatization of, 98; encountering, 152–153, 165, 174; as enriching, 53; erasing, 56, 109; between experience and

difference(s) *(continued)*
observation, 63; failure to accommodate, 159; in families, 128; in healthcare context, 248; identifying, 108; identity and, 166; in interpretations, 166; judgment of, 98; learning from, 130; lines of, 109; in looks, 75, 127; maintaining, 108; marginization and, 57; maximizing, 109; meaning of, 109; minimizing, 109; mistreatment for, 129; multifactorial nature of, 147; nursing and, 159; from others, norms, peer, 98; and parents, 96; physical, 65, 97; as precious, 140; reality of, 125; recognizing, 109; representation of, 98; resolving, 125; respect for, 141; silencing, 26; suffering and, 126; tension between sameness and, 98; thinking and, 127; value of, 140; way of working with, 52, 56; 155, 156

Differenz, 97
dignity, 113, 116
Dilthey, W., 141
Dingman, S., 22
Dinkins, C. S., xvi
diplomatic framework, 110
disability, xii; 63, 65, 98, 151; child with, 96; culture of, 100; experience of, 99; hiding, 98; judgment of, 98; learning, 23; reaction to, 98; representation of, 98; rights, 99; and thrownness, 98; visual, 98
disabled: caring for, 222; identity as, 98
disadvantaged groups, 222
disagreement: over meanings, 199
disassociation, 24, 32, 210; of body, 209
disciplines: applied, 12; health, 106
disclosedness, 14
disclosure, 11, 12, 17, 27, 28, 99, 107, 125, 127, 134, 232; of change, 248; understanding as, 5
discomfort: with thrownness, 233
discourse(s), xii, 5, 13, 14, 27, 34, 36; analysis of, 22, 34, 56; authoritative, 48; autoethnography and, 135; caring, 28, 29, 32; comfort with, 116; cultural, xii, 32; on diversity, 116; dominant, 21, 28; dominant rational, 45, 47, 48, 49, 50, 55, 56; education and practice and, 21; "essential," 50; between experience and naiveté, 49; feminist, 23, 24; function of, 33; of health, 28; hegemonic, 49; ideological, 136; influence of, 33; issues about, 135;

management and, 30, 39, 40, 44, 48; on multicultural education, 135; operational, 35; of outcomes, 28; in personal stories, 52; of professionization, 28; power of, 41, 43; practice and, 21, 37, 49, 56, 57; professional, 163; psychiatric, 41, 42, 44, 45, 48, 55; public moral, 29; of risk, 28, 30; social, 21, 32, 163; solution, 55; "totalizing," 50, 55, 56; of trauma, 23
discovering, 11, 16, 124; forced, 98
discrimination, 100, 150, 200
discussion, 117; in classroom, 199; of politics and culture, 131; of solutions, 55
disease(s), 22, 251; arthritis, 199, 200; communicable, 126; COPD, 214; organic, 23; process of, 43; stress of, 207
disfigured: face, 66; meaning of, 71
disfigurement, 65, 97
disharmony, 97
disorder: biosocial, 25; cultural, 25; personality, 27
disparity: maximizing, 109; minimizing, 109
disrespect, 109, 201
disruptions: of living, 64
dissonance, 98; feelings of, in practice, 158
distance, 32; difference and, 153; involvement at, 246; between professional and client, 32, 44, 163, 166, 186; recognition of, 166; reducing, 147; social, 11, 32, 214; from technology, 99. *See also* social distancing
distress, 188, 191; of abandonment, 65; of clients, 50; interpersonal, 41; power and, 53; psychological, 26; social, in nurse-patient relations, 166
district nursing, 148
distrust: of subjective feelings, 210
diverse populations, 221
diversity(ies), 114, 115, 116, 118, 140, 145; celebrating, 109; in community organizations, 115; convictions about, 118; education about, 114; in healthcare, 115; learning about, 116; maximizing, 109; of meanings of caring, 120; minimizing, 109; sensitivity to in caring, 116; teaching about, 115; in value of caring, 122; work, 115
doctoral studies, 119, 132, 133
doctors, 65, 66, 74; compassion and, 88, 96
doctrine of Christian love, 121
documentation, 249; of activities, 246

dogma: 54, 141; children and, 127; hidden, 56

doing: focus on, 207; for, 6; of striving, 161; struggle with being, 168; ways of, 161

domicile: place of, 153

dominance, 14; in culture, 26; in discourse, 28; medical, 10, 11, 158; practices, 27; teaching about, 118; of technology, 252

"Do no harm," 15

Dorothy, 120, 121, 122, 123

Dossey, B. M., 10

Douglas, M., 97

Doyle, M., 28

Draucker, C., xv

"Dr. Confidence," 73

"Dr. Doom," 72

dream: bizarre, 66; *not* a, 70; as truth, 64

dress, 153; Bengali, 131; national/provincial, 131; Pakistani, 131

dressing wounds, 242, 243

Dreyfus, H. L., 184, 187, 231

dualistic thinking: as illness, 136; opposites, 18; Western, 136

Dunlop, M. J., 185

Durie, M., 247

dwelling, 228; building, thinking, and, 227; journeying and, 229; with students, 230; in the world, thinking as, 229

dyadic encounter, 22

Dyck, I., 150

dying: caring for, 236

dynamic everyday tensions: culture as, 221

East, 130; Coast, 132; Middle, 129

Easter, 127

Eastern: beliefs and ideas, traditional, 113; cultures, 108; religions, 109; spirituality, 134; thought, 135

Easterners, 130

economic: advantage, 99; management, 30

economy: colonialism and, 110

Edmondson, R., 106

education, 30, 117, 130, 151, 153, 256; adult, 108, 129; affect of oppression on, 115; barriers to, 114; belief about, 238; bi-culturalism in, 150; for blind children, 75, 93, 95; caring literacy and, 50; clinical nurse, 238; colonialism and, 110; commitment to, 113; "concept package" of, 196; context of, 256; continuing, 114; critical, 49, 50; discourse and practice and, 21;

about diversity and multiculturalism, 114; engagement in, 50; gaps in, 219; general, 115; institution, 119, 249, 256, 257; and lectures, testing, cognitive gain, 196; level, 128; midwifery, 143; multicultural, 135; nurse, 119, 122, 123, 124, 125, 136; 181; nursing, 112, 117, 120, 121, 122, 143, 145, 148, 150, 151, 183, 192, 219, 248, 257; nursing, in India, 115; on-going, 135; own, 132; polytechnic, 239; power and, 56; practice and, 148; of preceptors, 255; professional, 169; programs, 114; progress, 117; role of, 114; self-harm program, 51, 56; vs. service, 222; service sectors and, 255; services of, 111; settings, diversity in, 115; special, 75; stories and, 52; system, 117, 118; transformation and, 49; undergraduate, 37, 51; value of, 128; Western, 113, 114; world of nursing, 254

Education: Department of, 150

educator(s): insensitive, 123; meanings of caring of, 120; perceptions of, 120; priorities of, 124

Edwards, S. D., 227

efficiency, 30, 34, 38, 51; costs of, 198

efficient causality, 191

Eggie, 84

Eliade, M.,134

elitism, 128

Ellis, C., 62, 63, 100, 105, 106, 107

emancipation: of ethnographic methodology, 127

emancipation/liberation: potential of knowl-edge, 11; strategies, 14

embarrassment, 159, 168, 170, 232

Ember, C. R., 98

Ember, M., 98

embodiment, 52, 63, 106, 188; of caring, 238; of experience, 243; intelligence, 191; of professional nursing, 252

emergency: contact, 51; room, 131

emerging: identity, 230; learning, 195, 200; partnerships, 248

Emma, 241

emotion(s), 25, 63, 106, 151, 165, 204; base-line, 25; caring and, 31; communicating, 247; detachment of, 31, 32; presence and, 214; stress and, 157

emotional: healing, 238; health, 247; needs, 168, 169

empathic stance, 62

empathy, 37, 51; being like patient, 162; failed, 11

empowerment, 51, 242; of females, 131

emptiness, 62

enabling, 51, 168, 189; caring and, 65; confidence as, 174; with stories, 199

encounter(s), 17, 63, 170; beauty in, 173; cross-cultural, 159, 160; with difference, 152, 174; dyadic, 22; of human beings, 187; interpretation of, 142; negative, 95; therapeutic, 11; with unfamiliar, 235

encouraging students, 230

enculturation, 3; to caring, 120

endorphins, 23

energy, 240; fourfold and, 227

engagement, 16, 49, 51, 52, 53, 54, 55, 63, 169, 173, 187; beauty of, 173; of being-in-the-world, 229; with doctoral studies, 119; non-, xii; with nursing practice, 235; of patient in learning process, 240, 241; point of, 100; reflective, 143; of students, 50; value of, 50. *See also* communication

Engebretson, J. C., 10

England, 111, 112, 148

Englehardt, J. H. T., 158

English, 161, 165; indigenous, 111; knowing, 128

enowning, 62

ensuring safety, 255

environment, 4, 7, 17, 24, 39, 110, 182, 190, 195; businesslike, 123; care, 29; clinical, 30, 35, 49; comfortable, 212; complexity of healthcare, 219; consumer-driven, 222; cultural, 182; healing, 221; healthcare, 7, 54; health service, 32; high-technology, 7; historical, 223; home, 129; hospital, 191, 223; isolating, 41; learning, 121, 191; managed, 30, 49; not conducive to learning, 239; problem-centered, 54; and risk management, 30; safe, respectful, 118–119, 140, 212; school, 121, 125; teaching-learning, 122; technology-driven, 222; workplace, 123

Episcopalian lay deacon, 128

epistemes, 34

epistemological: understanding, x; work, 106

equality, 68; "heavenly," 110; as illusion, 53; justice and, 145, 168; outcomes and, 143; in partnership, 150; and power, 53; sense of, 109

equipment (ready to hand), 229

esophageal cancer, 207

essays: personal, 63

essentialness of being, 99

Estefan, A., xi, 21, 24, 37, 264

ethical implications: of patient in learning process, 241

ethical-moral perspective, 118

Ethical Review Committee, 148

ethics, 51, 125, 141, 151; approach as, 212; of care, 184, 185; code of, 221; committee, 35, 148, 223; cultural safety and, 150; demands of, 160, 163; expertise and, 32; healthcare, 158; professional, 32; of relieving suffering, 205; workplace, 120

ethnicity, 10, 99, 109, 118, 126, 151; boundaries of, 171; culture and, 182; personal social network based in, 130; working with different, 163

ethnocentricity, 4, 169, 170

ethnographic: diaries, 63; inquiry, 121; memoirs, 63; study, 105, 120, 123; study of caring, 119, 120

ethnography, 107, 119, 120; autobiographical, 63; emancipated methodology, 127; of caring, 105; personal, 63; tension in, 135; themes in, 121

ethno-racial heritage, 129, 130

ethos, 202

Etter-Lewis, G., 63

Eurasian descent, 148

European, 113, 176; American, 120; clinic poster, 159; civil servants, 112; colonialism, 109; descent, New Zealanders of, 148

Europeanized culture, 113; name, 114; school, 113

evaluation, 83

evangelical: Christian, 121; Christianity, 123

Evans, B. C., 195

events: narrative as story of, 63; sociopolitical and religious, 115

Everett, B., 25

everyday: activities, 220; and everydayness, 98, 226, 232; experiences, interpreting, 225; practical, 16; representation of, 98

examination: self, 105, 106

excellence: demonstration of in nursing, 124

exclusion: of quality of life issues in healthcare, 207

exclusionary: approach, xii; caring as, 121
exemplars, 242; of caring, 136; of nursing practice, 253; from text, 212
exercises: academic, 125; imaginative, 55; observation and interview, 118
existential: embodiment of traditions, 164; overcoming, 99; struggle, 100
existentiale, 5, 6
existenticity, 225
existence, 65; authentic, 203; being and, 99; human, situated nature of; 141; language of, 226; mode of, 224; personal, 62
Exodus, 134
expectations, 64, 91, 97, 131, 174; diverging, 154; of clients, 154, 159, 161; of clients and providers, 158; of cure, 210; practice and, 143; research and, 144; societal, 210; unknown, 169
experience(s), xii, 4, 5, 7, 27, 253; ability to, 144; of abuse, 24; authority of, 45, 48; as befalling, striking, overcoming, transforming, 253; behavioral, 63; of body, 25; of care, 151, 181; of caring, 181; cherished, 159; clinical, 205, 222, 238, 239; of clinical instructors, 220; clinical learning, 219; of clinical placements, 219; and culture, xii; as diachronic, 135; of difference, 97, 152, 153; of disability, 99; early childhood, 120; emotional, 63; embodied, 243; fearing categorization of, 127; of feelings, 204; hegemonic, 123; illness, 208, 209, 210; individualized, 121; interpreting, 142, 149, 223, 225; intersubjective, 117; intimate, 63; knowledge from, 130; with language, 62; learning, 15, 186, 221; lessons of, 96; life, 122, 130, 133, 136; limitations of own, 114; lived, 3, 64, 97, 106, 191, 193, 197, 198, 223, 224, 231; of "lived" curriculum, 253; making sense of, 142; meaning of, 156; medicalization of, 65; narratives of personal, 63; of nurse preceptors, 219; nursing, 108, 142, 155, 156, 234; of nursing people of other cultures, 140, 158, 159, 174; objectification of, 65; as part of whole, 142; past, 161; of patients, 199, 241; personal, 106, 162; practical, 251; practice and, 143; of preceptors, 220, 223, 231; professional, 169; recollection of, 188; reflection of, 62, 202; relational, 106; research, 145; revealing, 62; at school, 112; of self, 5; shaping of,

63; sharing intimate, 63; stories and, 52, 62; story of lived, 191, 193, 201; of storyteller, 201; of students, 220, 241; subjective, 43, 52, 244; as teacher, 211; teacher/learner, 197, 198; of tension(s), 152, 153, 154, 159; over time, 106; totality of, 227; understanding, 106, 241; validating, 63; workplace, 49; writing, 63, 197
expertise, 15, 17, 188; acknowledging limits of, 119; ethics and, 32; of nurses, 158; pedagogical, 208; sharing, 54; in specialized areas, 52
explanation(s), 63, 106; maze of, 99; need for, 147
explicit: making contributions, 219
exploitation, 92; in relationships, 53
exposing: what matters, 63
expression, 110, 142; of caring, 17, 124; of compassion, 98; goals of, 106; story and, 173; of violence, 239
extinction: threat of, 98
eye(s): blind, 97; contact, 128; surgery, 112

faces, 98; assessment of, 83; disfigured, 66, 74; human, 65; new, 89, 92; socially acceptable, 98; unusual, 70
facial clefting syndrome, 83
facilitating, 13, 14; making meaningful, 254
facticity, 225
facts: as social constructions, 148; biological, 97; historical, 106; objective, 97
faculty, development of, 108
fairness, 110
faith, 63, 64, 99; in God, 76; simple, 65, 111
falling, 99; away, 108
familiarity, x; 5, 127, 145, 162, 188, 229, 244; loss of, 226; with nursing education, 254; un-, 98
family(ies), xii, 9, 12, 17, 22, 92, 98, 99, 108, 112, 132, 135, 152, 158, 159, 189; adopted, 89; African American, 68, 100; attachment to, 131; attitudes toward, 207; care and, 185, 247; caring relationships with, 165; culture of, 65; dying person and, 235; existence of, 99; extended (traditional), 64, 98, 111, 113; Gardner on, 63, 64, 70, 75, 98; harmonious, 99; immigrant, 108, 129; in healthcare context, 248; leaving, 207; Maori, 177, 246;

family(ies) *(continued)*
    meanings of, 6; model, 128, 129; names,
    128, 131; nuclear, 113; nurturing, 122;
    pain of, 166; of patient, 185; relationships
    with, 165, 232; rights of, 10; Samoan, 171;
    Sayeed Muslim, 108; support of, 75, 79;
    text, 100; traditions, 197; valuing of, 206
Farina, A., 98
farmers, 112
Farrell, G. A., 239
Farrugia, C., 27
fatal prognosis, 165, 666
fathers, 112, 127, 129, 234; daughter of,
    130; and determining role of mother,
    113, 127
Faustian choice, 98
Favazza, A., 23, 24, 25, 51
fear, 98; for personal safety, 147; of rejec-
    tion, 159
feeling(s): admiration, 159; alone, 248; anxi-
    ety, 231; cared for, 54; confident, good,
    238; dealing with, 79; experiential, 204;
    guilt, 237; at home, 188, 191; hurt, 206;
    injustice, 167; insecurity, 233; joy, 159;
    privileged, 159; regret, 173; safe in class-
    room, 208; satisfaction, 159; as subjective,
    distrust of, 210; toward, 17; understood,
    54; vulnerable, 98
female(s), 153; as caregivers, 183; Black,
    100; empowerment of, 131; improvisa-
    tions by, 130; professions, 133; respect
    and, 113; role, 130; self-harm and, 24; so-
    cialization, 24,108; status of in Western
    society, 134
feminism, 105; in autobiography, 63; dis-
    course of, 23, 24; literature of, 116; per-
    spective of, 185; in stories, 107; theories
    of, 24, 114, 116; writers, 107
Fenning, S., 23
Fessenden, T., 134
field accounts, 63
fieldwork, 120
film, 197
finding self, 98
Fink, E., 64
Finlayson, M. P., 218
fire-lighting, 28
first-person accounts, 63
First World,107
fiscal outcomes, 22
flexibility, 109, 146; to hear, 199

Florence, 242, 244, 245, 250, 251
Florida, 207
focused thinking, 236
food: Bengali, 131; Chinese, craved, 66; sto-
    ries and, 199
football, 86
forbearance, 6
forces: gathering of, 227
fore-conception, 227
fore-having, 227
foreknowledge, 4
fore-sight, 227
forestructure, 13; in interpretation, 227
forgetting, 64
Forrest, D.,166
Fosbinder, D., 22
fostering students, 230
Foucault, M., 25, 26, 34, 35
foundation: moral, of nursing practice, 253
fourfold (earth, sky, divinities, mortals), 227,
    228
fragility of body, 98
framework, 106; of cost-containment, 29; dip-
    lomatic, 110; ideological, 115; institutional,
    uncaring, 119; own, 127; therapeutic, 51; of
    time, 29; Western dualism, 136
framing problems, 194
France, 111
Frank, A. W., 202, 205, 208–211
Frank, G., 63, 65
Frankl, V. E., 203, 204
freedom: to care for others, 238; to choose
    to be, 255; irresponsible, 246; for learn-
    ing, 239; of transcendence, 134; "ulti-
    mate," 204
Freeman, M., 135
Freire, P., 39, 109, 134
Freund, P. E. S., 11
friede, 228, 229
friend(s), friendship(s), 68, 69, 78, 84, 93,
    94, 112, 132–135; being with, 206; coun-
    sel of, 133; female, 133; imaginary, 84,
    90; male, older, 130, 131; missionary, 113
frontier province, 111
frustration, 158, 159, 165
Fry, S. T., 140
fundamentalist background, 111
"fusion of horizons," 5, 11, 13
future, 6, 11, 117, 141, 225; making possi-
    ble, 13; of nursing education, 220; prepar-
    ing nurses for, 245, 250

Gadamer, H.-G., 3–7, 9–11, 13, 16–18, 65, 141–144, 163, 164, 173, 175, 176, 226; philosophy of, 143, 169
Gadow, S., 13
Gaines, A. D., 9
Gallop, R., 25
gap: between nursing and practitioners, 251–252; between practice and education, 251–251
gardeners, 111
Gardner family, 63, 98
Gardner, Jacqui, 65, 68, 86, 88, 92, 98, 99; mother of, 100; story of, 64, 65, 97–98, 99; writing of, 100
Gardner, Jamaal, 66–67, 70–72, 74–75, 78–81, 84, 86–91, 94, 100
Gardner, James, 65, 66, 67, 69, 71, 72, 74, 78–81, 83, 85, 86, 89–91, 97, 99
Gardner, Jermaine, 66, 68–98; as teacher, 78
Gasquoine, S., 146, 147
gathering(s): of forces, 227; in Indian community, 131; social, 112
Gaut, D., 124, 185
gaze: dialectical, 63
gender, 10, 24, 130, 151, 153, 154, 168; discussing, 116; generalizations about, 118; nursing and, 163; relations between, 129; religion and, 134; roles, 129
genealogy: discourse analysis and, 34
general education curriculum, 115
generalizations, deconstruction of, 118
General Motors Blue Cross and Blue Shield, 73
genes, 67
gentleness, 159
geographical orientation, 108
German, 73
gestures, 153; cultural, 98
getting it right, 161, 170, 175
ghetto, 94; thinking, 99
gift: of music, 98; of time to share, 238
Gilligan, C., 24
girlfriend: role of, 130
Gitlin, T., 36
give and take: in practice, 251
giving, 109; self, 116
Gladys, 69
Gnostic Christianity, 135
goals: dialogic and expressive, 106; educational, 120

god(s), God, 66, 99; asking for guidance of, 94, 96; begging, 77, 85; believing in, 86; communicating with, 121; damning, 67; faith in, 76, 96, 97; goddesses and, 134; grounding in, 99; hands of, 86; as male, 134; people who fear, 96; praising, 95; praying to, 85, 89, 91; single, 134; Sufis and, 135; thanking, 74, 86, 89, 90, 91, 97
Goffman, E., 98
Goldberg, D. T., 10
Good, M. J. D., 119
"good:" of other, own, general, 253; patient, 210
Gordon, D., 147
gospel song, 87
government, 109; civil servants, 112; principles of safety, 247; reforms in health and education, 219
Gower, S.E., 218
grades, 197; failing, 203, 204; unfair, 202
graduation, 94, 252; from nursing school, 218
Green, M., 108
grief: expression of, 236
grieving: therapeutic, 237
Ground, I., 22
groups: affiliation with, 128; care for minority, 223; cultural, 113, 163; interest, 10; occupational, 156; grounding: in God, 99
growth: mutual, 117; personal and professional, 115, 116; of practice, 243; self-, 133; spiritual, 123; student, 230, 242, 243
Gudykunst, W. B., 147, 157
guests, 110
guidelines: cultural safety, 247
guiding, 194, 199, 231; precepting as, 254; teaching as, 117, 119
Guignon, C. B., 225, 227
guilt, 25, 97, 98, 165, 167, 207; feelings of, 237
Guyette, M., 220
Guzzetta, C. E., 10

Haber, J., 122
Hahn, R. A., 9
hakims (healers), 111, 112
hallucinations, 28
hammer (ready to hand), 229
handicapped children: rights of, 92
Hankiss, A., 62
Hanson, P. A., 8

Harley, A., xv
harmony: being and, 99; family and, 99
Harrington, A., 143, 145, 148
Harris, L., 65
Hartman, C., 27, 31
Hartmann, S. M., 100
Hastrof, A., 98
Hayano, D., 106
Hazleton, M., 28, 29, 31, 32
Headley, J. A., 10
Heald, M., 28
healers (hakims), 111
healing, xi, xii, 3, 25, 65, 218, 237; caring as, 185; centrality of caring to, 219; curing and, 9; emotional, 236, 238; healthcare and, xiii; at margins, 100; music and, 98, 100; narratives and, xii; nursing and, 221; power of support, 235; practices, traditional, 222; processes, 216; rituals, 98; self, 98; support of, 106; symbols and, 100
health, 218, 256; of African American clients, 120; beliefs, 174; bicultural developments in, 150; centrality of caring to, 219; clinic, 167; components of holistic model, 247; consequences, 151; culture and, in teaching, 125; definition of, 150; disciplines, 106; discourse of, 28; habits, 213; holistic, 222; insurance, 73, 125; law, 135; need(s), 125, 157; outcomes, 257; paternalism in, 54; practices, complementary, 222; priorities, 56, 154; problems, personal, 198; professions, immigrants in, 114; professions, students in, xii; progress to, 154; promotion, 213, 257; reforms, 257; service environment, 32; services, rationalization of , 30; services, use of, 51; situations related to, 5; sociopolitical context of, 256; standards for, 10; women's, 167
healthcare, xiii, 151, 167, 213, 216, 218, 244, 253, 256; alternative and complementary practices, 135; articulating, 253; attitudes of workers of, 210; body-related in, 209; caring in, 96, 184, 185; changes in delivery, 31; colonialism and, 110; community, 108; context of, 22, 248; continual change in, 252; course in transcultural, 115; culture of, 26, 258; delivery, 226; discontent with, 119; diversity in, 115; environment, changes in, 219; equitable out-

comes and, 143; ethics, 158; healing and, xiii; hierarchy, teacher-student, 208; hospitals, 248; incorporating story in, 202; industry, 200; issues in, 208; intercultural, 116; interpretation and, 7; language of, xi; literature, caring in, 122; meaningful, service, 140; medical dominance of, 158; need for, 221, 258; needs of population groups, 222; negotiation, 222; primary, 223; professional, 253; professionals, disagreement among, 125; providers, xii; physicians, 8, 97; quality of life issues excluded in, 207; of refugees and asylum seekers, 135; respect in, 13; roles in, 205; services, 228, 247; settings, 10; stories of, 207; system, 125, 184, 207, 213, 252; teaching about culture and health in, 125; team, 8; tensions of, 18; transcultural, 108, 114; in U.S., 135; workers, 26, 27
hearing, 130; openness to (hearkening), 64
hearkening, 13, 64, 65
heart: managed, 31
Hebrew language, 129
Hegel: philosophy of history of, 100
hegemony, 10, 11, 26, 49, 53, 108, 109, 123
Heidegger, M., 3, 5–7, 11–18, 62, 64, 65, 97–99, 141, 144, 162, 187, 191, 193, 200, 224–229, 231–233, 244, 251–254, 258; hermeneutic phenomenology of, 220, 223; and hermeneutics, xii, 220, 223, 226
Heideggerian Hermeneutical Studies, Institute for, xv
Hekman, S. J., 142 , 149
Heliker, D., xv
Helminski, C., 107
helping students, 230
Hemmings, A., 26
Henderson, V., 155
heritage: English, 148; ethno-racial, 129, 130; Eurasian, 148; European, 148, 176; Irish, 148; Maori, 176; Maori/Pakeha, 148; Nga Puhi, 148, 176; Samoan, 148
Herman, J., 23
hermeneutic(s), xi, xii; 62, 224; analytical process, 223; circle, 4, 141, 143, 166, 187, 212; of conflict, 166; Heideggerian, xii, 220, 223, 226; inquiry, 176; institute for study, xv; interpretation, 142, 143, 147; language, of stories, 229; opening, 99; openness, 147; philosophy, 14, 141, 142, 154; process, 224; research, 144, 145,

146, 257; respect of, 160; response, 160; tradition, 14; understanding and misunderstanding and, 166

heroines, 100

Heron, J., 51

Hessmiller, J., xv

hierarchy: professions and, 133; of teacher and student, 195

Higgins, M., 182, 214

Hindu(s), 110, 112, 127, 131, 135; *darshan*, 121; Rama Krishna society, 131; religion, 127; socialization of, 112; ways, 131

Hirschmann, E., 110

historically black liberal arts college, 122

historicity, 14

history(ies), 63, 151; of American Indians (Native Americans), 115; biography and, 62; of concept of caring, 182; and culture, 98, 143; of destruction, 134; dialectics of, 141; facts of, 106; Hegel's philosophy of, 100; horizons in, 149; of hospital-based education, 222, 223; influences in, 228; language, 226; life, 63; of modern nursing, 119; moment of, 64; of New Zealand, 143; of nursing in context, 221; for preceptors, 228; of recollective pathways, 192; self, and, 107; shaping, 157; standing in, 3; as story, 107; of students in the culture of practice, 256; tensions of, 63

Hitchcock, Alfred, 84

"hitting reality," 245

Hochschild, A. R., 31

Hokianga region, 176

holding open and problematic, 193

holism, 5, 22, 33, 147, 150, 151; of world, 227

holistic: care, 9–10, 157, 183; health, 222; perspective, 247; practice, 160

Holland, 111

holocaust: American Indian (Native American), 134; ban on publications about, 134; history of, 134; Nazi, 134

home, 91, 95, 99, 107, 108, 112, 113, 114, 131; as haven, 78; parent's, 132

homelessness, 98

home-ness, 188

homicide, 28

"Homo hierarchicus," 108

Hones, D. F., 62

honesty, 100

hooks, b., 46, 50

Hooper-Kyriakidis, P., 15, 16, 235

hope, 70; symbol of, 100

horizon(s), 13, 170; conflicting, 166; cultural, 143, 149; fusion of, 5, 11, 13; historical, 142, 143, 149; limitations of, 164

horizontal violence, 239

Horsfall, J., 28, 41

hospital(s), 95, 111, 128, 171, 252; administrators, 10; agenda, 22; atrium of, 88, 90; bureaucracy, 10; as cocoon, 74; culture of, 188; education based in, history of, 222; environment, historical, 223; policy, 251; system, 54; teaching, 77

Hoult, S., 150

housing: safe, 222

Howarth, D., 34

Hultgren, F. H., 168

human(s): being, 141, 187, 225; beliefs of, 106; capacity to create meaning, 226; and care processes, 140, 166; as caring, 107; caring and, 32, 171; coexistence of, 140; communication among, 105, 164; as complex wholes, 120; diversity, 115; existence, situated nature of, 141; face, 65; interpretation among, 164; lives, intangibles of, 106; meaning and, 225; and other human beings, 225; passage, 134; possibilities, 4; potential, 11, 63, 100; respected, 113; as self-interpreting, 190

Humana Institutes, 87, 87–88

humanistic, 116, 134, 135, 150, 151; expressions of caring, 122

humanitarian philosophies, 143

humanities, 150

humanity, 97, 117, 225; of client, 45; crimes against, 134; dialectic and, 176; shared, 172

humanness, 145

human relations commission: county, 115

human science, 220; moral tradition in, 253

Human Sciences, Interpretive Studies in Healthcare and, 3

Hungler, B. F., 35

Hurston, Z. N., 64

husband(s), 66, 88, 95, 129, 131, 132, 133, 145, 167, 170, 186, 188, 190, 192, 194; choice of, 112; relationship with wife, 167; rights of, 168; social needs of, 131, 132; support by, 191

Husserl, E., 97
hypertelorism frontal nasal dysplasia, 83
hypothesis: Sapir-Whorf, 4

id, 203
ideals: egalitarian, 164; making visible, 173
ideas, 4; from data, 147; Eastern, 113;
    framework for, 115; weaving of, 105; writ-
    ing about, 145
identification: of risk, 28
identity(ies), 98; as blind and disabled, 98;
    changing, 109; confidence in, 174; creat-
    ing, 99; devalued, 98; deviant, 98; dual,
    107; emerging, 230, 234; evolving, 109;
    flawed or spoiled, 98; as lived experience,
    208; name and ethnicity and, 126; profes-
    sional, 32; reconstructing, 99; self and,
    32; of society, 97; stable, 109
ideology, 115; caring, 122, 124; discourse
    and, 136; disunity of, 136; of nursing, 32;
    of practice, 32; professional, 123
Ignelzi, J., 28
ignorance: feelings of, 159; maintaining, 109
"I/it" relationship, 116, 117
illiteracy, 110, 111
illness(es), 10, 154, 172, 173, 214, 215, 257;
    acute, 165; ambivalence about people
    with, 210; care about, 119, 223; critical,
    17; culture of, 214; dualistic thinking as,
    136; experience with, 209, 213; fatal, 196;
    life with, 209; meaning of, 213, 214; men-
    tal, xi, 28, 223; as metaphorical loss of
    destination, 211; model, 55; story of, 210;
    stress of, 191, 192
illusions: of scientific mastery, 106
image: mythical, 134; personal, 105; of self,
    62; welcoming, 107
imagination, 55, 161, 162; links with con-
    cern, 192
immersion: in culture, 254; learning practice
    by, 221
immigrants, 108, 158, 199; assimilation and,
    118; and Catholic church, 115; challenges
    to, 114; families, 108; in healthcare profes-
    sions, 114; oppression of, 115; outreach
    services for, 115; from postcolonial re-
    gions, 114; in U.S., 114
impartiality, 130
imperative: moral, 154
impersonality, 130
impetigo, 154

imposition: cultural, 11; of preceptors' role,
    254
improvisation, 130, 131
inauthenticity, 231
inbetweenness, 252, 254, 259
inclusivity: perspective of, 118
incompetent: rights of, 198
Incredible Journey, The, 96
independence, 93, 128
India, 108, 110, 111, 126, 128, 131; Agra,
    112; as British colony, 111; northern, 108;
    nursing education in, 115; partitioning of,
    108; postcolonial, 108
Indian(s): Bengali, 131, 133; in New
    Zealand, 153–154, 159; subcontinent,
    110; in United States, 108, 131, 133
indigenous: culture, 113; language, 111; of
    New Zealand, 149, 151, 152; peoples, op-
    pression of, 115
indignities: suffering, 98
individual(s), 130; acknowledging, 130; car-
    ing and, 185; caring situations, 214, 215;
    Christian-born, 109; emphasis on, 10;
    groups of, 163; Jewish-born, 109; mean-
    ing to, 203; needs of, 21, 175; psychopa-
    thology, 25; shared interpretations and,
    200; spiritual care of, 203; uniqueness of,
    106; value of in treatment, 210; whole-
    ness of, 203
individualism: "invisible hand" of, 135; shap-
    ing experience and, 63
induction: rhetorical, 106
inequalities: social, 143
inexperience: benefits of, 49
infancy: music and, 99
infections: chlamydia, 167; eye, 112
influence(s): cultural, 228; fourfold and,
    227; historical, 228; personal, 228; socio-
    political, 228
information: making meaningful, 254; need
    for, 213
informed consent, 200, 211
Inhaber, R., 220
inhibition: cultural, 108
injury, 23
injustice: feelings of, 167
in-laws, 132
inner peace, 120
inquirer: beliefs and behaviors of, 64; ob-
    served and as observer, 63; as phenome-
    non, 64; sensitizing of, 136

inquiry, 124, 125, 136; ethnographic, 121; forms of meaningful, 216

insecurity, 233

insensitivity, ix, xi, 7, 27, 131

insight(s), 229; preceptors', 224

Institute for Heideggerian Hermeneutical Studies, xv

institutions: change in, 257; educational, 249, 256, 257; frameworks, uncaring in, 119; healthcare, 158; multicultural, 108, 115, 125, 133, 135; review board in, 211; social, 253

instruction, 256; clinical, 220; practices, xiii

instructors, 55, 214; experience of, 220. *See also* teaching

instrumentation, 17. *See also* technology

insurance: health, 73, 125

integration: family, 128, 130; in practice, 255; of self and caring, 129

integration, social, 65

intellectual knowing, 204

intelligence: embodied, 190; evolutionary, 108

intensions: in caring, x

intensive care unit, 171, 209

interaction(s): clinical, 16; cultural, 14, 147, 158; interpersonal, 9; learning and, 197; nurse–client, 55; painful, 69; of past and present traditions, 142; among patients, students, nurse clinicians, teachers, xiii, 208; between practice and discourses, 21; praxis and, 136; proactive, 31; between researcher and data, 144; between self and others, 105; with situation, 193; social, 98; between story and participants, 200; understanding, 106

interdependence, 107

International Council of Nurses (ICN), 140, 141, 143, 163; Cranialfacial Foundation, 82, 90, 92

international home, 129

international students, 125

interpersonal: aspects of caring, 183; bridge, narrative as, 214, 215; interaction, 9; relationship(s), 6, 117, 159, 160; skills, 52; support, 98

interplay among client, clinician, context, 22

interpretation(s), 3, 5, 12, 14, 15, 135, 143, 144, 148, 166, 167, 176, 224; adequacy of, 142; alternative, 169; assumptions and, 227; authenticity, 227; circle of, 228; common, 197; communication and, 164; contextualizing and, 143; and culture, xi, 136, 149; of Dasein, 226; differing, 166; diverse, 197; of experience, 142, 149; forestructure of, 227; healthcare and, 7; hermeneutic, 142, 147; improvised, 130; individual, shared, 188, judgment and, 163; methodological, 146; mis-, 125; multiple, of caring, 124, 136, 181, 185; of name, 126; of narrative, 62; past and, 142; possibility of, 227; practice in, xi, 36; preontological, understanding of, 187; presuppositions and, 227; of self and story, 135, 225; shared, 191, 192, 197; of situation, 233; of subjective experience, 52; substantive, 146; teaching as, 119; textual, 143, 146; of themes, 120; of transcripts, 227; writing, 149

interpreter, 167, 200

interpretive: inquiry, 63, 64, 106, 141, 143, 146, 220; potency of, 64; practices, xii; research, 223; skills, xii

Interpretive Studies in Healthcare and the Human Sciences, 3

intersubjectivity, 45, 49, 51, 156; of experience, 117; of nature, 141

intervention(s), 14, 130; caring as therapeutic, 6; culturally congruent, 10; culture and, 9; extreme, 39; learning strategies, 99; listening as, 207; nursing, 157, 186, 187; professional healthcare, 125; reflective, 194; strategies, 15, 99; therapeutic, 42, 55

interventionist disciplines, 12

interview(s), 223, 224; data, 34, 35, 119, 146, 148, 149; exercises, 118; excerpts, 147; post-experience, semi-structured, 211

"I/Thou" relationship, 116, 117, 129, 134

intimate nature of care, 156

intolerance, 110

introspection: sociological, 105

intuition, 45; care and, 49

intuitive: knowing, 189

invisibility: of self to self, 115

inviting, 13

involvement, 17, 127, 163, 200, 235; cost of, 165; distant, 246; with other, 190; of patient, 241; with patients, 249; of self, 221

Inwood, M., 97, 227

IRB (institutional review board), 211

Ireland, 111
Irish ancestry, 148
Ironside, P., xv
Irving, J. O., 221
Islam, 110, 111, 112
isolation, 248; of preceptors, 249
Israel, 134
issues, 216; complex teaching, 241; cultural, nursing and, 150; quality of life, 207; of relatedness, control, desire in healthcare, 209; in stories, 201; understanding of, 235; writing about, 145

Jackson, J. E., 98
Jackson, P., 55
Jago, B., 63
Jane, 154, 159, 170, 172, 173, 175, 234, 243, 246–249
"Jane Crow," 100
Japan, 95
jargon, 83, 93
jazz, 96
Jehovah's Witnesses, 8, 9, 11
Jessie, 232, 233
Jesus, 121, 123
Jewell, D., 150
Jewish-born individuals, 109
Jo, 153, 154, 159
job(s), 131, 159
Johnson, J., 6
Johnson, M., xv
Johnstone, L., 26, 29, 33, 54
Jones, D. W., xv
Jones, E. E., 98
Josselson, R., 62
Jourad, S. M., 63
journal: reflexive, 145; researcher, 147
journey(s), 96, 105, 145; of care, 134; incredible, 97; mission, 110; in nursing practice, 229; personal, 106; self, 114, 115, 119, 133; spiritual, 114, 121, 134
Judaism, 134
judgment, 15, 79; diagnosis as, 205; of difference, 98; fear of, 35, 127; hearing and, 202; respect and, 202; unconscious, 163
judgmentalism, 238
Jung, C. G., 130
justice: equality and, 145, 168

Kaplan, A., 6
Karen, 71

Kavanagh, K. H., ix, xii, xv, 10, 13, 14, 15, 17, 62, 264
Kawa Whakaruruhau (cultural safety), 143, 144, 149
Kearns, R., 150
Keegan, L., 10
Keetie, 76
Kelly, D., 22
Kennedy Institute, 75, 79
Kennedy, P. H., 14
Kerby, A., 135
Kerényi, C., 130
Kersten, F., xv
Kess-Gardner, J., xii, 62, 97, 264
key terms, 152
Kim, Y. Y., 147, 157
kin, 63
King, J. E., 126
King, M., 226
kinship, 99; personal social network based in, 130
Kirmayer, L., 97
Kleinman, A., 65, 98, 100, 117, 134
knower: known and, 126
knowing, 136, 166, 169; concerning precepting, 220; fore-, 4; importance of, 237; intuitively, 189; not-, 166, 169; nurturing of, 99; shaping of, 105; thinking, 193; through use, 229; un-, 169; ways of, 45, 121, 220
Knowlden, V., ix, 7, 18, 265
knowledge, 27, 147, 152, 158; background, 235; calling forth, 228; clinical, 13; control of, 126; critical, 45; about culture care, 174; democratization of, 64; didactic, 124; differences in, 53; doubt of, 49; emancipatory potential of, 11; emerging, 195; experiential, 130; impressing with, 238; in mental health, 28; of multicultural concepts, 114; nursing, 124, 141, 145; from others, 226; practical, 241; practice and, 124, 252; production of, 126; scientific, 216; self-, 25, 115; about self-harm, 36, 37; of student, 242; theoretical, 124
Koch, T., 143, 145, 147, 148
Kolb, D., 227, 228
Kolker, A., 63
Kottak, C. P., 3, 5
KPMG Consulting, 223
Krieger, S., 63
Krishna: Hindu Rama, society, 131

labeling, 27, 35, 65, 77, 84; institutionalization of, 27
labor, 65; delivery and, 7
Lacan, J., 141
lack of preparation: preceptors', 255
Ladd, J., 11
Ladson-Billings, G., 126
Laing, R., 64
landscapes: cultural, 106
language(s), xi, 4, 5, 13, 98, 105, 153, 166, 172, 181, 182, 185, 214; Arabic, 129; Asian, 129; barriers to, 154; body, 159; caring and, 32; in clinical practice, 166; common, 50; culture and, 4, 182; dialectics of, 141; English, 111; experience with, 62; of health care, xi; Hebrew, 129; hermeneutic, 229; importance of, 226; imposition of, 111; indigenous, 111; learning and, 52, 111; meanings of, 142, 226; Mexican Spanish, 129; nature of, 226; preunderstandings and, 225; as prison, 98; tradition and, 5, 142
Lara, 154, 160, 161, 167, 168, 170
Lashley, M. E., 168
law: health, 135
Lawler, J., 155
Lazarus, Richard, 184
leadership: caring and, 193; oppression and, 134; power and, 53; in primary healthcare, 223; spiritual, 109
learning, 116, 136, 159; activities, 121; adult, 129; aids to, 52, 55, 56; about caring, 95, 181, 182, 212, 254; challenge of, 173; circle of, 200; clinical, 239; community, 195, 208, 209, 211; as concernful practice, 193; context, 258; culture, 3, 4, 108; from difference, 130; disabilities, 23; dwelling and, 230; effective, 245; emergence of, 195, 200, 211; environment conducive to, 239; experiences, 221; experiential, 15, 220; facilitating, 248; freedom for, 239; intervention strategies, 99; about letting go, letting be, 99; about loving, 95; needs, 255; to be nurses, 232; opportunities, 243; outcome-based, 208; personal and professional, 114; as praxis, 136; procedures, 241; process, 241; responsibility for, 231; by seeing, writing, speaking, 119; about self, 63; about self-harm, 36, 37, 56; shaping of, 105; situation, 241; skills, 250; source of, 170; from stories,

199; student, 195, 237, 240, 249, 256; teaching and, 115, 117, 183, 193, 214, 231, 237; theoretical, 239; vicarious, 247; ways of, 196, 222, 248; willingness toward, 116
Leary, J., 31, 32
Lebanese, 165
lecturers, 248; clinical, 219, 249, 255, 256
Lee, 249
legal: issues, 39, 51; safety, 150
Leininger, M. M., 10, 15, 32, 119, 122, 140, 150, 172, 182, 183, 184, 185
LeMone, P., 222
lenses, 106; of patients for caring, 181
Leonard, V., 182, 215, 226
letting: go, 65, 93, 99, 129; "let the other be," 170; "letting go and letting God," 99; students, grow, 242, 243, 245
leukemia, 210
leveling, 17
Levin, D. M., 63, 64, 65, 98, 99
Levinas, D., 160, 172
liability, 98
liberation/emancipation strategies, 14
library: public, and adult learning, 129
license to practice, 115
life: articulating experiences of, 106, 136; begging for, 85; Christian way of, 121; community, 97; daily, moral codes of, 110; experiences, significance of, 130, 133; explaining with writing, 62; fluidity of, 106; forces, 107; good, 66; histories, 63; improvised, 130, 131; meaning of, 135; middle class, 130; missionary, 110; personal, 108, 133; professional, 108; renegotiating, 98; representing everyday, 64; script, 108; sociopolitical and religious events of, 115; stories, 100, 106, 201, 214; stressful, 136; as teacher, 211; as whole, 142; young adult, 130
lifeworld, 65, 224; of practice, 230, 242; of preceptors of student nurses, 226; writing and, 105
likeness (sameness): understanding, 97
Lillis, C., 222
liminality, 126
limits of expertise, 119
Lindbergh Foundation: Charles A. and Anne Morrow, 18
Linde, C., 63
Lindeman, C., 184

lineage: Muslim, 114
Linehan, M., 25, 27, 41, 51
linguistic possibilities, 5
Linsay, G., xv
Lipson, J., 163
listening, 13, 65, 79, 175, 194, 200, 213,
    215, 237, 256; to call, 232; as interven-
    tion, 207; nonjudgmental, 205; to patient,
    197; to stories, 192, 212; as strategy, 199;
    supportive, 196, 204; as treatment, 207
Liszt, F., 91
literacy, 109; caring, 49, 50
literature, 145, 147, 149, 199; caring, xi;
    cross-cultural, 147; empirical, 220; femi-
    nist, 116; healthcare, caring in, 122; his-
    torical, 149; narrative and, 63; New
    Zealand, 143; nursing, 182; on preceptor-
    ship, 220; professional, 143; research-
    based, xi; sociological, 149
literature review, 34
lived: curriculum, 253; everyday, 224; experi-
    ences, 224; time and space, 227; world of
    nursing practice, 254
lives: authentic, 198; contextualized, 64; dis-
    rupted, 98; fulfilled, 198; intangibles of,
    106; respectful, 198; self-interpreting,
    228; story and, 105; women's, 64, 130;
    Zen Buddhist, 109
living, 136, 191, 193; experiences of, 193;
    possibilities for, 134, 225; with stories,
    202, 205; study of human, 105
locus of care, 222
Lofton, V., 28
logic, 55
Lopez, B., 141, 198, 199
loss, 24; of body part, 203; of control, 209;
    experience of, 204; of familiar, 226; learn-
    ing from, 204; magnification of, 98; mean-
    ing of, 203; response to, 204; symbolic,
    194
Loustaunau, M. O., 9
love, 71, 82, 88, 112, 172; doctrine of Chris-
    tian, 121; of god, 135; learning about, 95;
    "tough," 122
Lumby, J., 175
Lupton, D., 11, 28, 34
Lutheran: bishop, 111; Danish, mission, 111
Lyman, S. M., 126

Macgregor, F. C., 65
machines, 15, 171; breaking down, 244; care

and, 6, 7; comfort with, 244; concentrat-
    ing on, 244; living with, 244; mastering,
    244; as ready-to-hand, 244. See also tech-
    nology
Machoian, L., 24
magical control, 26
making: known, 14; room, 5
male(s): as curers, 183; God as, 134; Indian,
    153, 154; nurses, 153
malformation: craniofacial, hiding, 98
Malinowski, B., 63
"managed heart," 31; socialization of, 24
management: bureaucratic, 122; of client,
    33; crisis, 246; discourse of, 30; eco-
    nomic, 30; of environment, 29, 30; and
    nursing practice, 22, 30, 38; of patients
    and students, 251; of risk, 28, 29, 30, 31,
    34, 55; of self by nurses, 31
Mani, L., 110
manipulation, 43, 126
Maori, 145, 150, 152, 153, 154, 158, 159,
    162, 176, 177, 247; family, 246; and Pa-
    keha descent, 148; partnership and partici-
    pation, 151; recruitment and retention of
    nurses, 151
Mardan, 111
marginalization, 26, 28, 52, 57, 64, 94, 112;
    of diversity curriculum, 115; and silence,
    53
Markus, H., 98
marriage, 66, 113, 130, 131, 190; arranged,
    111–112; care about, 119; mixed, 119;
    name change with, 114
Mary, 120–124
Maryland School for the Blind, 75
Masius, J., 28
Mason, T., 29
massage, 222
Massey University, 148
matrifocality, 100
matters (mattering), 63, 100, 119, 146,
    189
maze: of explanation, 99
McAdoo, H. P., 100
McAllister, M., xi, 21, 24, 27, 37, 49, 55,
    265
McAra-Couper, J., 176
McAthie, M., 184
McCance, T. V., 221
McFarland, M. R., 10, 15, 119, 122
McGuire, M. B., 11

McKenna, H. P., 221

McKergow, M., 55

meaning(s), 3, 4, 14, 16, 26, 34, 130, 148, 153, 154, 155, 156, 165, 168, 173, 188; of ability, 100; apprehension of, 190; approximation of, 227; assigning, 226; authenticity of, 64; background, 189, 191; of being, 98, 224; of being thrown, 232; boundaries and, 64; of breathing, 100; of caring, 108, 115, 119, 120, 122, 124, 176, 181; choosing values as, 204; construction of, 144; in context, 142, 146; coping as recreation of, 240; creating, 226; cross-cultural, in nursing, 141, 142, 159, 160; cultural, 25, 100, 108, 149, 151; of death, 234; of difference, 109; disagreement over, 198; of "disfigured," 71; emerging, 204; experiential, 149; experimenting with, 149; exploration of, 142; of family, 6; hidden, 143; of human concerns, 223; of illness experience, 213; of improvised life story, 130, 201; of information, 254; integrating, 129; interpreting, 148, 149; language and, 142, 226; layers of, 142; of life, 135; of living with machinery, 244; making, 198, 203, 204, 205; in nursing, 141, 142, 159, 160, 173; of phenomenology, 190; possible, 176; of precepting, 223, 240; shared, 191, 213; situated, 223; of sound, 64; of stories, 196, 198; stress as disruption of, 240; structures of, 226; struggle for, 63, 64, 100; of tension, 232

measuring: care, 119, 184; outcomes, 30

mechanistic: approach, 190, 191

media, 29, 90, 91, 143, 145, 151; cultural safety and, 149; representation by, 28

medical: anthropology, influence of, 117; care, orthodox, 222; dominance, 10, 11; model, 26; practice, 183; profession, 11; science, 166; technology, 99, 166; treatment, 16

medicalization of experience, 65

medicine: Ayurvedic, 126, 135; bio-, 134, 135; body association and, 209; Chinese, 135; curative regime of, 253; natural sciences and, 253

meditation: place and, 127; spiritual, 107

Meleis, A. I., 163

memoir: ethnographic, 63

memories, 52; intrusive, 24; of past, 233; story and, 170, 199; unfolding of, 63

men: attitudes toward, 128; Indian, 128

Menninger, K., 23

mental health, 21; nursing, 21, 22, 28, 32, 34, 35, 37, 45, 47–49, 148

Mental Health Foundation, 24

mental illness, xi, 28

mentally ill: care for, 223

mentorship, 37, 48

Mercer, D., 29

Merleau-Ponty, M., 62, 184, 189

metaphor(s), 97; of hermeneutic circle, 141; sentient, 98; voice as, 201

Metcalf, T., 110

method(s), 145, 215, 223; explanatory, 220; hermeneutics as, 141; predictive, 220; writing as, 62

methodology: clarification of, 146; ethnography's, 127; hermeneutic, 141; pluralistic, xi; reflective, 182

Mexican: maitre d', 90; Spanish, 129

middle class: America, 136; life, 130

Middle East: cultures of, 113; immigrants from, 129

Midwest, 131

midwifery, 143, 148, 151

military service: nursing and, 122

millennium: healthcare in new, 216

Miller, B. K., 122

Miller, C., 110, 111

Miller, D., 24

Miller, D. T., 98

mind: knowing own, 63; state of, 12

mindfulness, x, xi, 64, 235, 236

mine-ness (authenticity), 254; of professional nurses, 252

Minichiello, V., 35, 36

Ministerial Task Force on Nursing, 219

minority: care for, 223; cultures, 51; groups, 125

miracle of music, 76

Misgeld, D., 119

misinterpretation, 125

missionaries, 110–114; activities of, 109; British, 110; care by, 111; Danish, 110; dual life of, 110; networking of, 112–113; promises of, 110; schools of, 111

mistakes: cost of, xi

model(s), 107; behavioral, 26; caring, 181; of conversion, 112; of culturally safe education, 150; Culture of Safety, 247; curriculum, 222; family, 128, 129; holistic

model(s) *(continued)*
    health, 247; illness, 55; of management,
    38; medical, 26; nursing, 32; of phenome-
    non, 194
modeling: storytelling, 203; with students,
    12; writing stories, 196. *See also* role-
    modeling
modernity: late, 28
moment: historical, 64
money, 128
monoculturalism, 151
monotheism: Western, 134
"Moonlight Sonata," 90
Moore, J. K., 9
Moore, T., 140
Moorhouse, G., 109, 110, 111
moral: agency, within situation, 236; codes,
    of daily life and work, 110; community,
    256; imperative, 154, 253; in nursing prac-
    tice, 253; perspective, 118; public, 29;
    sense, of healthcare, 253
morality, 130
Morieson, B., 218
Morley, P., 184
Morrison, T., 62
Morse, J. M., 6, 35, 119, 150
mother, 68, 108, 110, 112, 113, 199, 200; be-
    ing, 97; on drugs, 94; -in-law, 69, 136; Jac-
    qui's, 100; role of, 74, 99, 113, 130
motivation, 30, 190
movement between worlds, 231
Moyle, W., 27
Moyne, J., 107
Muir-Cochrane, E., 30
mullahs, 112
multiculturalism, xi, 10, 115; concepts of,
    114; in health care, study of, 114; insti-
    tute, 108, 115, 125, 133, 135; teaching
    about, 109; teaching and practicing, 127;
    topics in, 115; workshops about, 114
multiple: personalities, 83; perspectives,
    199
Munhall, P. L., 169
Munro, R., 28
Murchie, E. R., 151
Murray, Pauli, 99, 100
music, 64, 76, 80–82, 84, 85, 89, 90, 94–96,
    99, 112, 128; center in brain, 88; gift of,
    98; healing and, 98, 100; infancy and, 99;
    rituals, healing and, 98
Musick, J. L., 31

Muslim(s), 111; background, 114; conver-
    sion of, 110; lineage, 114; Sayeed, 108;
    surname, 114; teenage, 112
mutilation: religion and rite and passage
    and self-, 25
mutuality, 116
mythology, 127
myths: about self-harm, 26; personal, 99

naiveté: ambivalent, 108
names, 153; Bengali, 126; change with mar-
    riage, 114; Christian, European, 114; fam-
    ily, 131; interpretation of, 126
naming, 193
narrative(s), xii, 62, 63, 106, 231, 235, 238,
    239, 258; authenticity of, 64; descrip-
    tions, 147; experiential, 149; and healing,
    xii; of nurses, 149; paradigm, 234; peda-
    gogy, 192, 214; of personal experience,
    63, 105, 106; of preceptors, 230; in re-
    search, xii; of students, 182; of women's
    lives, 64
National Federation of the Blind, 76, 93
nationality(ies), 141, 143, 150, 154; disguise
    as other, 127; history of destruction, 134;
    Native American (American Indians), his-
    tory and status of, 115
natives: as illiterate, 110
naturalized citizen, 108
natural science: pedagogy and, 187; techno-
    logical practices and, 253
nature, 107; of real practice, 249
Nazi: concentration camp, meaning of, 203;
    holocaust, 134
Neal, M. T., 168
Neander, W. L., 6, 119
need(s), 16, 51, 127, 154; assessing learning,
    230; balancing, 240; as basis for service,
    33; caring, 64, 166, 183; for change in
    nursing education, 251; of clients, 52,
    146, 164; for control, 29; cultural, 146; of
    educational structures, 228; for fixing,
    210; for health promotion, 157, 257; holis-
    tic, 22; inability to meet, 158; individual,
    21; for information in practice, 213; inval-
    idating clients', 32; for learning, 255; nurs-
    ing, 174, 234; of others, 31; of patients,
    186, 228; of patients who self-harm, 22,
    29; of population groups, 222; of precep-
    tors, 240; seeing, 54; to see "the big pic-
    ture," 257; social, 131, 168, 169, 170; of

students, 125; to support, 166; to trust, 240; uniqueness of, 54; for understanding, 163

neem bark, 126

negative: being, 97; effect of scholarship, 126; focus on, 55; power relations, 56

neglect: benign, 110

negotiation, 12; educational, 150; of health-care, 222; between preceptors, patients and medical personnel, 241; social, 148

Negussie, B., xv

Nehls, H., 220

Neil, R. M., 185

Neonatal Intensive Care Unit (NICU); culture of, 8; nurses in, 7, 8; staff, 14, 16, 17

networks: of missionaries, 112–113; personal, 130; professional, 148

neurosurgeon, 86

newborns, 7

New, C., 99

New Delhi, 112

newspaper, 129

New Zealand, 141, 143, 148, 149, 150, 151, 152, 154, 158, 160, 161, 171, 176, 219, 220, 247, 255; history of, 143; Northern Region of, 153; nurses, 145, 150, 218, 220, 221; nursing organizations in, 221

New Zealand Education Act, 256

New Zealanders, 148

New Zealand Ministry of Health, 219

New Zealand Nurses' Organization, 221

Nga Puhi heritage, 148, 176

Nicholson, G., 119

NICU. *See* Neonatal Intensive Care Unit

Night Shift, The, 96

night: work at, 131

Nightingale, F., 221

Nikki, 85, 86

Niven, N., 32

Noah's ark, 128

No Blood—Medicine meets the challenge, 9

Nolan, P., 31

Noll, J. G., 26

non-caring, 122

non-engagement, xii; 63

nonjudgmentalism, 212

non-responsiveness: to patients, 213

nonverbal communication, 116

normality, 97; in appearance, 84

norm(s): checking in as, 197; classroom, 208; cultural, 112, 259; difference from,

98; everyday, 221; learning, 208; regional, 112; social, 17, 108, 130

North, N., 150

North Dakota, 115, 132

not being at home, 231

notes: observational, 212

novels: British, 128

novice, xii, 17; practitioners, 45, 47, 48, 52, 208, 244; transcultural nursing teachers, 115

numbers, reliability of, 210

nuptial arrangements, 112

nurse(s) (RNs), 17, 112, 140, 146; African American, 87; attitudes of, 210; Australian, 22, 162; authority of, 158; behavior of, 41; being-as-a-, 252, 258; being with, 228; as boss, 129; caring and, 48, 120, 121, 214; as chameleon, 162; charge, 236; Chinese American, 129; clinicians, 208; compassion and, 205; cultural sensitivity and, 146, 154, 166; culture of, 187; detachment between clients and, 32; developing, 238, 256; education, 257; educators, 119, 121–125, 136, 238; educators' meanings of caring, 120, 121; experienced, 45, 47; expertise of, 158, 235; frustrated, 38–39; as "good," 159; healing and, 221; hospitals and, 54; interactions with clinicians, students, patients, teachers, 208; interviews of, 119; intrapersonal responses of, 31; learning to be, 47, 232; male, 153; management of, 30, 31, 220; Maori, 151; mental health, 22, 34, 47; mine-ness of, 252; narratives of, 149; need to give care, provide support, 166; new, 45, 47–49, 218; New Zealand, 143, 145, 150–154, 158, 160, 161, 171, 176, 219–221; as "nice," 47, 85; in NICU, 7, 8; novice, 208, 244; power of, 124; practice of, 18, 32; preceptors, xii, 230; and prejudice, 164; professional, 31, 252, 257; quest for professional status of, 150; recruitment and retention of, 151, 218; response of, 54; responsibility of, 147; role(s) of, 31, 213, 218; satisfaction of cultural, 176; scholars, 124; self-care by, 31; shortage of, 218; social-philosophical dichotomies among, 136; staff, 249; students of, 205, 218, 235, 255; as teachers, 141, 144, 239; tension among, 143, 154, 163; thinking as, 229; trained, 111;

nurse(s) *(continued)*
  vicarious traumatization in, 31; as vulnerable, 45; women as, 164; working *with* clients, 54, 56, 166
nursing: accountability-based, 246; African
  American students, 120; baccalaureate
  programs in, 120; beliefs of, 254; building, 230; care processes, 166; caring and,
  21, 27, 32, 119, 151, 165, 172, 195, 213,
  214; communication and, 221; compassionate, 216; context, 223, 228; courses
  in, 108; cross-cultural, 141, 145, 146, 159,
  160; cultural conditioning in, 222; culturally congruent, 114, 140, 163, 166; culture of, 115, 120, 124, 219, 221, 232, 234,
  254; culture of practice, 240; demonstration of excellence in, 124; departments
  in, 118; discontent with, 119; distancing
  in, 166; district, 148; education, 112, 117,
  119, 143, 145, 148, 150, 181–183, 192,
  218, 248; education, changes in, 219;
  education, future of, 220; essence of, 160;
  experiences, 108, 142, 234; gap between
  practice and education, 251–251; give
  and take in, 251; history of modern, 119;
  hospital-based education in, 222; *hui,*
  150, 176; ideology, 32; in India, 115;
  indices, 220; literature of, 143, 150; lived
  world of, 254; meaning of caring in, 159,
  160; medical, 148; mental health, 21, 22,
  28, 32, 148; midwifery, 148; military service and, 122; models, 32; as moral endeavor, 158; moral imperative and, 253;
  in New Zealand, 149, 150; oppression
  and, 108, 115; overburdening in, 219; participation of new, 219; pedagogy, 215;
  pediatric, 114, 148; people from other cultures, 140–143, 146–154, 158–160, 174,
  254; philosophical basis of, 149, 151;
  practice(s), 29, 113, 119, 141, 145, 151,
  212, 225, 228, 230, 234, 246, 257; preceptors, 221; in private sector, 148; profession, 11, 119, 142, 221, 254, 258; profession, survival of, 231; profession, values
  of, 218; programs, 129; and public health,
  148; purpose of, 33; racism and, 145;
  reality of, 241, 246, 250, 255; risk and,
  30; safe, 151; safeguarding, 230, 254;
  school(s), 94, 95, 123, 194, 256; in social
  and political economy, 119; social distancing in, 166; spiritual care in, 121; staff,

26, 248; students, 117, 192, 200, 224,
  229, 231, 251; surgical, 148; symptoms
  and, 30; teaching reality, 230, 240; technical aspects of, 255; transcending cultural
  difference, 173; transcultural, 115, 150;
  transmission of culture by preceptors,
  254; uncaring, 214; uncertainty and, 176;
  values of, 254; violence in culture of,
  239
Nursing Council of New Zealand, 143, 151,
  176, 247, 255, 257
Nursing Ethics: Code of, 140
nurturing, 30, 99, 122; interactions, 9; practice, 99; students, 238

Oberlin Conservatory of Music, 96
object(s): body as socially influenced, 25; intertwining subject with, 64; motivation as,
  190; present-at-hand, 13; student as, 116;
  subject way, 191; as text analog, 142–143
objectifying, 6, 16, 32, 99; care, 16; of clients, 32, 49; experience, 65; with numbers, 117; of "other," 64; of students, 117;
  technology, 244
objectivity, 44, 52, 97
obligations: stories and, 199
obscurity: women and, 63
observation: behavioral, 184; exercises, 118;
  experience and, 63; inquiry and, 63; notes
  from, 212; participant, 106; skills of, 168,
  174; by students, 241
observer: participant-, 119
obstetric team, 65
Occidentals, 130
occupation, 131, 153, 156; prestige and,
  128
O'Donnell, J., 63
office: physician's, 199
Ogletree, T. W., 147
Ohio, 96
Oklahoma, 114, 115, 128; Tulsa, 129
O'Neill, J., 10
oneness of being, 136
one-size-fits-all, 195
Onions, C. T., 220
ontological: authenticity, 64; being, 225;
  function of beauty, 173; understanding, x;
  work, 144
opening: hermeneutic, 99; selves, 107
openness, 5, 11, 107, 169, 199, 232; attitude
  of, 199; being, 13; to dialogue, 13; to

hearing (hearkening), 64; hermeneutic, 147; listening as, 175; to others, 133, 161; to possibility, 193, 194; in practice, 174

operant conditioning, 23

operas, 128

opinion, 200

opportunities: learning, 243

opposites: dualistic, 18; movement between, 175; prejudicial, 176

oppression, 100, 108, 109, 116, 125, 126, 128; bureaucratic management and, 122; cultural, 108; cycle of, 134; dynamics of, 115; of immigrants, 115; of indigenous peoples, 115; nature of, 114; perception of, 181; progress confounded with, 126; social and cultural, 127, 128; writing about colonial, 115

order: of being, 107; "putting poems in," 198; role of managing, 31; "of things," 34, 35; world, 98

orderly, 86

ordinariness: value of, 32

organizations: cultures of, 122, 123, 258; diversity in community, 115; standards of, 231

"Orientals," 129, 130

orientation: academic and practice, integrated, 255; behavioral, xi, 42; biomedical, xii; client-focused, 48; cultural, 6, 108, 226; educational, 226; ethical, 212; ethical-moral, 118; exclusionary, xii, 121; future, 141; geographical, 108; hermeneutic, 212; holistic, 247; human science, 220; inclusive, 118; interpretive, 220; mechanistic, 190, 191; one-size-fits-all, 195; phenomenological, 191, 214, 215; postmodern, 55; post-structural, xi, xii, 36; problem-centered, 54, 55, 56; rational, 45, 47, 54; religious, 121; scientific, 191; social and political, 134; solution-focused, 55, 56; spiritual, 121; system-focused, 48; unreflective, 48; wellness, 55; Western dualism, 136; women's studies, 116, 133. *See also* paradigm

origins: cultural, 114

orphan, 111

orthodox: biomedicine, 9; care, 222

Osuch, E. A., 26

'other', others, 6, 11, 12, 13, 17, 22, 64, 97, 107, 109, 126, 127, 129, 130, 152, 153, 160, 169, 170, 225; being alongside, 225; being with, 228, 232; boundaries and, 126; caring for, 117, 238; commitment toward, 174; concernful being with, 231; cultures not your own, 140, 142, 144, 175; dialogue between self and, 117; difference from, 98; encountering, 170; face of, 160; good of, 253; human beings, 225; interaction with, 105; involvement with, 190; Levinas and, 160; needs of, 31; openness to, 133, 161; potential of, 109; preparing for, 117; questioning, 174; racial, 149; recognition of, 116; relationships with, 172; responsibility for, 126; self as, 133; as stranger, 147

othering, 115, 116, 129, 130

outcome(s), 34, 49, 173, 229, 256; assessment of, 195; desired, 123; of dialogue, 116; discourse of, 28; equitable, 143; fiscal, 22; health, 257; learning based in, 208; limited, 27; measures, 30; for patients, 16; of services, 30

outreach services for immigrants, 115

overcoming: existential, 99

Oxford English Dictionary, 97

Pacific: Islands, 153, 154, 159; Northwest, 207

pain, 66; of circumcision, 198; emotional, 24; of family, 166; of interaction, 69; judgment of, 186; of patients, 186, 187, 188, 189; physiological, 188, 193; of reality, 173; relief, medical, 200; symbol of, 193; of transformation, 62; of treatment, 27

Pakeha, 145, 148, 161, 171, 176; Pakeha/European, 153

Pakistan, 108

Pakistani, 127; anti-, views, 131; ban on publications, 134; clothes, 131; Peshawari, 131; woman, 128

Palmer, R. E., 226

Pamela, 158

Panadol, 240

paradigm(s): caring, 181; cure, 213; dominant, 50; narrative, 234; postmodern, 55; shifting and emergent, 18; unitary, 134

paradox, 140, 141, 146, 147, 152, 154, 159, 163, 164, 166, 169, 172, 174, 176, 215

Parent-Infant Stimulation Program, 75

Parent Teachers Association, 94

parent(s), 13, 15, 16, 108, 131, 132;

parent(s) *(continued)*
    attitudes toward, 206; education and, 128;
    of handicapped children, 81, 92, 96; inde-
    pendence and, 113; rights of, 8, 9, 11,
    12,93; role of, 206; shared culture of,
    114; surrogate, 97; worldview of, 12
parenting, 3
Parker, P., 141
participant(s), 35, 37, 49, 106, 142–144,
    146, 148, 149, 159, 160, 194, 195, 208,
    212, 214; community, 199; inquirer as,
    63; Maori, 151; personal lives of, 207; pre-
    ceptor, 223, 227; in Recollective Pathway
    course, 196, 201; stories of, 145, 207
participant-observer, 106, 119
participatory ways of working, 53
partnering: nurse-client, 54; nurse-hospital,
    54
partnership(s), 256, 257; emerging, 248;
    equal, 150; Maori, 151; marital, 113; Ne-
    gotiated and Equal, 151
passage from human to suprahuman, 134
past, 6, 108, 117, 141, 225; alive in present,
    106; communion of present and, 247; tra-
    ditions of, 142
paternalism, 51, 54
Paterson, B., 184
Paterson, J., 172, 173
Pathan, 110
patience, 32, 96
patient(s), xiii, 38, 97, 119, 153, 154, 158; ac-
    countability for, 250; advocacy of, 200; Af-
    rican American, 207; attending to, 244;
    being there for, 159; care for, 245, 246,
    249; caring centered on, 10, 185; culture
    of, 187; day-to-day practice with, 241;
    death of, 234, 235, 237; discontented,
    119; engaging in student learning, 240; ex-
    amination of, 209–210; experience of
    care, 151, 181; families of, 232; focusing
    on, 244; "generic," 187; "good," 210; ig-
    noring, 244; interaction with students,
    teachers, clinicians, 208; line between
    healthcare provider and, 117, 158; lis-
    tening to, 197; needs of, 29, 146, 185,
    228; not talking to, 244; as other, 152;
    outcomes of, 16; permission by, 241; post-
    operative, 191, 241; protecting, ix; real
    world of, 225; recovery by, 241; relation-
    ships with, 232; responsibility toward,
    147; safeguarding, 239, 256; satisfaction

of, 119; self-harm of, 22; students and,
    241, 244; trauma to, 241; voices of, 194,
    198; vulnerability of, 29. *See also* clients
Patients Voice, The, 197
patriarchy, 130; adjustment to, 130; dis-
    courses on, 136; oppressive side of, 131;
    personification of, 131; professions and
    traditional, 133
patronization, 128; perception of, 181
patterns: constitutive, 223
Payer, L., 9
Payne, S., 34
Peabody Institute, 66, 96
peace: inner, 120; sense of, 127
pedagogy, xii; cofounded, 193; content of
    caring, 122; conventional, 187, 195; exper-
    tise of, 208; history of, 192; narrative,
    192, 193, 214; nursing, 215; principles of,
    50, 56; Recollective Pathway, 182, 192; re-
    flective, 186; site-specific, 193
pediatric nursing, 114, 148
peer(s): difference from, 98; sighted, 93;
    support of, 50
people(s): of color, status of, 126; diverse,
    222; illiterate, 111; indigenous, oppression
    of, 115, 151; tribal, 110
perception(s): of caring, 117; of reality, 189;
    of ways of teaching, 120
Perego, M., 33
"perfect" baby(ies), 66, 71; child, 63; vs. "dif-
    ferent," 97
permission from patients, 241
Perry, C., 23
person: nurse as, 31; uniqueness of, 191
personal: beliefs, 123; development, 117;
    dialogue, 105; experiences, 106, 244;
    growth, 115; health problems, 198; iden-
    tity, devalued, 98; ideologies, 124; ill, 244;
    images, 105; influences, 228; interest
    groups, 10; journey, 106, 134; learning,
    114; meanings, 120, 168; myths, 99; narra-
    tive, 105, 106; in nursing practice, 253;
    philosophies of caring, 120; prejudices,
    168; and professional self, 105, 108;
    safety, fear for, 147; social networks, 130;
    story, 100, 136; subjectivity, 244
personalities, 132; caring and, 122; multiple,
    83
personality disorder, 27, 28, 42, 47
person-culture connection, 105
personnel: NICU, 16, 17

perspective(s), x; academic and practice, integrated, 255; awareness of, 116; behavioral, xi, 42; biomedical, xii, 25; biosocial, 25; client-focused, 48; critical, 14, 33; dichotomized, 29; ethical, 212; ethical and moral, 118; exclusionary, xii,121; hermeneutic, 212; holistic, 247; human science, 220; inclusive, 118; interpretive, 220; mechanistic, 190, 191; multiple, 148, 199; one-size-fits-all, 191; own, 235; of patient, 146; phenomenological, 32, 191, 214, 215; political, 134; postmodern, 32, 55; post-structural, xi, xii, 22, 33, 36; problem-centered, 54, 55, 56; problem-solving, 28; psychological, 25; rational, 45, 47, 54; scientific, 191; social, 134; solution-focused, 55, 56; system-focused, 48; unreflective, 48; varied, 116; wellness, 55; Western, 128, 134, 136; women's studies, 116, 133. *See also* paradigm

Peshawar: city of, 113
Peshkin, A., 145, 172
Peterson, A., 28
Pfifferling, J. H., 10
Phaedrus, 173
phenomenology, xii, 187, 223, 224; concern and, 190; Heideggerian hermeneutic, 220; interpretive, xii; meaning of, 190; as perspective, 187, 214; philosophy of, 32; view from, 182, 190
phenomenon (phenomena), 130, 149, 215; caring as, 185, 216; conception of, 227; discussion about, 131; experiential, 142; inquirer as, 64; instinctual, 203; interpretation of, 185; meanings of, 120, 142; model of, 194; of nursing people from cultures other than your own, 141, 146, 160, 163; of oppression, 109; psychotic, 23; sharing meaning of caring as, 124; spiritual, 203; story as, 197; of strangeness, 147; understanding, 227
phenotype, 129, 150
Phillips, S. S., 185
philosophers, xv
philosophy(ies), 109, 136, 185; biomedical, 9; of caring, 120, 121, 122, 124; of cultural safety, 141; Eastern Taoist, 120; Gadamerian, 143, 169; Hegel's of history, 100; hermeneutic, 14, 141, 142, 146, 154; holistic, 147; humanitarian, 143, 147; personal, 120; phenomenological, 32; scientific, 9; Sufi, 107; teaching and learning, 120

physical: abuse, 24; characteristics, 150; differences, 153; health, 247; safety, 157
physician(s), 65, 68, 97, 112, 209, 210; behavior of, 200, 201; caring and, 96; power of, 158
piano, 66, 80, 81, 82, 84, 85, 88, 89, 90, 91, 95
Picasso, 86
place, 99, 128
placement(s), 232; clinical, 219, 221, 251
plastic surgeon, 82, 88
Plato, 173
play, 175
pleasure of transformation, 62
pluralism, xi; methodological, xi
pluralistic methodology, xi
poetry, 147, 198; Sufi, 107; writing, 81
Pöggeler, O., 229
policies: anger at, 203; culture and, 8; hospital, 251; Israeli toward Arabs, 134; of social institutions, 253; standardized, 29, 30; uncaring, 119; university, 195
Polit, D. F., 35
politics, 141, 143; awareness of, 222; context of, culture and, xii; discussion of, 131; and economy, 119; events of, 114
Polkinghorne, D., 64
pollution, 97
Polytechnic, 248
Pomare, E. W., 153
population(s): aging, 221; clinical, 52; diverse, 221; healthcare needs of groups, 222; New Zealand, 153
Portugal, 111
position: dichotomous, 108; vulnerable, 66
positive reinforcement, 238
possibility(ies), 12, 136, 140, 152, 164, 169, 174, 175; for change, 33, 163; human, 4; imagining, 192; linguistic, 5; openness, 193
post-colonial regions: India, 108; immigrants from, 114
posthumanist: age, 55
post-modernism, 32, 33, 55
post-operative recovery, 186, 187, 188
post-structural: approach, xi, xii, 22, 33, 36
post traumatic stress disorder (PTSD), 23
potential: of being, 6, 12; emancipatory, of knowledge, 11; human, 100; of other, 109

poverty: background of, 207

power, 24, 34, 36, 54, 151; of biomedicine, 10; of choices, 204; clients and, 53; control in, 54; of curriculum, 117; issues of, 53; knowledge and, 124; leadership and, 53; nonjudgmental, 98; of nurses to instigate change, 124; in practice, 56; of providers, 158; as resource, 26; of stories, 201, 211, 212; of support, 98, 235; sense of, 25; shared, 54; teaching about, 118; using, 53, 54, 57; of voice, 223

powerlessness, 12, 24, 159, 200, 201

practical: activity (ready to hand), 229; everyday, 16; experience, 251; knowledge, 241

practice(s), 15, 130, 176, 242, 259; accepting, 54; accountability of professional, 258; advocacy, 13, 92, 96, 97; alternative and complementary healthcare, 135, 222; analyzing conversations, 195; appropriating, 4; attending to, 12; attitudes about nursing, 29; being fully present, 9; of biomedicine, 134; building of, 240; calling or pulling back, 166; calling out stories, 196; care, 55, 181; care-based foundation in, 253; caring, 21, 22, 33, 47, 56, 96, 181, 184, 195, 197, 198, 208; caring nursing, 195; certainty of, 150; changing needs in, 255; checking in, 197; client-focused, 48, 162; clinical, 13, 50, 51, 123, 124, 166, 207, 242; comforting, 30; coming to know, 167, 169; community, 193; community-centered, 195, 208; competence in, 14, 123, 252; concernful, 193, 195; context of, 22, 27; critique of, 151; cultural, 185, 187, 225, 236, 240; cultural safety in, 145, 247; day-to-day, xiii; demands of safety in, 258; dialectic and, 41, 176; discourse(s) and, 21, 34, 37, 56; discovering, 11, 98; discriminatory, 150; dominant, 27; education and, 21, 49, 56, 148; encountering difference, 152; engagement in, 50, 56, 235; everyday, stories and, 52, 187; expectations and values, and, 143; experiences and, 35, 45, 143; expert, 15, 45; facilitating, 13; gap between education and practice, 251–252; gathering conversations, 195; getting it right, 170, 175; giving, 109; growing, 243; guiding, 194; health-caredelivery, 226; holistic, 160; ideology of, 32; imperatives of, 50; incorporating story in, 202; influence in, 48; influence of stories on, 213; interpretations of, x, xii, 158; inviting, 13; journeying within, 229; of keeping students in mind, 238; knowledge and, 124; language in, 166; learning to, 221; license to, 115; life world of, 230; listening, 194, 195; making sense of world, 4, 5, 163; management and, 38; moral and personal, 253; motivating, 30; of multiculturalism, 127; nature of caring, 21; nature of real, 249; need for information in, 213; negotiated, 13; negotiating, 12; new, 252; nursing, 18, 32, 56, 113, 119, 125, 126, 141, 145, 158, 174, 184, 211, 212, 216, 221, 222, 225, 228, 235, 240, 244, 256–258; nurse-patient relationship in, 160, 162; nurturing, 99; opportunities, 252; outcomes, 216; paternalistic, 51; patronizing, 51; with people who self-harm, 37, 44–45; perpetuating, 4; practicality of, 22; private, 113; protecting, 29; quality of, 231; questioning, 98, 146; reaching out, 166; readiness to, 251; reading, 146; real and ideal, 141; reflective, xi, 56, 200, 255; relationship with knowledge, 252; resistance to, 43; respectful, 140, 194; responsive, 49, 54; revealing, 12; role of culture in assessing, 182; safe, 252; safe-guarding, 229–231, 254; safety in, 256, 258; scope of, 257; self-formative, 64; self-harm and, 51; setting, 208, 232; shaping, 47; showing, 147; situations, 243; skillful, 193; skills for nursing, 223, 243, 241; solution-focused, 55, 56; spiritual, 64; standards of, 50, 160; stories about, 207; storytelling and, 53; striving, 146, 152, 158, 159, 160; supporting, 30; system-focused, 48; taken-for-granted, 50, 56, 156; teaching, xii, 30, 52, 231; teaching-learning, 195; teaching nursing, 52; technology in nursing, 252, 253; telling, 147; tension between theory and, 152, 252; as theory, 185; therapeutic, 41; thinking, 146, 193; touching, 8; traditional healing, 222; transforming, 26, 252; uncovering, 11; understanding and, 14; unexpectedness in, 246; unhelpful, 50; ways of, 44; witnessing, 194; working with clients, 54; in workplaces, 30; writing, 146 practitioner(s), 226; beginning, 243; of client care, 253; competence of new, 252; developing competent, 245; novice, 45, 47; preceptors as, 240; reflective, 141; safety of new, 252; situation and, 193

praeceptum: meaning of, 220

pragmatism: scientific, 99

praxis, 16, 136

precept: meaning of, 220

preceptee/preceptor: growing together, 239; working together, 239

precepting, 248; as double accountability, 236; knowing concerning, 220; lack of support for, 249; meaning of, 220; time consuming, 250; willingness to, 232

preceptor(s), 48, 218, 226, 247, 249, 252, 256; as backup, 243; being as, 221, 223, 224, 227, 230, 238, 248, 254, 257, 258; being vigilant, 239; as builders of nursing practice, 230, 240; care for, 252; caring for students, 238, 240, 254; caring role of, 235, 253; challenging, 243; communication to student, 242; context of, 228; crisis management by, 246; day-to-day, 259; demands on, 250; dialogue between preceptees and, 253; diversity and flexibility of, 257; double accountability of, 239, 245, 249, 250; experience of, 220, 223, 224; as facilitators of making meaning, 254; focus of, 241; imposition of role of, 254; isolation of, 249; keeping student in mind, 234; lack of preparation of, 255; letting students grow, 242; life world of, 226; management of situation by, 241; meaning of, 220, 221, 240; as model, 234; need to trust students, 240; nurse, xii; of patients, 254; payment of, 256; practice of, 223, 259; as practitioners, 240; and preceptee, 223, 225, 239; preparation of, 254, 255, 256; roles of, 223, 255, 258; safeguarding patients, 242; safeguarding students, 252; services of, 256; and skill learning, 223; student and, 242; support by, 243; and talking through, 241, 242; toll on, 240; as transmitter of culture of nursing, 254; uncertainty of, 249, 250; undervaluing of, 249; vigilance of, 240; voices of, 219

preceptorship, 220; significance of, 224

preconceptions, 15

predictability of body functions, 209

preferences, 4

pregnancy, 66, 68; reliving, 67; 167, 168

prejudice(s)/prejudgment(s), 4, 13, 28, 140, 142, 144, 145, 152, 163–165, 168, 170, 174–176; distance, 189; expression of, 131; of nurses, 176; personal and professional, 168, 169; "true," 164

preparation: need for change in, 256

prereflexive mode, 226

presence, 99; emotional, 214; giving self through, 116; unified, 227; visible, 99

present, 6, 100, 117, 225; communion of past and, 247; relevance of past to, 50, 106; traditions and, 142

"present-at-hand," 65, 99; objects, 13

presentation(s): improvised, 130; oral, 118; of self, 131

preserving from harm, 228

"Presidents, The," 68, 80

prestige, 99, 128, 141, 143

presuppositions: interpretation of, 227

pre-understandings, 64, 142, 144, 225

primary healthcare: nurses as leaders in, 223

principles, 110, 247

Priscilla, 68, 100

prison: language as, 98

private sector nursing, 148

privilege, 99; nurses and, 158; teaching about, 118

proactive interaction, 31

problem-centered orientation, 54, 55, 56

problems: isolating, 55; of students, 125; search for, 55; unanticipated, 125

problem-solving approach, 28

procedures, 242; confidence with, 243; learning, 241; standard, 22

process: learning, 241

prodigy, 89

productivity, 182; investment in, 210

profession(s), 106; advancement of nursing, 220; diversity and, 114; female, 133; health, xii; immigrants in health, 114; nursing, 254, 257; practice-based, 125; sharing meaning of caring in, 124; survival of nursing, 231

professional(s): accountability, 230; community, 221; dialogue, 176; disagreement among, in healthcare, 125; education and experience, 169; ethics, 32; expectations of being, 131; growth, 115; identity, 32; journey, 134; learning, 114; life, 108, 130;

professional(s) *(continued)*
literature, meanings, 120; medical, 11; networks, 148; nurse as, 31, 252; nursing, 11, 142, 140, 143; personal self, 105; posture, 115; prejudices, 168; responsibility, 147, 162, 245; satisfaction, 245; socialization, 120, 123; standards of practice, 160; support of, 133; women, 133
professionalization: discourse of, 28
professor: university, 108
prognosis: fatal, 165, 166; grim, 207
program(s): cultural safety, 151; educational, 114; immigrant, 115; nursing, 129; nursing baccalaureate, 120; nursing education, 222; outreach service, 115; preceptorship, 220; religious education, 128; self-harm education, 51; of study, 205; Unitarian Universalist, 128
progress: educational, 117; and oppression, 126; Western education and, 113
promises: false, 99
prompting, 242
property: ownership of, 128
protection of self, 209
protocols, 40, 48, 93; in practice, 247
Providence, 28
providers: caring and, 185; healthcare, xii; line between clients and, 117; power of, 158
Psalm 119, 220
pseudonyms, 148, 212
psychiatry, 26, 153, 203; Australian, 26
psychoanalytic theory: understanding, 24
psychodynamic theories, 23
psychologists, 83; clinical, 119
psychology: "discount store," 94; and distress, 26; and perspective, 25; relational, 24; theory, 25
psychopathology: individual, 25
psychosocial needs, 186
psychotic phenomena, 23
PTSD (post traumatic stress disorder), 23
public: attitudes of, 28; health nursing, 149; moral discourse, 29; policy, caring and, 185; school system, 92; self, 107; university, 121
publications: ban on, Holocaust, 134
publishing about oppression, 115
pulling back, 166
Pushto, 131
Putnam, F. W., 26

qualitative inquiry: spirit of, 148
quality of life: issues of, 207
queen of the house, 66
question(s), 4, 98, 147, 149, 154, 156, 174, 201, 208; about assumptions, 195; of choice, 190; constructing, 193; critical, 34, 143; critical thinking and, 196; data collection, 35; about nurses leaving nursing, 218; open-ended, 148; process of asking, 242; research, 144; situation, 249; spiral, 224; stories and, 196; understanding and, 142, 144; of what is happening, 202; of "why," 190
Quigley, D., 108

race, 10, 99, 129, 141, 143, 150; culture, 118; discussing, 116; generalizations about, 118; heritage of, 120, 130; relations, 149; as taboo topic, 126; teaching about, 120; theory of, critical, 126
racial other, 149
racism, 200; and nursing practice, 145; as taboo topic in American culture, 118
rage, 64
Rahiri, 176
Raia, J., 28
Raj (rule): British, 110; healthcare and, 110
Ramsden, I., 141, 143, 151, 163, 247
Rapp, C., 51, 55
Rapunzel, 79
Rather, M., 220, 229
rationality, 45, 55; technical, 193
rationalization of health services, 30
Ray, M. A., 185
reaching out, 166
reaction: instinctual, 203; meaning and, 203
reader: trust of, 63
readiness to practice, 251
reading(s), 146, 149, 223; assigned, 199; caring and, 198; data, 35, 36; 130; meaning of, 198
ready-to-hand, 6, 15, 16, 229; un-, 229
reality(ies), 14, 27, 66; of academic culture, 123; awareness of, 99; concrete, 117; construction of, 107; of difference, 125; "hitting," 245; ideal and, 173; imagining, 192; as known, 4; language as, 226; "my," 107; of nursing, 230, 240, 241, 245, 250, 255; objective, 36; pain of, 173; patients', 197, 202; perception of, 189; physical, 64; of practice, 249; practice oriented in, 254;

revealed and shared, 63; subjective, 52; talking, thinking, writing about, 27; teaching, 240; understanding, 194

Reason, P., 175

reasoning: clinical, 16, 55; creative, 51

Rebecca, 238, 240, 248, 249

rebirthing, 99

recidivism, 44

reciprocity, 116, 117, 142, 256; storytelling and, 206

recollective: thinking, 195

Recollective Pathway, 182, 193, 194, 215; course in, 195

records: medical, 77

recovering: by clients, 21, 241; students, 123

Reed, J., 22

Reed-Danahay, D., 63

Reeder, F., 13

reflection, xi, 51, 62, 106, 108, 124, 142, 147, 148, 186, 204, 215, 246; caring and, 181, 196; on clinical relationships, 192; critical, 21, 212; dialectic and, 176; and experience, 135; of experience, 62; on experience, 202; -in-action, 193; participation and, 106; pedagogy and, 187; philosophical, 185; practice and, xi, 141; in representation, 98; in research, 212; self-, 125; on self, 63; on situation, 192; on story, 193, 196, 199, 203, 211; by student, 191; teaching caring and, 182, 192; upon practice, 255

reflective: activity, 193; intervention, 194; mode of everydayness, un-, 232; practice, 200; process, caring as, 185–186; thinking, 196

reflectivity, 56, 64, 105, 107; anthropology and, 105; engagement and, 143; journal and, 145; pre-, 142; and unreflectivity, 48

reflexivity, 14

reflexology, 222

reform(s): contemporary, 193; government and healthcare, 248, 257

reframing, 51; seeing self-harm differently, 54

refugees, 135, 158

registered nurses (RNs). *See* nurses

rehabilitation, 257

Reichard, G. A., 98

reinforcement: positive, 238

Reinharz, S., 63

reinterpreting, xi

rejection, 100, 112, 154; fear of, 159; risk of, 63

relatedness: of body in healthcare, 209; as issue, 208

relational psychology, 24

relations: race, 149

relationship(s), 24, 100; caring, 50; between clinicians and clinical practice, 124; community of, 228; cultural, 26, 158, 162; equal, 53; experiences and, 106, 116; between identity and difference, 166; interpersonal, 6, 117; "I/Thou," 116, 117; between language and culture, 4; as dialogue, 116; marital, 131; mutual, 56; negative power, 56; nurse-client, 56, 154, 158, 160; one-to-one, 221; with others, 172; part-whole, 4, 142; with patients and families, 232; reciprocal, 117; reflecting on, 192; socially distancing, 166; stories of, 206; student-teacher, 53, 116; therapeutic, 154

release: sense of, 238

releasement, 64, 99

religion(s), 8, 9; and beliefs, 110; caring and, 122; ceremonies, 127; community, 127; dimension of, 118; Eastern, 109; educational programs, 128; events, 115; genderized, 134; Hindu Rama Krishna, 131; imposition of, 111; nursing orders and, 183; self-mutilation and, 25; story and, 110; teachings of, 118, 136; values and, 120; Western Christian, 121

remembering: forgetting and, 64; stories, 199

reports: written, 118

representation(s): cultural, 98; of disabled, 98; of everyday life, 64; by media, 28; reflection and, 98; in research, 152

research, xi, xii, 106, 142, 147, 152, 158, 250; action, 257; caring, 181; clinically focused, 158; context, 232; healthcare, 135; hermeneutic, 141, 144, 145, 257; interpretation of, 143, 146, 223, 227; journal, 147; literature based on, xi; narratives in, xii; nursing education; 219; product, plausibility of, 148; prejudices in, 144; rigor in hermeneutic, 147, 148; story as, 202; subjective, 107; and values, 202; writing and, 147

resilience, 33, 51, 52, 56

resistance, 24; to conversion, 110; to and in practice, 43, 44, 45, 48, 49
resources, 56, 75; allocation of, 29; education, 219; of social workers, 96
respect, 44, 54, 63, 113, 116, 131, 160, 161, 194, 202; attitudes of, in practice, 174; for difference, 141; for experience, 212; female and, 113; in healthcare, 13; lack of, 109; for stories, 199, 203, 215; "talking back" to, 199; for voice, 212; want of, 113
respectful: listening to stories, 206; lives, 198
responses: to story, 206
responsibility(ies), 99, 248, 259; caring, 160, 185; Dasein, 225; double, 249, 255; to employees, 231; ethical, 156, 185; of nurses, 146, 185, 239; patient care, 246; professional, 162; for self and others, 126; for students, 252, 258; for teaching and learning, 231; tension and, 157
"restless to and from between yes and no," 251
rethinking, xi
revealing, 12, 145; disclosure and, 125; of experience, 62; of meanings, 119; practices, 208, 253; self, 12, 107
review of literature, 34
rewarding patients, 210
Reynolds, B., 32
rhetorical induction, 106
Richardson, L., 63, 105
Richman, J., 29
rights, 9; beliefs about, 160; disability, 99; of families, 10; of husbands, 168; of incompetent, 198; to justice, 170; parental, 8, 9, 11, 12, 77, 92, 93; women's, 170
rigor: in research, 147; of work, 148
risk, 28, 48, 54; assessment of, 51; from clients, 29; containing, nurses' role of, 31; dialectic of trust and, 29; discourse of, 28, 30; identification of, 28; management of, 28, 29, 30, 31, 34, 55; nursing and, 30; to society, 29; in storytelling, 99; symptoms and, 30
Ritchie, J., 152
Ritchie, Lionel, 76
rite of passage: self mutilation as, 25
ritual(s), 45; healing and music, 98
RNs. See nurses
Roach, M. S., 32

Robinson, R., 27
Rodgers, J., 164
Rogers, A., 24
role(s): ambiguity of, 31; assisting, 228; caring, of preceptors, 235; clinical, 131; conflict, 113; daughter-in-law, 130; empathetic, 162; enhancing, 148; female, 130; gender, 129; girlfriend, 130; guiding, 228; healthcare, 205; mother, 99, 130; nurses', 29, 213, 228; of preceptors, 258; of risk containment, 31; sister-in-law, 130; supporting, 228; teaching, 228, 255; wife, 130
role-modeling, 120, 124, 125, 230
Ronai, C. R., 63
"Rondo," 83
Roseman, M., 98
Rosenberg, A., 100
Rosenberg, R., 136
Rothenberg, P., 117
routine, 40, 45
Rowan, J., 175
Rowe, J., xi, 21, 265
rules: change of, 129; rigor in research and, 148; routines and, 40
Rumi, Jelaluddin, 107
Rummel, L. G., xii, 219, 223, 265

sacred and profane, 134
sadness, 192; focus on, 194
safeguarding, 228, 258; practices, 229, 230, 231; students and patients, 239, 242
safety, 28, 29, 40; cultural, 141, 143, 144, 145, 149, 150, 151, 157, 176, 222, 245, 247, 258; emotional, 151; learning and, 212, 208; legal-ethical, 151; need for, 250; of patients and students, 240, 251, 256; patient's view of, 258; personal, 147; physical, 151, 157; practice, 255
St. Pierre, E. A., 62
sameness: difference and, 98; recognizing, 109
Samoa, 148, 154, 159, 171
sampling: convenience, 35
Samu, 171, 172
Sandelowski, M., 148
Sapir-Whorf hypothesis, 4
Sarah, 245, 246, 252
Sarason, S. B., 124
Saroyan, W., 140
satisfaction: of clients/patients, 119; of preceptors, 245; with services, 22

Sayeed Muslim, 108, 111
Schirato, T., 34, 35
schizophrenia, 28
Schliessmann, L., 15
scholars, xv, xvi, 184; achievements of, 124;
    community of, 198, 211; nurse, 124
scholarship, 106; Sufis and, 135; understand-
    ing and, 125, 126
Schon, D.A., 193, 200
school(s), 95, 114, 198; administrators, 93;
    for adults, 129; African American stu-
    dents in nursing, 120; assignments in,
    117; caring and, 123, 184; challenge of,
    205; and community, 209; and concernful
    practice, 193; culture of, 123; elementary,
    93; environment, 121; Europeanized In-
    dian, 113; experience at, 112; graduate,
    114; high, 108; language, 111; middle, 93,
    94; mission, 111; nursing, 94, 95, 120,
    123, 184, 194, 256; policy, 203; private
    European day, 113; public, 92, 93
Schutz, A., 147
Schwass, M., 150
science(s), 16, 63, 99, 135; and caring, 183,
    184; dialectic and, 176; human, 220, 253;
    knowledge of, 216; mastery of, 106; moral
    tradition in, 253; natural, 187, 220; prag-
    matism of, 99; relationship with service,
    166; social, 150; technological practices
    in, 253
scientism, 4
Scott, R. A., 98
script: life, 108
Scudder, J. R., 155, 158, 185, 253
Scupin, R., 4
search for caring, 125
seclusion, 41, 45, 135
sects, 110
security, 29; sense of, 122
"seeing," 97; learning by, 119
seekers of asylum, 135
self (selves), 64; appraisal of, 145; assess-
    ment of, 14; authentic, 115, 203; aware-
    ness of, 49, 115, 133, 161; care for, 6, 18,
    31, 117, 123, 167; consciousness of, 63,
    106, 231; culture and, 14, 105, 107; devel-
    opment of, 175; dialogue with other, 117;
    doubt of, 64; examination of, 105, 106; ex-
    istence of, 203; expression of, voice and,
    54; finding of, 98; growth of, 133; harm-
    ing of (*see* self-harm); healing, 98; history

and, 107; identity and, 32; image of, 62;
    inquiry of, 107; integrating, 129; interpret-
    ing of, 187, 188, 189, 190, 210, 225, 228;
    invisibility to, 115; involvement of, 221;
    knowledge of, 25, 115; management of,
    31; narratives of, 63; opening, 107; and
    other, 126, 133; personal/professional,
    105; presentation of, 131; protection of,
    209; public and private, 107; reclaiming
    of, 63; reflecting on, 63, 125; revealing
    of, 12, 107; sacrifice of, 123, 132; sense of,
    25; sheltering, 62; social, 25; society and,
    107; soothing, 23; stigma and, 51; stimula-
    tion of, 26; stories and, 52, 135; theories
    of, 51; understanding of, 106, 147, 231;
    writing the, 62
self-harm, xi, xii, 21–23, 25, 27, 28, 33, 41,
    42, 45, 50–54; adolescence and, 24; age
    and, 24; behaviors, 23; among clients, 36,
    40, 41, 45, 47, 48, 50, 56; clinical path-
    ways for, 51; coping and, 24; costs of, 23;
    diagnostic categories and, 51; education
    about, 37, 49; females and, 24; function
    of, 45; myths about, 26; practice skills
    and, 52; religion and, 25; response to,
    39–40, 43; rite of passage and, 25; theo-
    ries of, 23; therapy and, 23; understand-
    ing, 170; worth, 174
Sen, S., 110
sensitivity, 9, 51, 57, 96; caring behaviors
    and, 121; cultural, 14, 51, 109, 115, 123,
    146; to diversity, 116; to emotion, 25; per-
    sonal, 114; to race, 120; training, 94
sensory being, 64
separateness, 97, 98; in-, from universe, 136
servants: civil, 111; government, 112
service(s): church, 127, 128; educational,
    111, 255; focus on nursing, 222; health,
    32; healthcare, 228, 247; meaningful, 140;
    mental health, 37; need as basis for, 33;
    of nurse, 147, 164, 219, 228, 254; as nurs-
    ing priority, 222; of occupational thera-
    pist, 75; outcomes of, 30; to patients, 253;
    of physical therapist, 75; providing, 143,
    219; rationalization of health, 30; relation-
    ship with science, 166; satisfaction with,
    22; settings, 256; of social worker, 75; of
    teachers, 254
setting(s): acute care, 219, 226, 231, 232;
    classroom, 199; educational, 256; employ-
    ment, 148; healthcare, 10; hospital, 157,

setting(s) *(continued)*
226; polytechnic, 239; practice, 208, 232; service, 256; ward, 226
settlers in New Zealand, 149
Severtsen, B. M., xii, 181, 195, 266
sex, 141, 143
sexism, 51
Shabatay, V., 160
shame, 69, 98, 167, 170
Shamian, J., 220
shaping by caring and culture, 105
shared world, 233
sharing: culture, 98; experiences, 63; meaning of caring, 124; time, 238
Sharma, U., 135
Shaw, N., 23, 24, 33
Sheehan, T., xv
Sherman, M. E., 28
Sherrard, I., 150
Shibayama, Z., 64
showing, 147, 148
siblings, 132
sick, 154; care of, 257
significant others, 22
sign(s), 97; exemplars of caring as, 136
silence, 13, 52, 53, 64, 107; clearing, 99; of care, x; and difference, 26; students and, 125; of voice, 24
similarities: differences and, in nursing, 140
Simmel, G., 147
Sims, S., xv
Sinclair, A., 53
Singapore, 148
Singha, R., 110
sisters-in-law, 136
Sisters of Charity, 120
situation(s), 16, 26, 99, 187; attunement to, 236; awareness of, 203, 204; being in the world of the, 187; blame for, 98; caring and uncaring, 196, 214; challenging, 245; of client, 33, 52; clinical, 52; context and, 185; health-related, 5; individual, 185, 214; interaction with, 193, 194; interactive, 16; interpretation of, 197, 203, 233; and learning, 117, 201, 241; making sense of, 142; management of by preceptor, 241; meaning of, 188, 191, 192; of the moment, 4; moral agency within, 236; portraying, 202; practice, 243; real, 242; response to, 235; safe, 241; shared interpretation of, 197, 233; significance of,

203; stories in, 195, 201; supervised, 241; and teaching, 117; thinking and, 199
skill(s), 208; applying, 52; calling forth, 228; caring, 21, 52, 56; clinical, 15; communication, 222, 252; demand for, 219; engagement, 54; having, 96; interpersonal, 52; interpretive, xii; learning, 250; of observation, 168, 174; of physicians, 97; practicing, 241, 243; story as, 200; technical, 7, 15, 175; understanding, 14; for working *with*, 54
skin color, 153
Slayer, Kenneth, 82, 83, 91
Slayer, Marcie, 82, 84, 86, 88, 90
Sloan, R., xv
Slunt, E. T., 173
smallpox epidemic, 111
smile: baby and, 76
Smith, D., 107
Smith, E. B., 9
Smith, J. K., 148
Smythe, E., 146
Smythe, L., 176
Snider, J., 221
Soares, J., 31
Sobo, E. J., 9
social: acceptability, 26, 98; beings, 3, 98; competence, 26; connections, 22; constructions, facts as, 148; control, nurse and, 29; dialogue and negotiation, 148; discourse, 21, 32; distance, 32, 166, 214; and emotional needs, 168, 169; gatherings, 112; groups, 10, 130; inequalities, 143; institutions, culture and politics of, 253; integration, 65; interaction, 98; needs, husband's, 131; norms, 17, 108, 130; oppression, 127; and political economy, 119; roles, teaching about, 118; rules, 156; science, 150, 118; self, 25; status, 141, 143; structures, 150; suffering, 100; taboo, 23; transactions, 117; unacceptability, 65; worker(s), 75, 79, 81, 83, 94, 96, 119
social distancing (marginalizing, ostracizing), 11, 51, 52, 65, 94; between client and nurse, 163, 166; silence and, 53
socialization, 3, 49, 128, 130; caring and early, 121; and celebration, 189; divergent, 131; female, 24, 108; Hindu, 112; male, 24; of students, 123; professional, 120

social-philosophical dichotomies, 136
society(ies), 108; American, 10; beauty-oriented, 74; biomedicine in non-Western, 134; change and, 148; expectations of, for ill person, 210; identity of, 97; New Zealand, 145, 247; nursing and, 158; prescribed roles of, 130; response by, 65; risk to, 29; rural, 154; self and, 107; sociopolitical dimensions, 118; urban, 154
sociological introspection, 105
sociologist, 145
sociopolitical: context, health and, 256; influences, 228
"sojourner" (sojourners), 121, 134
Solberg, S., 6, 119
solicitude, 6, 13, 15
solution: finding a, 239; orientation toward, 55, 56; searching for, 55
Somali family, 158
son, 66
song: gospel, 87
Sonata, 84
Sorrell, J., xvi
sound: meaning of, 64
Sourial, S., 46
Southern Methodist University, 86
space(s): continuum, 117; creation of, 49; culture and, 182; lived, 227; resources or constraints in, 226; for teaching, 246; time and, 62; unity of time and, 229; between worlds, 230
Spanish: Mexican, 129
sparing, 229
speaking: learning by, 119
Special Education Department, 75, 93
speech: understanding meaning through, 142
speech therapist, 83
Spence, D., xii, 140, 141, 144, 145, 146, 149, 152, 156, 163, 176, 266
spiral of change, 257
spirit, 100; art and, 65; of qualitative inquiry, 148; strength of, 54
spirituality, 106; beliefs and, 123; caring and, 121, 123, 203; course on, 123; development of, 121; Eastern, 134; growth of, 123; and health, 247; journeys, 114; and leadership, 109; meaning of, 203; and meditation, 107; practice of, 64; realm of, dialogue and, 117; respect of, 140; teach-ing about, 118; understanding, 135; un-wellness and, 154; views of, 136
Spoonley, P., 151
Stack, C. B., 100
staffing, 29, 248; of NICU, 14, 16, 17; nurse, 26; responses, 218; short, 249; of wards, 232
standard(s): of care, 17, 161; of healthcare, 10; of nursing graduates, 219; organizational, 231; of practice, 160; procedures, 22; of social institution, 253
"standing reserve," 15
Stannard, D., 15, 16, 235
state: church and, 112; of mind, 12
status, 98, 99, 151; of American Indians (Native Americans), 115; educational, 131; female, in Western culture, 134; master, 98; as model family, 129; of people of color, 126, 129; professional, 150; social, 141, 143; student, 246
Stein, H. F., 10
step-mother, 112
stereotyping, 77, 99, 127, 129, 130, 200; positive, 129
Stetson, B., xvi
Stewart, E. C., 10
stigma, 28, 98; loss of control and, 209; and self-harm, 51
Stinson, B., 28
Stokes, E., 110
Stordheur, S., 31
story(ies), 7, 27, 157, 165, 166, 170, 172, 173, 174; academic and personal, 136; accuracy of, 202; analyzing, 192; as anecdotes, 206; asking for, 211; authentic, 202; autoethnographic, 105; calling out, 196; of caring, 165, 181, 205; children and, 127; as chronicles, 206; of class participants, 207; of clinical practice, 207; as communication, 211; complete, 202; context and, 211; converging, 200, 204, 206; as conversation, 195, 208; as creation, 62; cultivating, 201; as dangerous, 201; development of, 204; embedded in situations, 195; emerging, 204; of family, 129; of fatal illness, 196; feminist, 107; gathering, 192; give and take of, 198; "good," 127; of healthcare system, 207; helping to articulate, 205; as hermeneutic language, 229; historical, 107; and how of thinking, 229; idea of reflecting on, 193;

story(ies) *(continued)*
  illness and, 208, 210; improvised, 130; influence on practice, 213; instructors', 206;
  interpreting self and, 135; Jacqui's, 64,
  97–99; of lack of support, 207; learning
  from, 199, 201, 206; life, 62, 63, 100,
  105, 106, 130, 191, 214; listening to, 192,
  212; living with, 202, 205; as meaning
  making, 199, 201, 203; memory and, 170;
  narrative and, 63; original, 200; about
  others, 206; paradigm, 186; of participants, 145; permission to tell, 105; personal, 52, 62, 100; as phenomenon, 197;
  power of, 191, 211; questions and, 197;
  readable as, 63; reading and discussing,
  196; reciprocity and, 206; reflexive, 105,
  107; religion and, 110; remembering, 199;
  respect of, 63, 203, 206, 215; retelling,
  200; rhythm of, 197; sad, 214; sharing,
  130, 192, 199; sides to, 110; situations
  of, 200–202; of students, 186, 187, 188,
  200, 204, 207, 229; students wanting,
  127; about teens, 207; themes of, 192;
  theorized, 106; thinking *about*, 201, 202;
  thinking *with*, 201, 202; traditional, 107;
  as trip, 199; understanding, 192, 194; unfolding of, 201; urgency of, 197; whole,
  202; about work, 206; writing, 127, 149,
  208
storytelling, 53, 63, 100, 106, 193, 196,
  199–201, 203; risk in, 99
strangeness, 147
stranger, 147; *danger*, 147
strategy(ies): coping, 240; emancipation/lib-
  eration, 14; intervention, 15, 99; of listening, 199; for rigor in research, 148
Street, A. F., 124
Street, F., 162
strength, 33, 65; building, 53; exposing hidden, 56; seeing, 54, 55, 56
stress, 32, 122, 136, 156, 238, 239; of disease, 207; as disruption in meaning, 240;
  of preceptors, 240, 248; work-related, 31,
  158
striving: being and doing of, 161; as hermeneutic response, 160, 162, 168, 169, 173,
  174; *toward right*, 152, 159
struggle, 62, 113, 160; between being and
  doing, 168; with breast cancer, 197; for
  coherence, 63; with differences, 113, 163;
  existential, 100; with health concerns,

208; for meaning, 63, 100; retrospective
  and prospective, 162
student(s), xii, 54–57, 119, 214, 243, 245,
  247, 251; accounting for, 250; adult, 256;
  African American nursing, 120; ages of,
  118; aggressive, 118; assessing, 230, 239;
  being, 248; beliefs and values of, 120,
  121; caring, 183; caring about, 119, 121,
  123, 232, 236, 238; challenging, 243;
  Christian, 121, 123; coaching of, 124; as
  creative and rebellious, 112; cultivating,
  230; culture and, 254; demands of, 125;
  distress of, 235; dwelling with, 230; encouraging, 230; experiences of, 220, 241,
  248, 253; graduate, 122; growth in, 123,
  230; health needs of, 125; helping, 230;
  hierarchy and, 208; history of practice
  culture of, 256; hysteria of, 237; importance of, 237; interaction with patients,
  clinicians, teachers, 208; international,
  125, 129; as interpreter, 200; keeping in
  mind, 230; knowledge of, 237, 242; lack
  of caring toward, 239; learning, 181,
  256; learning by, 240; learning from, 116,
  248, 249; learning of, 203, 254; letting
  grow, 242, 243; lifeworld of, 226; lived
  curriculum and, 253; Maori, 150; in medicine, 77; minority, in America, 125; needs
  of nursing, 235; need to trust, 240; need
  to see "big picture," 257; negative, 118;
  nurses, undergraduate, 218, 219, 224;
  nursing, 117, 186–189, 192, 200, 205,
  221, 226, 238, 255; nurturing, 230; as object, 116; opportunity to practice, 252;
  and parents, 128; pedagogy and, 193; as
  people, 258; as preceptee, 234; preceptors and, 242, 254; preparation of, for possibilities, 252; privileged, 238; problems
  of, 125; progress of, 117; reaction to, 236;
  real world of, 225; reception of, 219; recovering, 123; reflective, 191; responsibility for, 258; safeguarding, 239; as "sojourners," 121; status of, 246; stories and,
  127, 200, 207; teachers and, 116, 125,
  127, 208, 230, 237; as "there," 231;
  thoughts of, 118; time needed by, 244;
  transforming, 254; undergraduate, 114,
  122, 218, 219, 224, 231, 249; use
  of stories by, 206; Vietnamese, 201;
  voices of, 194, 195, 199; worldviews of,
  118

study: of caring, 21; descriptive, 145; doctoral, 119; ethnographic of caring, 119, hermeneutic phenomenological, 124, 223; of human living, 105; of multiculturalism, 114
Stuhlmiller, C., 41
Stuhlmiller, C. M., 63
Styles, M., 166
Subcontinent: Indian, 108, 110, 111, 126, 131
subculture, 189
subject: intertwining object with, 64; to object dialogue, 116, 190; object way, 191
subjectifying of "other," 64
subjectivity, 25, 45, 52, 53, 156, 224; distrust of feelings of, 210; of experience, 244; as gathering place, 227; research and, 107
subordination: teaching about, 118
success, 128
suffering, 65, 130, 170; human, 117, 126; indignities, 98; relief of, 205; social, 100; students and, 125
Sufis, 107, 135
Sufism, 109
Sugarman, J., 9
suicidality, 23
suicide, 24, 50; planning, 79–80
Sulu, 171, 173
supervision, 251; of clients, 30; clinical, 51
support, 30, 37, 80, 125, 150, 166, 249; of administrators, 118; bureaucratic, caring and, 122; of charitable causes, 129; of colleagues, 115; of community, 204; of family, 69, 75, 85, 132, 177; of friends, 84; of group, 75, 92; of healing, 106; instrumental, 98; interpersonal, 98; lack of, 207; listening as, 196; need to give, 166; nonjudgmental, 98; of parents with different children, 97; of peer, 49; power of, 98, 235; preceptor and, 48, 243; by professional women, 133; spiritual, 98; by staff, 88; in workplace, 157
suppression: cultural, 108
suprahuman: passage to, 134
surgeons, 83, 240
surgery, 82, 83, 86, 88, 89, 91, 92, 200, 209; night before, 85; observation and care, 241
surrogate parent, 97
surveillance: role of nurse, 29

survival, 54, 65, 99, 110
sussed (understood), 177
syllabus, 195, 196
symbolic: loss, 194; pain and, 193; thinking, 4
symbol(s): cupcake as, 186; death as, 234; healing and, 100; of hope, 100; writing as, 100
sympathy, 15; for students, 232
symptoms: ignoring subjective, 210; reporting, 210
system: belief, 121; educational, 117, 118
Szwed, J. F., 100

taboo: against discussion of race, 118; social, 23
tactics: survival, 99
tales: confessional, 63
talking: in clinical context, 28; about reality, 27
"talking through," 241, 255
tangi (Maori burial ceremony), 247
Tanner, C. A., 13, 16, 147, 212, 225, 235, 236
Taoism, 120–122, 136
tape-recording, 148, 211, 223
Tapp, D., xvi
Tara, 159, 161
tasks: measurable, 38
Taylor, B., 32, 166, 172, 175
Taylor, C., 141, 142, 169, 170, 220, 222, 226
teacher(s), 112, 116, 128, 202; anger at, 203; blind, 93; experiences of, 211; as guide, 117; and hierarchy with students, 208; at historically black liberal arts college, 122; insensitive, 93; nurse, 144, 239; nurturing and loving, 122; pedagogy and, 192; role of, 254, 255; students and, 116, 125, 181, 186, 208; voices of, 194, 195
teaching(s), xii, 12, 51–52, 55, 56, 99, 126, 127; blind children, 75, 95; care about, 119; about caring, 105, 120, 123, 181, 182, 185, 195; in classroom, 222; clinical, 122, 257; conceptual, 208; as concernful practice, 193; about culture and health, 125; about diversity, 114, 115; as guiding and interpreting, 119; and learning, 115, 117, 120, 121, 182, 186, 193, 214, 231, 237; about multiculturalism, 109, 127;

teaching(s) *(continued)*
  nurses to care, 218; practice and, 231; preceptor, 241; about race, 120; reality of nursing, 230, 240; reflection, 192; responsibility for, 231; rewards of, 123; students, 219, 230, 237; styles of, 120; taking time for, 246, Taoist, 136; theoretical, 219; time and space for, 248; transcultural nursing, 114; Unitarian, 136; university, 114; ways of, 120
techne, 16
technicians: operating room, 88
Technodrome, 84
technology, 7, 15–17, 135, 166, 172, 175; demands of, 10; distancing from, 99; dominance of, 252; environment driven by, 222; Heidegger and, 244; high, 7; medical, 99; nursing and, 255; practices of, 253; rationality and, 193; relationship with service, 166; tools of, 99
Tedlock, B., 63, 64, 106
teenagers, 206; Muslim, 112; story of, 207; in U.S., 128
teeth: neem and, 126
telling, 147, 148
temperature and other vital signs, 240
temporality, 223; Dasein and, 225
tender loving care, 8, 172
tension(s), 12, 16, 17, 22, 29, 31, 33, 66, 147, 156–159, 165, 168, 169, 174–176, 221, 259; confidence and, 174; day-to-day, 22; between difference and sameness, 98; between discourses, 42, 49; dynamic, 63; in ethnography, 135; everyday, 221; examining through stories, 52, 64; experiencing, 152, 154; healthcare and, 18; memory of, 232; among nurses, 143; between people from different cultures, 162, 174; in practice and work, 37–38; in preparing nurses, 250; between society and nursing, 158; in teaching, 118; between theory and practice, 252
Terri, 92
test(s), 67, 202; diagnostic, 210; of learning, 211
Te Taha Hinengaro (emotional), 247
Te Taha Tinana (physical), 247
Te Taha Wairua (spiritual), 247
Te Taha Whanau (family), 247
Texas, 83, 88; Dallas, 83
textbooks on tape, 95

text(s), 34, 106, 107, 143, 147, 149, 212; authentic interpretation of, 227; connecting, 63, 100; exemplars from, 212; family, 100; interpretation of, 143, 146, 226; object as analog of, 143; story, 52
texture: cultural, 97
"them:" *other* and, 109; "us" and, 116, 129, 130
thematic patterns, 224
theme(s), 36, 120, 123, 149, 152, 160, 200, 201, 204, 218, 251; developing, 212; identifying, relational, 223; of inquiry, 121; making visible, 165; relational, 230, 234; story, 201; *striving*, 146, 160
theory(ies): activity of (unready to hand), 229; behavioral, 23; biomedical, 9; of care, 184; critical racial, 126; cultural, 26; of culture care, 150; feminist, 24, 114, 116; lack of, in autoethnography, 135; learning, 239; of motivation, 190; postmodern, 55; as practice, 185; practice versus, 252; psychoanalytic, 24; psychodynamic, 23; psychological, 25; scientific, 9; of self-harm, 23, 51; story and, 106, 192; trauma, 23
therapeutic(s), 98; encounter, 11; framework, 51; grieving, 237; intervention, 6; listening, 207
therapy, 240; occupational, 75; physical, 75; self-harm and, 23; speech, 83; writing as, 63, 97
Theresa, 154, 157, 160
thing(s): in world, 227
thinking, 5, 50, 56, 146; being and, 229; building, 227; critical, 51; deductive, 55; difference and, 127; dualistic, as illness, 136; as dwelling in the world, 229; focused, 236; ghetto, 99; *how* of, 229; inductive, 55; knowing and, 193; lateral, 51, 55; out loud, 256; as nurses, 229; about reality, 27; recollective, 195; reflective, 196; about situation, 199; with stories, 201; symbolic, 4; writing and, 147
Third World, 107
Thomas, B., 30
Thomsen, S., 31
Thorsen, R., 63
"Thou:" "I" and, 129, 134
thought(s), 107; Eastern, 135, 136; nondualistic, 136; of students, 118; Western, 108

threat of extinction, 98

thrownness, 7, 14, 17, 65, 99, 225; disability and, 98; discomfort with, 233; precepting and, 231, 232

Tibbles, P., 30

Tilah, M., 158

Tilley, J. L., 28

Tillman-Healy, L., 63, 106

time, 6, 141, 167, 182; changing, 126; communion of past and present, 247; constraints, 163, 226; consuming, precepting as, 249, 250; cross-cultural communication and, 159; Dasein and, 225; demands of linear, 228; embracing, 65; framework of, 29; future, 6; gathering, 65; interpreting practice and, 36; linear, 6; lived, 227; for machinery, 244; metaphysical, 239; past and present, 6, 50, 56, 106, 108; as preceptor, 223; present, 64, 106, 108; resources and, 226; revealing with, 62; to share, 238; space and, 62, 117, 229; spent with patients, 47, 48; traditions and, 142; understanding and, 6, 142

Timewell, E., 35, 36

Toland, D., 28

tolerance, xii, 15, 24, 99; problems and, 55

Tolman, D., 24

Tolstoy, L., 196

tomorrow, 70

tones, 98

tools, 16, 99. *See also* technology

topics: framing of, 118

topography, 110

totality, 99

touching, 8

"tough love," 122

tradition(s), 4, 5, 45, 136; authority and, 4; of care, 135; cultural, 133; hermeneutic, 14; interaction of, 142; language and, 142; peace and familiarity and, 127; story and, 107

traditional: tribe, 111; ways, 126; ways of knowing, 220

traditionalism, 108, 131

tragedy, 64, 75

training: nurses in hospitals, 222

transactions: social, 117

transcendence, 17, 99, 134, 135

transcription, 212

transcripts, 34, 35, 36, 149, 223, 224; interpretation of, 227

transcultural healthcare: course, 108, 115; teaching, 114

transcultural nursing, 150, 153; course in, 115

transformation, 64, 125; with education, 49; with knowledge and practice, 252; pain and pleasure, of, 62; of students, 253–254; of views, 119

transformative: curriculum, 117; practices, 4, 26

transhistorical world, 63

transmission: of culture by preceptor, 254

transpersonal world, 63

trauma, 241; discourse of, 23; theory, 23

traumatization, 27; vicarious, 31

Travelbee, J., 145, 172, 183

treatment, 26, 27, 30; aggressive, 11; attitudes toward, 210; choice of, 210; financial burden of, 207; medical, 16; options, 200; pain of, 27; protocols, 198; stress of, 207; values of individual in, 210

Treaty of Waitangi, 150, 151, 152, 153, 176, 247

tribe: coping and, 114; people in, 110; traditional, 111; woman in, 113

triggers: emotional, 237

troops (visitors), 157

trust, 44, 63, 154; ability of patients to, 205; dialectic between risk and, 29; distrust, 210; interpersonal, 174; need for in preceptor-student relationship, 240; in power to change, 123

truth, 5, 97, 100, 144, 173; dream as, 64; living, 117; paradigmatic, 134

trying, 159

Tulsa, Oklahoma, 129

Turner, B. S., 10

"turning around:" as change, 15

tutor, 237, 238; clinical, 251; tech, 248

"Twinkle, twinkle, little star," 90

Tymieniecka, 253

Uggie, 84

Ulin, R. C., 4, 14

"ultimate freedom," 204

umheimlich (unsettledness), 231, 233

uncaring, 213

uncertainty, 154, 159, 175, 176, 193, 248; of preceptors, 250, 254; problems and, 193

uncle, 111, 112

unconcealment, 65; of being, 99, 233

uncovering, 11
undergraduate: student nurses, 224, 231, 249, 255, 257
understanding(s), 4, 5, 11–15, 33, 107, 110, 145, 149, 166, 174–176, 188; as active, 136; background, 144, 187; being, 37, 99; of caring, 124, 125, 129; challenge to, 170; changing, 126, 146, 169, 170; competence in practice, 14; of constraints, 201; cross-cultural, 165, 166; culturally safe practice, 247; culture, x, 151, 152, 166; cyclical, 141; Dasein and, 226; as disclosedness, 5; "distortive," 170; empathetic, 214, 215; epistemological, x; experience(s), 106, 224; extension of, 146; feelings, 54, 165; forestructure of, 227; "good," 253; of healthcare providers, xii; hermeneutic circle of, 143; humanistic, 39; implicit, 170; interactions, 106; issues, 235; language and, 142, 226; learning as, 119; likeness, 97; mis-, 154, 166; multiple, 124; mutual, 166; nature of, 164; need for, 54, 124, 163; new, 169; nursing practice, 212; oneness of being, 136; ontological, x; of other, 253; patient experience, 241; patterns, 3; practical, 229; pre-, 142, 170; preceptors and, 219; preconceived, 227; preontological, 187; prior, 163; provisional, 142; psychoanalytic, 24; scholarship and, 125; search for, 64; self, 106, 114, 147, 170, 231, 253; shared, 173, 194; situation, 14, 161; spirituality, 135; stories and, 53, 196; striving for, 142; sussing, 177; teaching as guiding toward, 119; temporal nature of, 144; theoretical, 36, 45, 48; time and, 6, 142; uniqueness, 191; universal, 134, 140; ways of, 163
unexpectedness in practice, 246
uniqueness, 191
Unitarian Universalist: program, 128; teachings of, 136
United States, 17, 108, 109, 128, 134, 136, 150, 199, 220; immigrants in, 114, 115, 129, 135; international students in, 125; teenagers in, 128
unity: of dwelling and journeying, 229; of space and time, 229; of world, 227
universal: caring as, 107; meaning of caring, 124, 125; paradigm, 134; patriarchy as, 130; wholeness, 107
universalities, 140

universalizability, 130, 134
universe: inseparability from, 107, 136
university, 248; community, 135; Massey, 148; multicultural institute in, 115; policy, 194; professor, 108; public, 121; teaching in, 114; Washington State, 194; of Wisconsin–Madison, xv
unready to hand, 229, 244
unreflectivity, 48
unrelatedness, 97
Unschuld, P., 134, 135
unsettleness (umheimlich), 231, 233
upbringing: religious, 67
Uris, L., 134
"us" and "them," 116, 129, 130; other and, 109
use: knowing through, 229

value(s), 9, 13, 15, 34, 128, 143, 168–170, 175; adoption of, 108; beliefs and, 64; of caring, 49, 56, 120, 122, 124, 221; as caught, 218; of clinical nursing practice, 124; conflicting, 168; conviction of superiority of, 150; cultural, 17, 108, 130, 174, 182, 187, 221; of difference, 140; of education, 128; everyday, 221; of family, 206; free choosing of, 204; of ill persons, 209; of individual in treatment, 210; of New Zealand nurses, 145; of nursing practice, 254; of ordinariness, 32; personal and professional, 221; representing, 202; respect of, 140; of self worth, 174; transmission of, 218; of wedding anniversary, 189; Western Christian religious, 120
Vandenberghe, C., 31
Van der Kolk, B., 23, 24, 51, 54
Van Maanen, J., 63
Van Manen, M., 100, 105, 147, 148, 160, 224
Vaughan, P., 23
verbal: abuse, 24; communication, 116
Verbrugge, L. M., 98
verfallen, 225
Veronica, 121, 122, 123
Vetlesen, A. J., 130
victimization, 94
Victoria, Australia, 218
Victorian: neo-, upbringing, 128
Vidich, A. J., 126
Viennese, 205
Vietnam: PTSD and, 23

Vietnamese, 200; student, 201
vigilance of preceptors, 239, 240, 245
violence: horizontal, 239
visible: making care practice, 208; making
   ideal, 173; making invisible, 165
vision quest, 198
visual disability, 98
visualization: strategies of, 161
vital signs: observations and, 239
Vivekananda, K., 23
voice(s), 52, 54, 64, 84, 107, 193, 194; authenticity of, 108; diverse, 199; lack of,
   223; learning to use, 54; as metaphor,
   201; of nurse clinicians, 198; of patients,
   198; of patients, clinicians, teachers, and
   students, 195; of preceptors, 219; rebellious, 133; respect for, 212; shifting, 135;
   silencing, 24, 26; stories and, 53; of storyteller, 201, 205
vulnerability, 24, 66, 98, 146, 154, 174; in
   care, 29; of patients, 29

Wachterhauser, B. R., 141
Waitangi, Treaty of, 150–153, 176
waiting and acting, 50
Walker, D. R., 153
Walker, J., 218
Walsh, K., 49
ward(s), 226, 242; familiarity with, 232; hos-
   pital, 148, 226; staffing of, 232
Warnick, M., 22
Washington, 78; State University College of
   Nursing, 194
watching: learning by, 247
Watson, J., 6, 8, 18, 32, 110, 119, 166, 172,
   184, 185, 216, 221, 253
Watson, K., 110
Watts, R., 185
Waugh, R. A., 9
way(s): of being, caring as, 214; of being in
   the world, 185; of knowing, 220; of learning, 195, 196, 212, 222; of life, Christian,
   121; of preceptors, 254; of striving, 161;
   subject-object, 191; of teaching caring,
   120
Webb, C., xvi
Webb, J., 34, 35
welcoming, 232; of tools of technology, 99
well-being, 160, 169, 221; of clients, 50
wellness orientation, 55
Welton, M., 55

West, 108, 130
Western: acculturation, 118, 128; authors,
   130; culture(s), 6, 108; education, appreciation for, 114; gender roles, 134; monotheism, 134; promise of culture, 113;
   thought, 108, 135, 136; toothpaste, 126;
   value of difference in, 140; world, 147
Western Christian: culture, 113; religious
   values, 120
Westerners, 129, 130
Westernization, 114, 126
whanau room, 163, 171, 176
what *matters*, 100
White House, 82
Whitten, N. E., Jr., 100
whole(s): dialectic between part and, 12; human as complex, 120; relationship to part,
   4; sense of, 149
wholeness, 5, 64, 164; fourfold as, 227; spiritual care of, 203; universal, 107
Whorf hypothesis: Sapir-, 4
why?, 67, 88
wife: relationship with husband, 167; role
   of, 130
Wilkin, P., 33, 44, 54
will, 99
Willett, C., 10
Williams, M., 22
Williams, W. C., 199
willingness, 161; to precept, 232; to learn,
   116
Wisconsin–Madison: University of, xv
wisdom, 25, 49, 64; clinical, 15; dialectic
   and practical, 176
witnessing, 112, 194; by caregivers, 205; patients' concern, 208
Wittgenstein, L., 4
woman/women, 239; advantaged, 99; blind,
   93; as bossed, 129; forgetting and, 64;
   and health, 167; lives of, 130; Maori, 145;
   narratives of, 64; as nurses, 164; obscurity
   and, 63; professional, 133; respect and,
   113; self-harm and, 24; status of in Western culture, 134; successful, 133; tribal,
   strong, 113; studies of, 116; white, 88
Wonder, Stevie, 69, 76, 82
Wood, P. J., 150
words, 98, 147, 152, 159, 161, 173; exploring, 146; learning and, 52
work: intrapersonal response to, 31; load,
   249; moral code of daily life and, 110;

work *(continued)*
  nature of, 159; relationships, 136; rigor
    of, 148; settings, 148
working: together, student and preceptor,
    239, 242; *with*, 54
workplace(s), 21, 29, 35, 199; culture of, 49;
    discontentment in, 119; entering, 243; en-
    vironment, 123, 158; ethics, 120; health-
    care, 26, 27, 200; hegemony in, 49; prac-
    tices in, 30; risk management in, 29;
    stress in, 31, 32
workshops: continuing education, 114; diver-
    sity, 115
world(s), 98; academic and practice, 255; be-
    ing between, 259; being-in-the-, 5, 6, 14,
    62, 99, 141, 169, 187, 194, 200, 216,
    225–229, 233, 238, 244, 254, 258; bureau-
    cratic, 131; coming into, 191; concrete,
    117; connections in, 223; constituted by,
    191; corporeal, 98; cruel, 69; different,
    171; dwelling in, 229; everyday, 163; ex-
    pectations of common, 97; First, 107; im-
    mersion in, 5; life, 230; local moral, 117;
    made unknown, 98; making sense of, 4,
    5; meaning-saturated, 224; mediating, 62;
    objective, 97; nursing crises around, 218;
    of nursing education, 254; of nursing prac-
    tice, 229, 234, 235, 239, 244, 254, 255,
    258; order, 98; of patients, 181, 191, 192,
    225; of preceptors, 223, 254; personal,
    116; predefined, 191; real, 75, 225; rela-
    tional, 225; restlessness between, 231; sci-
    entific, 99; shaping, 98, 105; shared, 233;
    situated, 228; social, 226; space between,
    230; of students, 225; temporal, 228;
    Third, 107; transhistorical, 63; transper-
    sonal, 63; uncertain, 62, 100; Western,
    147
World Health Organization, 150
worldhood, 5, 8
worldview(s), 5, 14, 17, 18, 97, 133; dif-

fering, 99; of parents, 12; representing of
    in story, 202; student, 118
worrying: about machines, 244; caring as,
    160
wounds: dressing, 243; showing, 54
writer: birth of, 62; "invisible hand" of, 135;
    stories and, 62
writing(s), 106, 130, 146, 149, 153, 185,
    198; analytical vs. kinder, 63; books, 96;
    about colonial oppression, 115; consents,
    for student observations, 241; the experi-
    ence, 63; about ideas and issues, 145; ill-
    ness and story, 208; as inquiry, 62, 64; in-
    terpretations, 149; Jacqui's, 100; layers of,
    106; learning and teaching through, 119;
    lifeworld and, 105; poem, 81; about real-
    ity, 27; reports, 118, 245; and research,
    147, 148; and rewriting, 146, 149; the
    self, 62; sociological, 143; story(ies), 127,
    149, 196; symbols, 100; teaching with,
    117; as therapy, 63, 97
Wrubel, J., 32, 124, 158, 172, 185, 186,
    188–191, 215, 223, 226, 228
wunian, 228
Wyatt, S., xvi

x-ray, 199

Yalom, I., 51
Yamada, K., 65
yielding, 64
yoga, 135
Young, P., xvi
Young-Mason, J., 197
youth, 134; values and, 128

Zalumas, J., 17
Zborowski, M., 150
Zderad, L., 172, 173
Zen, 51, 109
Zussman, R., 209